THEORY
OF
HEARING

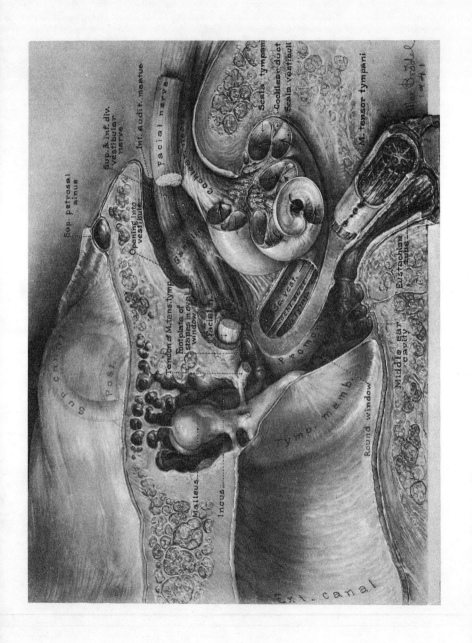

Theory of
HEARING

Ernest Glen Wever

Professor of Psychology
Princeton University

DOVER PUBLICATIONS, INC.
NEW YORK

Published in Canada by General Publishing Company, Ltd., 30 Lesmill Road, Don Mills, Toronto, Ontario.
Published in the United Kingdom by Constable and Company, Ltd., 10 Orange Street, London WC 2.

This Dover edition, first published in 1970, is an unabridged republication, with minor corrections, of the work originally published in 1949 by John Wiley & Sons, Inc.

Standard Book Number: 486-62399-8
Library of Congress Catalog Card Number: 74-93199

Manufactured in the United States of America
Dover Publications, Inc.
180 Varick Street
New York, N.Y. 10014

*To my associates
in the study of the ear*

PREFACE

At the time, a little over two decades ago, that my interest began to be aroused in auditory theory, a particularly intriguing situation had developed, in which the old differences between the two main types of theory—the place and frequency theories—had been brought to a new peak of opposition. The freshly discovered facts about sensory nerve action had forced important revisions in these rival theories, and in their revised forms the theories were found to be even farther apart than they had been earlier in their assumptions about the neural representations of sounds. Indeed, in their assumptions as to the actions of the auditory nerve in representing the fundamental properties of pitch and loudness the two types of theory had come to be almost diametrically opposed.

This situation obviously set the stage for an experimental test to decide between the two forms of explanation. And the means for the test was at hand; the electrophysiological techniques that were proving their worth in providing the basic evidence on sensory nerve action had only to be applied directly to this problem. This was the occasion for the studies that Dr. C. W. Bray and I began on the nature of auditory nerve impulses.

When we planned our experiments we took it as obvious that observations on the nature of the impulses produced in the auditory nerve in response to sounds would give proof of one or the other of the rival theories. The matter turned out otherwise, for as soon as the first results were at hand we perceived what no doubt should have been apparent before: that the representation of pitch in terms of place in the cochlea and the nerve and its representation in terms of the frequency of nerve impulses are not in any essential conflict. We came to see that the new evidence, and all of the old as well, could be reconciled with both these forms of representation. And so we were led to adopt a kind of fusion or compromise of the two rival hypotheses: a dual theory that seeks to retain the better features of each of the traditional explanations and to avoid their difficulties.

Since this theoretical suggestion was offered we have experienced a new wave of activity in the auditory field, with the electrophysiological method in particular providing many additions to our fund of information. It is my belief, in contemplation of the accumulated evidence, that our early position is fully justified, and that a proper understanding of the process of hearing is to be gained by way of the fusion and compromise of principles just referred to. The development of this view constitutes the principal theme of this book.

The treatment begins in Part I with the earliest groping speculations about the ear and follows the gradual rise of the anatomical knowledge out of which the theories of hearing were developed. These theories are then taken up one by one, mostly in the order of their appearance from the beginning of the seventeenth century to the present, and with special attention to the ones that have had the major influence on subsequent thought. In this treatment it has been my intention to give to each theory as full and unprejudiced and even sympathetic an account as possible and then, on occasion, to add a suggestion or two about the theory's more serious shortcomings.

In Part II the two principal types of explanation, the resonance type of place theory and the simple frequency theory, come in for a more searching consideration. Here these theories are developed in their most modern forms and are made to stand in the face of the present evidence. This critical treatment brings out the virtues and the faults of each type of theory, and it also points the way to the compromise position—the volley theory—by which the old conflicts can be resolved.

Part III deals in detail with the volley theory. It gives a description of the framework of the theory and its basic assumptions, and it then reviews the primary evidence on which this theoretical structure rests: the physical, physiological, clinical, and other evidence relevant to the representation of sounds by both spatial and temporal processes in the acoustic nervous action. Finally, in the later chapters, comes the true testing of the theory as it is brought to grips with the various facts of auditory experience and is made to relate and explain them.

The treatment of the auditory phenomena is not exhaustive. Some of the phenomena are covered fully, others sketchily, and a few not at all. The decision rests upon the relevance to theory. Sometimes, too, particular facts have remained untreated when their explanation follows so closely the pattern already laid down in dealing with others of the same class that it has seemed unnecessary to enlarge the discussion further. Certain other limitations also are deliberately imposed. I have given little attention to the observations made on mechanical models of the cochlea, a very great many of which have been devised and manipulated in support of particular theories. It has seemed to me that each model only reflects the properties built into it, and its performance testifies rather to the mechanical ingenuity of its inventor than to the correctness of his views about the ear. Likewise, and for much the same reason, I have given little credence to the mathematical formulations of the theories. They are only models of a formal, symbolic sort, and they give an illusion of precision to ideas that on account of the limitations in our knowledge cannot really be precise. Like the mechanical models, they appear, at the present stage of our theorizing, quite as likely to confuse and mislead as to inform. In this connection I point out that I have accepted the hazard of translating into plain language—or language as plain as may be—certain of the theoretical conceptions that have been formulated only in elaborate mathematical terms; and I can only trust that in this process I have not done too much violence to their authors' intentions.

The historical form of treatment in the first part of the book serves a double purpose. It brings to light the earlier conceptions that have an interest in their own right and that foreshadowed what was to come; and also it provides an opportunity for introducing in relatively simple terms many of the fundamental concepts that have to be treated more elaborately later on.

Near the end of the book is a short list of terms, abbreviations, and symbols, with explanations that will be of help to readers unfamiliar with the more technical language of this field.

Appended also is a list of references. For practical reasons its length has been held to a minimum. Included are the sources specifically cited and a few others chosen largely for their guidance to the further literature. The student wishing to pursue

particular topics will find a starting point in the sources given,
and in consulting them he will quickly acquire a working bibliography.

I am indebted to many colleagues and friends for their help
in connection with this work. I am especially grateful to Dr.
Stacy R. Guild and Dr. W. A. Munson for examining portions of
the manuscript, and to Dr. Merle Lawrence, Dr. Herbert S.
Langfeld, and Dr. Frank A. Geldard for a critical reading of the
whole of it. My further thanks are due to Dr. Guild and the
Johns Hopkins Otological Research Laboratory for making available to me the special anatomical material used in the measurements of the human cochlea reported in Chapters 5 and 11.

The frontispiece is from "Three Unpublished Drawings of the
Anatomy of the Human Ear," by the late Max Brödel, reproduced
with the kind permission of the publishers, the W. B. Saunders
Company. Short quotations made from Helmholtz at several
points in the text are taken from Ellis' translation of his work
On the Sensations of Tone with the permission of Longmans,
Green and Company.* Accompanying certain of the figures
throughout the book are my acknowledgments to the many other
authors and publishers who have extended me the courtesy of
reproducing their drawings.

My special thanks are to my wife, Suzanne Wever, who
assumed the long and exacting task of typing the manuscript.

ERNEST GLEN WEVER

Princeton, N. J.
May 1949

---

* The Ellis translation has been reprinted by Dover.

CONTENTS

Part I: The Classical Theories

1. THE BEGINNINGS OF AUDITORY THEORY   3
2. THE HELMHOLTZ RESONANCE THEORY   25
3. THE PLACE THEORIES AFTER HELMHOLTZ   43
4. THE FREQUENCY THEORIES   76

Part II: The Modern Developments

5. MODERN DEVELOPMENTS OF THE CLASSICAL THEORIES   97
6. AUDITORY NERVE RESPONSES   121
7. FREQUENCY REPRESENTATION IN THE AUDITORY NERVE   157
8. THE VOLLEY PRINCIPLE   166

Part III: The Volley Theory

9. THE VOLLEY THEORY: THE BASIC EVIDENCE   189
10. FURTHER EVIDENCE ON COCHLEAR LOCALIZATION: THE ACOUSTIC NEUROLOGY   221
11. SENSITIVITY   268
12. LOUDNESS AND FATIGUE   299
13. PITCH AND PITCH DISCRIMINATION   327
14. AUDITORY ABNORMALITIES   354
15. THE PRODUCTS OF TONAL INTERACTION   375
16. TEMPORAL PHENOMENA OF AUDITORY PERCEPTION   399
17. BINAURAL PHENOMENA   424
18. THE VOLLEY THEORY IN REVIEW; CONCLUDING OBSERVATIONS   435
    DEFINITIONS AND SYMBOLS   443
    REFERENCES   447
    INDEX   471

Part I
The Classical Theories

CHAPTER 1

THE BEGINNINGS OF AUDITORY THEORY

Auditory theory lies in the unsettled ground between two vast and flourishing fields. On the one hand is the field of physical acoustics, greatly expanded in modern times in the eventful developments of electronics and provided with a great array of instruments and techniques. On the other hand is the psychology of hearing, which treats of our experiences and actions as a result of the stimulation of the ears, and is now richly benefited by the tools of stimulation and control that the new acoustics has provided.

Our contemplation of the progress made in these two fields gives us good reason for satisfaction. About the physics of sound we know a great deal. About the subjective phenomena we know only a little less. But at this point our complacency is disturbed. We have not progressed as far as we should like in our further task, which is to relate these two and to say how the physical stimulus acts upon our sensory and neural mechanisms and through its actions there becomes translated into auditory impressions.

Converging on this task are many lines of endeavor. In our study of the anatomy of the ear we discover the forms and natures of its several parts. In sensory physiology we treat of the more peripheral of the processes in which these parts are concerned, and in the neurology of the acoustic and broader cerebral systems we learn of the more remote consequences of these processes. It is noteworthy that of late the usual techniques of these sciences have been augmented in the development and refinement of the electrophysiological method, which examines the functions of cells by means of their electrical activities. This method is being applied most energetically in the study of the sensory and neural processes and is contributing abundantly to our knowledge of them. Contributing too is the clinical study of hearing and its aberrations. Still, with all these

3

ways of approaching the problem and their truly prolific yield of information, we find much that we lack in understanding. This is the reason for a theory. Specifically, the theory seeks to bring together what is known, to establish lines of relationship within this knowledge, and to chart the areas of obscurity. Such is its first purpose; and in carrying out this purpose it will also accomplish the second, of no lesser importance, which is to point out the ways of further exploration.

Earlier, and extending back as far as we know, the need for orienting theory was likewise felt; and perhaps even more poignantly then, for though curiosity was quite as keen as now the knowledge was less.

The theory of hearing has a long history. Its beginning stage was simply the development of ideas as to how sounds enter the head and make their presence felt. Only later came the conception that has formed the center of speculation in this area ever since—the conception that sounds are analyzed and otherwise worked upon within the peripheral receptor.

It is easy to understand why the first theorizings were on a simple level. Early considerations of sensation in general accorded to the mind only a passive role; the belief was that the mind received direct impressions from the world outside and that the objects perceived were as they truly existed. It took many centuries of observation and thought to gain for us the modern view that the perceiver has much to do with the things of his perceiving: that he takes in the variations of stimulus and puts them through a series of transforming processes to derive what we call a sensory experience, and that the internal processes are quite as important in determining the qualities of the experienced objects as the external cues that arouse them.

The ancient Greek philosophers developed theories of sensation in the course of their search for the sources of knowledge. They began by accepting the naive view that perception is a mirroring of the external world, yet they soon found it necessary to complicate this outlook in order to account for the obvious differences among the senses. They solved this problem of sensory variety by reference to the magic formula that 'like is perceived by like.' This is a formula handed down from primitive thought, just as the mirroring principle was; and though it may have seemed a more sophisticated idea at the time, it still was an expression of the same elementary kind of thinking, in which all things are accounted for by direct analogies. We are perhaps most familiar with the medical version of the principle, as the homeopathic doctrine that 'like is cured by like'—by which the hair of the dog is hopefully applied to the wound caused by his bite.

The formula was applied generally in the theory of the sources of knowledge, with the assertion that a universal reason finds entrance into man through his senses, but makes its entrance only under the condition that there is a reason or soul within him so that the outer activity shall be met by one of a corresponding kind. The doctrine achieves an explanation of the variety of experience by the assumption of a multiplicity of qualities in man, each accessible to one corresponding in the outer world.

The specific applications of this principle of resemblances are most clearly understood in the sensory theory of Empedocles, who lived in the fifth century B.C. Sensation, Empedocles said, always requires an immediate contact between the object and its perceiver. There are material emanations from the object, exact copies of it, that enter the sense organ through its pores, provided that these pores are appropriate in size. To have an effect there, and impress themselves upon the mind, the emanations must encounter a substance of the same nature as themselves. So for vision there is a light in the eye by which we perceive the external light, and for hearing there is an internal air by which we perceive the moving air that constitutes a sound.

We find that Empedocles and the others of his day knew something of the nature of sound as a propagated series of aerial disturbances. They had also an elementary knowledge of the anatomy of the ear, including the easily visible parts of the external ear and some features of the middle ear. They knew about the drum membrane, and the tympanic cavity beyond it, and the fact that this cavity is filled with air. It was this tympanic air that they considered the essential substance by which aerial vibrations are perceived.

The tympanic air they thought of as similar to ordinary air, yet not precisely the same. It was a highly refined substance, particularly tenuous and pure; and it was a permanent part of the sense organ. Its origin posed a problem, and Plato suggested that it was implanted during uterine development. This idea of the 'implanted air' was destined to haunt the theory of hearing for two thousand years and more.

Further advances of theory had to await the accretion of anatomical knowledge. Galen * (about A.D. 175) spoke at length of the uses of the external ear, which in man he regarded as mainly ornamental, and saw in the tortuous course of the auditory passages a protection for the delicate 'neural membrane' within, which he conceived as the receptive tissue. He made no mention of the tympanic membrane, and very likely did not see it; indeed, it may have been absent in the old, badly preserved specimens that no doubt he had to use for study. The 'obliquely twisted passages' to which he referred must have included the external meatus and its expansion into the tympanic cavity. His comparison of their form to a labyrinth is not to be taken as evidence that he knew anything about the inner ear or what we call the labyrinth nowadays.

In contrast to his indefiniteness about the deeper cochlear structures, Galen showed a familiarity with the auditory nerve region. He saw the bundle of nerves passing from the brain into the internal auditory meatus and named them collectively the fifth cranial pair, following his teacher Marinus in this, as he said. He distinguished two branches: one, the larger, that he called 'soft' he identified as going to the ear, and the other that he called 'hard' he traced to the muscles. These branches are of course the auditory and facial nerves, which we now recognize as independent and number as the eighth and seventh cranial pairs.

---

* For Galen's works, in Latin translation, see the list of references at the end of the book.

In general, this list is to be consulted for original sources whenever an author's name is mentioned. When more than one title appears under an author's name, each is given a number, and a particular one is referred to in the text by adding its number after the name. Sometimes an author's name is given without any number even though the listing will be found to include two or more titles; then all the titles are pertinent to the point under discussion.

Soon after Galen's time, as we know, science in general went into decline. Political and social upheavals at first and then a dominating theology combined to throttle further empirical adventures and in the Mediterranean area even to submerge the gains already made. For further developments in audition we must look beyond the empty spaces of the Middle Ages to the labors of the great anatomists of the sixteenth century.

In the anatomical advancements of this new scientific age the ear like every other bodily organ came in for a share of painstaking study. Nonetheless, on account of the special difficulties that this structure presents, progress at first was halting and was concerned in the main with parts of the middle ear.

DISCOVERY OF THE CONDUCTIVE MECHANISM

Berengario da Carpi in 1514 mentioned two tympanic ossicles, which evidently had been discovered earlier; but it remained for Vesalius (1543) to describe them accurately and give them their modern names of malleus and incus. A little later Ingrassia (1546) discovered the stapes and also the two windows of the cochlea.

Fallopius (1561) described the ossicles and their articulations in detail. He recognized the two principal divisions of the inner ear and called them as we do now the labyrinth and cochlea.

Eustachius (1564) gave a good description of the tensor tympani muscle and indicated its function. It had been seen before by Vesalius and others but had not been recognized as a muscle. Another structure vaguely known earlier but first accurately described by Eustachius is the tube connecting the tympanic space with the pharynx and now known by his name. The second tympanic muscle, the stapedius, was first clearly described by Varolius (1591).

Now the essential structures of the conductive system were revealed, and it was possible for Coiter (1566) to write the first book dealing specifically with the ear, his *De auditus instrumento*, and in it to present a systematic account of the transmission of sound. He traced the vibrations from their entrance into the external auditory meatus through the tympanic membrane and ossicles, and by way of the cochlea and labyrinth to the auditory

It was through this interest in acoustic efficiency that resonance theories arose. The physical basis—the phenomenon of resonance —is a matter of common experience. It is easy to observe that various enclosures, like narrow halls and domed towers, have special acoustic properties, reverberating the sounds introduced into them; and the similar behavior of smaller cavities and tubes is only a little less obvious. Work with musical instruments having tuned strings shows that these strings readily pick up motions of the air and come themselves to vibrate. Also, it is soon made clear that such mechanisms are specific in their actions: for any one condition of tuning they respond favorably to some sounds and remain insensible to others.

The first observations of resonance are unknown; but Galileo in 1638 formally discussed the phenomenon and set forth its principles. He stated the laws of the pendulum and saw that similar relations hold in the behavior of vibrating strings. He observed not only the sympathetic vibration of bodies tuned in unison, but also those related in simple intervals like the octave and the fifth. Later Kircher (1673) carried out a number of experiments in investigation of the phenomena.

THE FIRST RESONANCE THEORY: BAUHIN IN 1605

The first resonance theory of hearing was formulated in 1605 by Caspar Bauhin, a student of medicine and Professor of Anatomy in the University of Basle, in Switzerland. It was cavity resonance that he spoke of. Consider the date, which precedes the clear understanding of the inner ear structures. The deeper cavities were known, but only vaguely, and were thought to contain air (as very likely they did in the poorly preserved or dry bones that served as objects of study). When the aerial waves beat upon the ear, Bauhin said, there is resonance in its various tubules and spaces, in the depths of which the auditory nerve lies. The resonance is selective, for the cavities contain openings of different sizes, lengths, and forms.

The grave sounds are received in the large, roomy spaces, and the acute sounds in the small, narrow ones. Thereby the different kinds of sounds are accommodated.

Bauhin found a difficulty, as did others of the time, in locating the actual receptive process. Because he accepted the implanted-air hypothesis he was inclined to believe that the true seat of hearing was the tympanic space where he thought this air was; but he did not altogether deny a receptive function to the labyrinthine and cochlear spaces as well. He suggested a little hesitatingly that these innermost cavities might aid the receptive process in an indirect way by damping the sound waves and thereby preventing undesirable reflections from getting back to the tympanic space.

This theory, in a somewhat modified form, was still held a good deal later in the century. In 1672 Willis gave a detailed presentation of it. By then the anatomy of the ear, especially its deeper parts, was much better known, although the passages still were believed to be air-filled. On the basis of this increased knowledge Willis was able to give an account of sound transmission that is remarkable for its time. As he described it, the external ear gathers together the sonorous particles that constitute a sound and directs them inward by way of turning and twisting passages to the most intimate recess where a thin membrane is placed. The sound, shaking this membrane like a drum, delivers the impression to the sonorous particles planted beyond. These particles lie in the cavity where the ancients placed the implanted air, "which thing indeed is not unlikely," he added. Beyond, in the petrous bone, is the cochlea (by which he meant a chamber shaped like a snail's shell), and into it the sound is propagated. In fact, he said, there are two cochleas. One, near the chief oval hole, tapers down gradually and ends in a small cavity. The other progressively expands and ends with a large aperture into another chamber, without any membrane covering it. This description of two 'cochleas' perhaps represents a confused knowledge of the two cochlear scalae and, I think, the opening of one of them into the vestibule.

Willis knew about the three auditory ossicles and one of the tympanic muscles. To the muscle he assigned the function of adjusting the tension of the drum membrane according to the strength of sound stimulating it; to the ossicles he gave no particular role.

This is a cavity-resonance theory which is generally like that of Bauhin but, curiously enough, without any reference to a selective treatment of high and low tones.

A little later, in 1680, Perrault gave a description of the process of hearing which followed that of Willis in most respects. However, as already mentioned, Perrault differed from his predecessors in placing the implanted air within the cochlea. Although he regarded the bony spiral lamina as the peripheral organ of hearing, it was this inner cavity that he regarded as finally set in vibration by the sounds and as responsible for stimulation of the nerve fibers. Also, in his account, just as in the views of Bauhin and Willis, it was in the air passages that an augmentation of sounds by resonance was presumed to occur.

It is of incidental interest that this theory of cavity resonance still persists in modern times, as for example in the speculations of Lucae.

DU VERNEY'S RESONANCE THEORY IN 1683

Presently we find a new departure, a resonance theory almost modern in form. This is the theory of Joseph Guichard DuVerney, first presented in 1683 in his *Traité de l'organe de l'ouie,* the second known treatise dealing exclusively with the ear.

DuVerney was a physician of prominence in Paris; he was Professor of Anatomy and Surgery at the Jardin Royal des Plantes, a medical counsellor to the King, and a member of the Academie Royale des Sciences. He was an intimate of Edme Mariotte, also a court physician with scientific interests (famed as discoverer of the blind spot of the retina), and with whom he evidently discussed many of his ideas. In introducing his treatment of auditory functions he paid a generous tribute to his friend as sharing the responsibility for "a good part of what herein will be found most remarkable."

DuVerney presented a good general account of the anatomy of the ear. He described in detail, and largely correctly, the various parts of the external, middle, and inner ear: the auricle and meatus, with the drum membrane below; the tympanic cavity and its contents; and the three divisions of the inner ear. He traced the transmission of sounds through the drum membrane and ossicular chain to the cochlea, and he believed also in a second route, through the air of the tympanic cavity and the round window.

The cochlea he considered the principal organ of hearing, but he believed that the remaining parts of the inner ear, the vestibule and the semicircular canals, served this function also. His reasons were plausible: he noted that some animals, like fishes and (he thought) birds also, lack the cochlea and have only these other parts, yet they hear; and all three divisions of the inner ear are served by the same nerve which ought to have a single function. He argued further that the tortuous passages of the labyrinth should act like the tubes of trumpets and similar

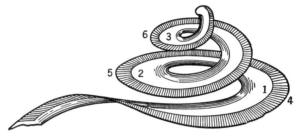

FIG. 1. DuVerney's drawing of the spiral organ of the cochlea. The part of the ribbon marked 1, 2, 3 is the bony lamina, and the part marked 4, 5, 6 is the membranous lamina.

musical instruments to augment the sounds passing into them and thereby aid the excitation of the nerve expansions within. Bear in mind that he still believed, as had his predecessors, that all the bony spaces were filled with air, the classical 'implanted air.'

DuVerney described the cochlea as divided lengthwise into two passages by a partition consisting of the bony spiral lamina and a membrane extending from the bony lamina to the outer cochlear wall. Thus, he saw the basilar membrane perhaps more clearly than anyone had before; certainly his is the first figure portraying it. He described it as a very thin membrane, thinner than the bony lamina and dark in color, which is clear evidence that he saw the membrane itself. However, he did not conceive for it any function distinct from the spiral ligament but regarded the whole as a suspensory structure.

He believed, as Perrault had done, that the auditory nerve fibers were distributed to the bony lamina, and he regarded this lamina therefore as the true receptive apparatus. Sounds, he thought, are made to strike upon the spiral lamina from two sides simultaneously by way of the oval and round windows. The bony spiral lamina is admirably suited to respond to sounds because it is "hard, dry, slender, and brittle"—the properties that he deemed requisite to this function.

The bony lamina he regarded as a selective mechanism. Because it is broader at the basal end than toward its extremity, the different kinds of sounds are distributed along its extent. Here are his concluding statements, in translation. "In short, this lamina is not only capable of receiving the aerial vibrations, but its structure makes it seem likely that it is capable of responding to all their various characteristics; for since it is larger at the beginning of the first turn than at the extremity of the last one (where it ends at a point), and its other parts diminish proportionately in size, we may declare that the larger parts can be vibrated by themselves alone, and are capable of being agitated only slowly and hence respond to the grave tones; and that on the contrary the narrower portions on being agitated are more rapid in their movements and respond to the acute tones. It is the same as in a steel spring, whose larger parts give slow vibrations and respond to deep tones, whereas the narrower parts give faster and more lively vibrations and respond to acute tones. The result is that by virtue of the different vibrations of the spiral lamina, the spirits of the nerve (the nerve which is distributed over the substance of the lamina) receive different impressions which represent in the brain the various characteristics of tones."

Note that the localization of low tones at the base and high tones at the apex is contrary to modern theory; but this form of localization is reasonable for the osseous spiral lamina because that structure narrows as it ascends the cochlea.

This is a theory of the peripheral analysis of sounds by resonance—and, be it noted, two centuries in advance of Helmholtz.

THE RESONANCE THEORY AFTER DU VERNEY

The further development of auditory theory is distinguished by a continuing inquiry as to the identity of the cochlear resonators. DuVerney considered a thin, firm plate like the osseous spiral lamina ideally suited to vibration, but two influences led away from this structure and toward the softer parts. One was a classical bias, dating from Galen, in favor of a delicate 'nervous' membrane as a percipient agency; the other was a growing appreciation of the nature of resonance and the virtues of stretched strings as vibrating elements.

Valsalva (1707) seems to have been swayed by the ancient theory. He maintained, in a way reminiscent of the early principle of resemblances, that the 'soft' part of the auditory nerve ought to supply the soft parts of the inner ear. His observations hardly go beyond DuVerney's. He verified the fact that the auditory nerve after entering the internal auditory meatus breaks up into a great many fine filaments which then pass through minute holes in the bony walls. It is doubtful that he was able to follow these filaments farther, but he believed (quite correctly as it turns out) that they expand not upon the bone but over the membranous zones of the cochlea, vestibule, and semicircular canals, which he called the 'zonae sonorae.' The part in the cochlea he distinguished as 'zona cochleae,' his name for the membranous spiral lamina.

The further interest in the process of resonance and in the specific action of the ear led, for a time, only to a refinement of DuVerney's formulation. DuVerney had spoken of the vibration of the bony lamina in general terms, with tones distributed over its length. Later this lamina was described, quite improperly of course from an anatomical standpoint, as made up of a series of transverse strings in independent motion. Thus Haller in 1751, in reporting the opinion current in his day, described the osseous lamina as "an indefinite number of cords, continually shortening in their lengths, and by that means adapted to harmonic consonance with the great variety of acute and grave sounds so as to vibrate sympathetically with the most of them; namely, with the longest in the base of the cochlea with the grave sounds, and the shortest nearer the apex with the acute sounds." A little later, anticipating an issue of a century yet to come, he went on to say that "the distinction of sounds no doubt depends upon the rapidity of the tremors in the acoustic nerve, accordingly as they succeed one another frequently or slowly in a brief time. For this, it is not necessary that the tremors be numbered by the mind, but only that their numbers be different and that this difference excite changes in our perceptions."

With Cotugno (1760) the theory takes a turn to the now familiar form, for he accepted both the above variations: he took from Valsalva the idea of a sensory membrane, the 'zona cochleae,' and he conceived this membrane as made up of a series of vibrating strings. Though not the first to do so—it seems to have been general at this time—he used the analogy of a stringed musical instrument to represent the action. He compared the inner ear with a cymbalo (an instrument something like a harp placed horizontally and played with hammers) as containing a series of parallel strings under tension and varying in lengths from one end to the other. Because he knew, as Valsalva did also, that the membranous lamina grows wider as it ascends the cochlea, he placed the low tones in the apex and the high tones at the base. This reverses the localization that had its source in DuVerney and brings us to the modern type.

In the latter part of the eighteenth century this theory of cochlear resonance was as familiar to students of the ear as it is today, and as general in acceptance. That is to say, it was the current theory, claiming the center of attention, yet having on occasion to face opposition.

Cramer (1741) objected that the strings of the spiral lamina were too short to vibrate suitably. Esteve (1751) saw several difficulties. He doubted that the strings ran parallel to one another and kept sufficient independence to move singly. He did not believe that they could be maintained in the proper tension. He pointed out also (as had Galileo earlier) that stretched strings respond in segments as well as in their total lengths, and this ought to give a confusion of harmonic tones.

At the end of the century the theory had come to be regarded with much uncertainty. Thomas Young (1807) sketched it briefly, with the comment, which certainly lacks enthusiasm, that "the opinion does not appear to be wholly improbable." Magendie was more uncompromising, with the statement that "the osseo-membranous partition, which separates the two scalae of the cochlea, has given rise to a hypothesis that no one believes

(the limbus and the part below the rods) "like a drumstick on a drum." This action seemed to him necessary to excite the nerve fibers, which he followed only a little way beyond the bony channels and so believed to be below the dentate band.

Corti saw the cells that we know as the hair cells, but he had only a distorted idea of them. The inner row he took as part of the innermost segment of his rods, and the three outer rows he pictured as attached to the outermost segments.

It is of interest that Scarpa probably had dimly seen Corti's rods, for he described, at the free edge of the bony spiral lamina, a number of threads running out with open spaces between them. Likewise, Huschke had seen the hair cells as "cne or several rows of yellowish, irregularly arranged bodies."

Kölliker, who had followed Corti's work with enthusiasm, added a number of amplifying details. He traced the nerve fibers out through the edge of the bony lamina to the vestibular surface (not the tympanic as had been believed), and from there he supposed them to run outward to end at Corti's rods, which he judged accordingly to be a neural apparatus. The separateness of these fibers and their endings led him to surmise that they acted individually to represent different sensations. Hearing he attributed to the vestibule and ampullae as well as the cochlea, but he considered that only in the last is tonal discrimination possible.

Kölliker's observation of the rods was no improvement over Corti's. A little later, Claudius (1856) was convinced that they were anchored to the basilar membrane at their outer as well as their inner ends and sketched them as crudely arched in shape. It remained for Deiters (1860) to see them in their true position and form. The term 'organ of Corti' at first referred only to the 'rods' or what we now call the arches of Corti; but as other details of the sensory apparatus were revealed the term came to be applied to the whole, a practice that now serves as a fitting recognition of Corti's part in opening up this aspect of cochlear anatomy.

Deiters not only saw the true forms of Corti's arches but also made out their connections in support of the reticular membrane and the hair cells. He further discovered other supporting members between the reticular and basilar membranes, though he failed to work out their true details. He described the hair cells as resting on little stalks rising from a footing on the basilar membrane, and considered these stalks an outgrowth of the cells themselves. Actually, as Nuel firmly contended against consid-

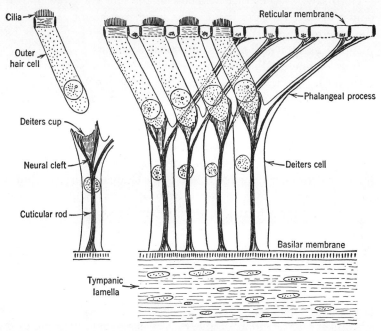

FIG. 6. The supporting mechanism for the outer hair cells. The Deiters cells are shown below, with their supporting cups and their phalangeal processes running obliquely up to the reticular membrane. On the left the hair cell and its Deiters cell are shown as separated. The neural cleft passes the nerve fibers to the lower end of the hair cell. The view is from the axis of the cochlea. From Held, in Bethe's *Handbuch der normalen und pathologischen Physiologie*, Vol. 11, 1926, J. Springer, Berlin.

erable opposition at the time, these stalks belong to separate cells. These latter cells, which came finally to be called the Deiters cells or phalangeal cells, are most remarkable structures, whose details Held (3) finally made clear.

As shown in Fig. 6, these cells have two parts, a main body that rises from the basilar membrane to the lower level of the hair cells, and a side arm given off thereabouts that reaches up to the reticular membrane. The main body contains a cuticular rod whose foot rests on the basilar membrane and whose head arborizes into a cup that snugly nestles the lower end of an outer hair cell. The ascending arm also contains a cuticular rod, a branch of the main one, that runs a little distance apicalward and then expands to form a headplate in the reticular surface. Actually, the reticular membrane is no independent structure but merely a mosaic formed by the headplates of these cells together with similar expansions formed by Corti's rods. Cuticular collars embrace the upper ends of the hair cells and provide the openings through which their cilia or 'hairs' protrude. The hair cells thus are firmly sustained by the Deiters cells at both their ends.

Still other accessory cells are named from their discoverers. Most important are the cells of Hensen—tall columnar cells that form an outer buttress to the hair cells and the Deiters cells. Beyond these are the more cuboidal cells of Claudius, lying among the other cells that cover the outer portion of the basilar membrane and line the external sulcus. Still farther outward, covering the vestibular portion of the spiral ligament, is a highly vascular band, observed by Huschke and carefully described by Corti, who gave it its name of stria vascularis. Corti noted that this band has the appearance of a secretory tissue, and he suggested that its function is the formation of the endolymph of the cochlea, a view still held at the present day (cf. Guild, 3).

A task yet remaining was the disclosure of the complete courses of the auditory nerve fibers. Kölliker had erroneously found them ending at Corti's rods. Schultze satisfied himself that these rods are not nervous by observing their staining reactions and resistance to reagents. He went on to work out many of the true connections. He saw some fibers in association with cells under the inner rods of Corti (evidently the inner hair cells) and others running out to cells regularly spaced under the outer rods (the outer hair cells). Most of the fibers that he saw ran into (or near) the tunnel and along it in a spiral direction. Nuel also saw these spiral fibers and followed them some distance in their courses. He found them running under about 60 rods and then turning in a radial direction. He traced them for a little distance outward between the outer rods, above the level of the basilar membrane, but there he lost sight of them. Retzius (2, 3) observed further the outward courses of these fibers and their actual endings at the hair cells, and Held (2, 4) elaborated their further details. This work finally identifies the hair cells as the actual sensory elements, and denotes all the other structures as accessory in function.

Inevitably this development of anatomical knowledge led to a revival of interest in auditory function.

DuVerney's hypothesis, which had continued to be preserved in a torpid state, in the form in which Haller's textbook presentation had molded it, now came to be re-examined with a critical eye, with a view toward amplifying its details and identifying the actual resonators. We have seen how Huschke and Corti commented in passing as to the vibratory possibilities of the specialized structures that they found. Now in the more inclusive and more insistent speculations of Helmholtz these questions of theory were to be raised to a new level of scientific concern.

CHAPTER 2

THE HELMHOLTZ RESONANCE THEORY

The year 1857 marks the beginning of the modern period of auditory theory, for in that year Hermann L. F. Helmholtz in a public lecture on the scientific foundations of music offered the first formulation of his resonance theory.

Helmholtz at that time was Professor of Physiology at the University of Bonn and had already begun to be recognized as one of the leading figures of his age. He was then in the early stages of the work that appeared six years later and was destined to become the classic in its field; this was *Die Lehre von den Tonempfindungen*, or *Sensations of Tone* as it was entitled in Ellis' translation into English of the third edition. Here he presented his theory in full.

The appearance of this theory was a historical event of high consequence, and this despite the fact, brought out in the preceding chapter, that basically the theory was nothing new: the idea of cochlear resonance was by then two centuries old. For two principal reasons Helmholtz's theory captured the immediate and enthusiastic attention of the public and scientific world alike and has continued through the ninety years of its history to dominate its field.

The first reason for the success of the theory lay in the manner and skill of its presentation. It was developed in connection with problems of musical harmony and musical perception in general, and thus it served to illuminate a domain of broad popular interest. Though it was a technical matter of great complexity, it nevertheless was presented with model simplicity and clarity and with a deft disregard of possible difficulties.

The second reason is more important for the scientific life of the theory and reflects Helmholtz's peculiar genius for bringing together in a meaningful way a number of ideas previously only loosely related. He integrated the concept of resonance with three other important developments of the period. These were

25

Ohm's law of auditory analysis, Müller's doctrine of specific energies of nerves, and the important anatomical discoveries of Corti.

AUDITORY ANALYSIS AND OHM'S LAW

It is not difficult for anyone with musical training, and for many others not formally schooled, to recognize by hearing alone that a musical chord is complex—that it is made up of several notes sounded together. More than that, it is possible to observe that a single note, when formed on almost any of the usual musical instruments, is itself decomposable into a fundamental tone and one or more overtones.

This ability of the ear to analyze complex sounds was first made into a formal principle by G. S. Ohm in 1843—the same Ohm who is known for his elementary law of electricity. It is pertinent to note in this connection that Ohm not only asserted the fact of analysis but that he specified the form that the analysis must take. Here he was guided by a mathematical theorem formulated a few years earlier by Fourier.

Fourier developed his theorem in connection with a study of the conduction of heat through solids, a subject curiously remote from the area of acoustics. Yet the principle that he worked out, as he himself was aware, is quite a general one and is applicable to all kinds of periodic motion. Indeed, it has become one of the most far-reaching ideas in the field of wave mechanics. The implications for sound are brought out in the following statements:

1. Any periodic sound wave may be considered analytically as the sum of a series of simple pendular waves, whose frequencies bear to one another the ratios of the integers 1, 2, 3, 4, and so on. (These pendular waves are usually represented as sine waves, though cosine waves, which have the same shape, will do just as well, or a formula may conveniently include both sine and cosine terms. For simplicity the following discussion mentions only sine waves, and the reader may bear in mind that the same statements hold for cosine waves and combinations of these two trigonometric forms.) We speak of a series of sine waves whose frequencies follow a consecutive pattern of this kind as a Fourier series. For an illustration of this type of

analysis, see Fig. 7, which shows first a complex wave and then the two sine waves into which it may be resolved.

2. For any complex wave, this analytical treatment yields a unique result. The series of sine waves, with their particular amplitude and phase relations, are absolutely determined, and no other series of sine waves of whatever amplitudes and phases can issue from the decomposition of the original wave. It should be added, however, that this analysis of complex waves into sine waves is not the only possible form of analysis. Indeed, analysis might take an indefinite number of forms, but no one yet has demonstrated a form that mathematically is as simple and convenient as that of Fourier.

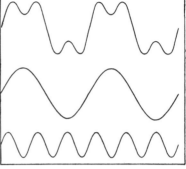

Fig. 7. Wave analysis. A complex wave is shown above, and below are shown the two sine waves into which it may be analyzed. Considered conversely, this figure also represents synthesis: the upper curve results when point by point we add the amplitudes of the two lower ones. A composite curve of different form results when we maintain the two simple curves in their frequencies and amplitudes but shift one with respect to the other along the time axis, i.e., alter their phase relations.

3. Synthesis follows a law that is the corollary of the law of analysis: simple waves may be added to form a complex wave, and the result of such a combination is unique for any given series when amplitudes and phases are specified for every member of the series.

The exact statement of Ohm's law of auditory analysis is that the ear performs the type of analysis defined by Fourier's theorem. For example, when a complex note is sounded whose fundamental frequency is 1000 ~, we should be able, after suitable training, to recognize not only the 1000 ~ component but also the overtones of frequencies 2000 ~, 3000 ~, 4000 ~, and so on. Of course, the amplitude of a component may be too small to permit us to identify it, or the amplitude may even be zero; but such variations do not impair the validity of the law.

On the same rule, a simple vibration, one that follows the form of a sine curve, is always heard as a single tone, and is not susceptible to analysis into other elements.

Helmholtz was greatly impressed by the fact that the ear analyzes sounds, and by the further consideration that it does so (as he believed) in the particular fashion stated in Ohm's law. This performance he designated as the most striking and distinctive achievement of the ear. He made it the foundation of his theory, and from it derived what to him was a conclusive argument for the presence of selective resonators in the ear. For, he said, the only known mechanical system by which a complex sound can be resolved into the elements described by Fourier's theorem is a series of resonators tuned to progressively different frequencies. In his words, "When we look about in nature for an analogue of such analysis of periodic motion we find none other than the phenomenon of sympathetic vibration."

Helmholtz obtained additional evidence for his hypothesis from his experiments on the synthesis of vowels and other complex sounds. He showed that such sounds could be imitated by exciting simultaneously a number of tuning forks suitably chosen in frequency and intensity. Only frequency and intensity were significant variables here; the phase relations could be changed at will without noticeable alteration of what he referred to as the musical quality. This ineffectiveness of phase, in Helmholtz's view, was the result of the fact that the ear analyzes the sound into its component simple tones, and phase relations are lost in the process.

As has already been shown, many others before Helmholtz, even as early as Bauhin in the beginning of the seventeenth century, had conceived of resonators in the ear; but in these earlier theories the concept of resonance was derived simply as a means by which the ear could receive sounds and achieve the necessary degree of sensitivity to them. The idea of analysis was implicit, it is true, but it was never developed as a basic principle. It was Helmholtz's particular contribution to the resonance hypothesis to claim for the process of resonance a unique status as the only possible means of accounting for the kind of analysis shown in auditory perception. He could take this step because the way had been opened for him by the contributions of Fourier and Ohm.

THE DOCTRINE OF SPECIFIC NERVE ENERGIES

Although the experiential basis of Helmholtz's theory was auditory analysis, its theoretical background was Johannes Müller's doctrine of specific energies of nerves. This doctrine represented an attempt to solve the very ancient problem of the nature of our sensory phenomena and their relations to the external world. Müller took the view that our experiences of quality—tones, colors, odors, and the like—are not direct appreciations of the properties of physical objects but are effects produced within ourselves under the influence of external forces.

This conception of the nature of sensation was not original with Müller; but he made it into a formal doctrine, gave it a name, and lent it consequence. Aristotle and others of the Greek period had expressed this same idea in opposing the earlier notion that the mind is in direct contact with the external world, or receives material emanations from objects. Much later, the British empiricists developed the idea more explicitly in their assertion that experience depends upon bodily processes, and finally in 1811 Charles Bell anticipated Müller by stating it in a clear form and adducing evidence for its validity.

Müller first presented his doctrine in 1826 and then elaborated it further in his famous textbook, the *Handbuch der Physiologie,* in 1838. His principal statement was that "sensation consists in the sensorium receiving through the medium of the nerves, and as the result of the action of an external cause, a knowledge of certain qualities or conditions, not of external bodies, but of the nerves of sense themselves." The relationship between nerves and their qualities he regarded as a specific one: there are five kinds of nerves, one for each of the 'five' senses; and one nerve can determine only its own kind of sensation.

Müller indicated two main lines of evidence in support of his doctrine. A given type of physical energy may affect different nerves and in doing so may give rise to different qualities of sensation. For example, pressure on the eyeball may produce spots of light, and a blow on the head may make the ears ring.

Then we have the counterpart of this: various physical causes when brought to bear upon one sensory nerve always give rise to one quality, that peculiar to the nerve concerned. Thus we may excite the optic nerve with light, or pressure, or an electric current, and the result always is visual sensation.

Müller left open the question of the precise place of origin of the sensory quality in the nervous system; and this problem remained as a challenge to subsequent investigation.

Helmholtz was influenced by Müller, who was his teacher and associate, and he considered the resonance theory to be an expression of Müller's doctrine. Actually, however, Helmholtz's theory extended the doctrine well beyond anything that Müller had conceived. Müller ended with the distinction of general fields of sense: vision, hearing, and the others. Then Natanson suggested certain subdivisions within some of these fields: in touch he distinguished three forms of specificity, and in hearing two, which were tone and clang. Volkmann carried this subdivision further, suggesting, for example, a specificity for every distinguishable pitch of the auditory range. Every fiber of the auditory nerve, he said, gives on stimulation its own peculiar effect. Helmholtz accepted this extensive multiplication of auditory specificities; and his resonance theory was an attempt to indicate concretely the nature of the processes, physical and physiological, on which these specificities depend.

CORTI'S ANATOMICAL CONTRIBUTIONS

For the objective support of his assumption of resonators in the ear, Helmholtz in the first presentation of his theory called attention to Corti's observations on the minute anatomy of the cochlea, which had appeared in 1851, six years earlier. Corti's researches, he said, had revealed the probable resonators.

It is a curious fact, in view of the importance to his theory, that Helmholtz at this time had only the vaguest appreciation of Corti's observations, and this despite the easy accessibility of the published results. We have to conclude that he knew of them only from others and not at first hand. In his 1857 lecture he spoke of Corti's newly discovered elements as 'little plates' and again in a similar discussion a year later as 'elastic plates and hairs,' whereas Corti referred to his structures as 'teeth' and described them as long, thin rods anchored at one end. Undoubtedly, Helmholtz or his informants confused the structures that Corti had discovered in the cochlea with others already known in the endings of the utricle, saccule, and semicircular canals. This confusion was cleared up in Helmholtz's later presentation of his theory in 1863.

THE IDENTITY OF THE RESONATORS

Claudius in 1856 had seen the arches of Corti, which Kölliker later named, and Deiters in 1860 represented their true detail. Helmholtz was aware of these developments and also of Kölliker's assertion, later proved erroneous, that the auditory nerve fibers had their terminations on the arches themselves. In 1863, therefore, the claim that Corti had made for his elements as the resonators seemed well supported. Helmholtz suggested further that the external segments of the arch, the outer rods of Corti, were the resonators proper, for, he said, they seem to be under tension, and they have their feet on the free, movable part of the basilar membrane. The inner rods, on the contrary, rest on the fibrous edge of the limbus where the basilar membrane is anchored and seem less favorably situated for movement. The outer rods vary in length throughout the cochlea, with those at the apex somewhat longer than those at the base, and this variation, perhaps together with variation in the tension or stiffness of the rods, could give the necessary differentiation of resonance characteristics.

On this basis, indefinite from the anatomical aspect as it admittedly was, Helmholtz established his conception of a series of progressively tuned resonators in the ear, with high tones located in the base of the cochlea and low tones in the apex. His analogy, now familiar to all, was the piano with dampers raised, which will echo a note sung loudly into it because those strings are set in motion that are tuned to the simple tones constituting the sound. An analysis is obtained if some record is made of the particular strings that are set in motion.

In the ear it is likewise necessary that there be an appreciation of what cochlear elements are in vibration at any instant.

This result is achieved by the provision of a separate nerve fiber for every cochlear element. Whenever the resonator responds its specific fiber is excited and the result is the perception of a tone of particular pitch.

THE REVISED THEORY

Helmholtz later was forced to make a new choice of anatomical elements to play the part of resonators, as a result of the definitive researches of Hensen and Hasse.

Hensen carried out the first careful measurements of cochlear structures. He observed first of all that the outer rods of Corti vary in length only about twofold throughout the entire extent of the cochlea, and he pointed out that this degree of variation is slight in view of the range of resonance characteristics required in the hearing of several octaves of tones. He then indicated the basilar membrane as a more likely resonant structure, for its width varies more markedly—according to his observations about 12-fold—from base to apex.

Hensen's objections to the arches of Corti as the resonators were strengthened when Schultze showed that the auditory nerve fibers do not end upon them but upon the hair cells; and these objections became practically overwhelming as a result of Hasse's studies on the cochlea of birds. Hasse found that in the bird there is a short cochlea that contains parts analogous to practically all those found in the mammalian cochlea, except for the arches of Corti. Arches are entirely lacking. Now, no one can doubt that birds hear and discriminate sounds with reasonable keenness. All—except perhaps the ones that utter only isolated chirps or whistles—must learn their patterns of song by ear. The canary and the mocking bird are notable performers in this respect. Hence it is certain that the arches of Corti are not essential to the functioning of the ear.

First in 1869, and again in detail in the third edition of his *Sensations of Tone* in 1870, Helmholtz recognized the force of Hensen's and Hasse's evidence and revised his theory in agreement with Hensen's suggestions, with the transverse fibers of the basilar membrane as the resonators. By this change the theory returned to a form more like that of earlier times, as in the formulations of DuVerney and his followers.

Helmholtz in the earlier formulations of his theory made a distinction in the mode of representation of tones and noises. The resonating mechanism of the cochlea, as we have seen, served for tonal reception. Noises, on the other hand, he ascribed to other parts of the inner ear; probably, he said, they depend upon the cilia of the ampullary and macular organs. Exner, however, objected to this distinction, pointing out that tones and noises have many features in common and that there are all stages between the two: most tones are impure, and nearly all noises have a definable pitch. Helmholtz recognized the force of this argument, and in 1877, in the fourth edition of his book, he modified his position by admitting the responsiveness of the cochlear resonators to abrupt and irregular vibrations. He still believed, however, that the ampullary and macular cilia were probably the receptors for the most rapid vibrations and therefore were the mediators of the "squeaking, hissing, chirping, and crackling sensations."

THE EVIDENCE FOR RESONATOR ACTION

As we have seen, it was Helmholtz's fundamental contention that the phenomenon of auditory analysis, and likewise that of the synthesis of complex sounds, can be explained on the assumption of a system of resonators in the ear, and on no other basis. The strength of this position, as he knew, depends in important measure on the possibility of identifying the appropriate anatomical elements, and the foregoing discussion shows how this aspect of the problem was treated.

More than this, however, the assumption of resonators in the ear carries with it rather specific implications as to the characteristics and mode of operation of the auditory mechanism. Resonators exhibit certain properties, and it is necessary to demonstrate that the ear reflects these properties and in general operates in a manner consistent with the physical principles and limitations governing resonator action.

The conditions that Helmholtz specifically considered are (1) the degree of independence of the resonators, (2) their graduation with respect to frequency, (3) their number in relation to the ability to distinguish pitch, and (4) their selectivity and persistence of action.

DEGREE OF INDEPENDENCE OF THE COCHLEAR RESONATORS

In the first place, as Helmholtz was aware, the acceptance in his later theory of the transverse fibers of the basilar membrane as the resonators brought in a difficulty that was not present, or at least was less apparent, in the original theory. The transverse fibers of this membrane are not anatomically separate and free, as the rods of Corti had been taken to be, but are embedded in the matrix of the membrane. It was necessary therefore to assume for this membrane certain unusual properties in order that the transverse fibers might act as though they were independent, or practically so, despite the presence of cross connections. The fundamental assumption is that the transverse tension is great and the longitudinal tension is 'vanishingly small.'

In his consideration of this feature Helmholtz examined a basilar membrane and reported that he found practically no tension in either the transverse or longitudinal directions. He concluded, however, that the possibility remained that in life a transverse tension was present, as demanded by the theory. This position he considered to be upheld by an observation made first by Todd and Bowman and later by Nuel that the membrane tears more readily along the lines of its transverse fibers than across the fibers.

The cross connections, according to Helmholtz, are too weak to interfere with the essentially independent movement of the fibers, yet have the advantage of providing a surface against which the fluid pressure can operate.

THE TUNING OF THE RESONATORS

A second requirement of the theory is that the resonators be graduated in characteristics to a degree corresponding to the range of discriminable pitches. In this relation Helmholtz referred only to the evidence of Hensen that the transverse fibers of the basilar membrane show a progressive variation in length, yet his discussion clearly indicates that he had in mind the possibility of variations also in the other conditions that determine the tuning of vibrating strings, namely, tension and mass. However, he had no evidence regarding these conditions and did not attempt to treat them explicitly.

THE NUMBER OF RESONATORS

A further requirement is that the number of resonators be sufficient. If the simple sensations of pitch arise separately and independently in the action of the cochlea, then there ought to be a resonant element for every discriminable tone, and the total number of elements should be at least as large as all the distinguishable tones throughout the audible range.

Helmholtz first approached this problem in his earlier discussion of 1863, when the rods of Corti were taken as the resonators. Then he attempted to correlate Kölliker's observations of the number of these structures with Weber's measurements of pitch discrimination. Kölliker had estimated that there were 3000 rods of Corti in the human cochlea. Of these, Helmholtz allotted 200 to the 'non-musical' ends of the scale where discrimination is poor, and the remaining 2800 to the middle seven octaves where discrimination is keen.

This allocation gave 400 rods to the octave or 33⅓ for each semitone in the middle region. Weber had shown that practiced musicians can discriminate tones of 1000 and 1001 ⌣, or about 64 steps in a semitone, which meant that there were about twice as many discriminable pitches as available elements.

Later when Waldeyer had revised the count of outer rods of Corti to 4500 the situation was little better, for by then Preyer had demonstrated even finer pitch discrimination. Waldeyer's figure made it possible, in the middle range, to assign 600 elements to the octave, or 50 per semitone, yet Preyer's results showed 1000 discriminable pitches to the octave, or 83 to the semitone.

Curiously enough, Helmholtz seemed not at all disturbed by this insufficiency of elements and did not regard it as any obstacle to his theory. He got around the difficulty by the following ingenious argument. A tone of a frequency midway between the tones proper to two adjacent rods of Corti will affect both of them at once, and this kind of action will be interpreted in perception as a tone of intermediate pitch. Indeed, many intermediates may be heard, because the relative degree of excitation of two resonators will vary with the nearness of the frequency to the one or the other; and the possible number of intermediate pitches will depend ultimately only on the delicacy with which we can apprehend the relative strengths of excitation. It is this situation, he suggested, that causes us to hear a steadily rising frequency like the tone of a siren as continuous in pitch rather than as ascending by discrete steps.

In the development of his later theory, in which the transverse fibers of the basilar membrane became the resonators, Helmholtz might have found a simpler solution to his problem, for the basilar membrane fibers are much more numerous than the rods of Corti. There are some 10,500 of them, enough to account directly for the full number of specificities as calculated. He did not adopt this solution, however, but maintained his belief in the importance of the arches of Corti. Now he accorded the arches the role of intermediaries between the resonating basilar membrane fibers and the auditory nerve terminations. He said that the arches first were affected by the movements of the basilar membrane fibers and that they in turn communicated the effects to the hair cells. His reasoning was that the movements of the membrane could more readily be transmitted to the endings in the hair cells by firm structures like the arches than simply by the soft mass of the intervening cells. A consequence of this view is that there can be no greater number of basic specificities than there are arches, and so he retained his special argument for the rise of intermediate pitches.

THE SELECTIVITY AND PERSISTENCE OF THE COCHLEAR RESONATORS

In first presenting his theory Helmholtz spoke of a resonator as allocated to every pitch and, contrariwise, of a particular tone as affecting only its proper resonator. This formulation may have served only a didactic purpose; but it is likely that Helmholtz himself a good part of the time thought of his theory in these simple terms. At any rate, as we have seen, he soon found it necessary to complicate the picture in order to reconcile the number of discriminable pitches with the available number of arches of Corti. He complicated it further when he came to the question of the selectivity of the cochlear resonators. He was thoroughly aware of the physical principles involved. No resonance is wholly specific. A resonator acts most vigorously in response to the frequency to which it is tuned, and to a lesser degree to frequencies above and below this frequency. The extent to which the neighboring frequencies are discriminated against is referred to as the selectivity of the resonator; a high degree of selectivity means that the amplitude of the response falls off rapidly with even slight departures from the tuned frequency, whereas a low degree of selectivity means that frequencies some distance away will still have an appreciable effect. Alternatively we speak of the range of resonance, which expresses this same property in a converse sense: the range of resonance is the width of the band of frequencies that produce an appreciable response. The range is broad when the selectivity is low, as then many frequencies are operative; while the range is narrow when the selectivity is great, and only frequencies closely similar to the tuned frequency have an effect.

The selectivity depends upon the damping, which is an expression for the degree to which the vibratory motion is opposed by frictional forces. These frictional forces are always present in some amount, both within the vibrating body and external to it, and they play a significant part in determining the nature of the vibration. If the damping is low, then the selectivity is high, and conversely. For example, a tuning fork in air is but lightly damped and can be set in sympathetic vibration only by frequencies that closely approach the frequency to which it is tuned. On the other hand, the same fork if immersed in water will respond to a wide range of tones: its selectivity will then be reduced on account of the greater frictional resistance imposed by the liquid medium.

The damping also determines the persistence of action of a resonator after its excitation has ceased. When the damping is low the energy that has been imparted to the resonator is dissipated only at a gradual rate, largely as acoustic energy, so that the movement persists for a long time. On the other hand, when the damping is great the energy is extracted quickly, much of it being reduced to heat, and the movement soon dies away. A tuning fork in air will speak for a long time after it is struck; but if immersed in water will come to rest after only a few vibrations.

It will be evident that, since selectivity and persistence are mutual effects of damping, they must vary concurrently. A high degree of selectivity is associated with long persistence, and low selectivity with slight persistence.

Helmholtz discussed the significance of these properties in the process of hearing and tried to work out a definite conception of their effects. A rough idea may be based on ordinary experience. It is obvious, he pointed out, that the damping of the cochlear resonators cannot be so low as that of a tuning fork, whose response persists for many seconds, for such long persistence would interfere with our ability to distinguish notes that follow one another in close succession. Since notes are separately perceived in rather rapid passages of music, it seems evident that the persistence is of the order of a small fraction of a second. On the other hand, the persistence cannot be assumed to be negligibly small, advantageous though that might be from the standpoint of perceiving rapid changes of pitch. The reason is that to have short persistence we must have high damping, and the high damping would so reduce the selectivity of the resonators as to impair our ability to distinguish one pitch from another. With high damping any one tone would excite a great array of resonators, perhaps almost the entire series, and we should hear only an utter confusion of sound. Evidently— so he argued—some intermediate degree of damping must prevail.

Helmholtz sought a more precise answer to this question in his study of 'musical shakes.' A 'shake' is executed by sounding two adjacent notes at a rapid rate. Helmholtz, working with the piano, found that in the region of $A = 110 \sim$ two notes remained distinct when struck alternately at the rate of 10 per second. This result he took to mean that in the time of $\frac{1}{10}$ sec the vibration of the cochlear resonator corresponding to one of the notes had fallen to so low a level as to be negligible in comparison with the vibration of the other resonator which now was set in action.

This observation of the persistence of vibrations will give a numerical value for the damping and the selectivity only with the aid of two further items of information. It must first be determined just how low an amplitude must be reached for the vibration of a resonator to become inappreciable. Helmholtz had no measure of this function and could only offer an estimate. He supposed that the action of a resonator would become inappreciable when its amplitude fell to $\frac{1}{10}$ its original value. It must further be considered, in speaking of the range of resonance, at what point the response of a resonator to a frequency different from its natural frequency may be considered negligible, and here again Helmholtz took the figure of $\frac{1}{10}$. With these assumptions and the observation that in $\frac{1}{10}$ sec the response had fallen to the point where it did not blur the next note, Helmholtz calculated the range of resonance as about one semitone on either side of the tuned resonator, or as a whole tone over all.

Helmholtz conceded that this result was only a rough approximation but considered that it afforded a concrete conception of the action of the ear. He added that "when we hereafter speak of individual parts of the ear vibrating sympathetically with a determinate tone, we mean that they are set into strongest motion by that tone, but are also set into vibration less strongly by tones of nearly the same pitch, and that this sympathetic vibration is still sensible for the interval of a Semitone." This important feature of Helmholtz's theory is often lost sight of because during most of his presentation he emphasized the distinctness of the action of the cochlear elements, and it is always simpler to think of a separate resonator for every distinguishable pitch. Helmholtz himself was not at all clear regarding the implications of this idea for his theory. He failed to see that when the resonators no longer act separately they cease to obey the law of specific energies. We shall return to this problem later.

THE RECEPTION OF THE THEORY

From the beginning, as we have noted, Helmholtz's theory had a welcome reception. Moreover, its fame was enhanced rather than dulled after the revision forced upon it by Hensen's and Hasse's discoveries. By then it seemed to have met and overcome its most serious obstacles, so that during the next decade it reached its highest level of scientific popularity. In 1874 it was possible for Buck to speak of it as enjoying universal acceptance among physiologists.

Later, doubts and criticisms began to appear, largely as a result of a closer study of cochlear structures and a realization of the severe anatomical requirements issuing from the physical assumptions of the theory. Once the revulsion began it developed rapidly and led to a number of proposals for revision and the emergence of rival hypotheses.

The first serious criticism of Helmholtz's theory came from Rinne as early as 1865, but the most weighty opposition was that of Rutherford in 1886, in which the basic concept of peripheral analysis was attacked and an alternative theory was proposed. Then in quick succession came the theories of Waller (1891), Hurst (1895), and Bonnier (1895) and near the close of the century those of Meyer, Ewald, and ter Kuile, all of which set forth new conceptions of the action of the ear to take the place of the resonance principle. By this time, as the new century began, Helmholtz's theory had swung completely away from its former position of almost unchallenged eminence. It was criticized on every hand, and many considered its faults to be overwhelming, and like von Ebner were disposed, although reluctantly, to give it up altogether.

The divergences from Helmholtz's conception took various forms. The mildest grew out of doubts concerning the presence of stretched strings in the ear and led to the proposal that there is differential resonance of a suspended membrane; such were the theories of Hasse and Ewald. More serious was the objection to the principle of resonance itself, as voiced by Hurst, ter Kuile, and Watt, yet with retention of the concept of place representation based on other considerations. Most radical of all was the rejection of the place principle together with the idea of peripheral analysis, and the proposal of a new 'frequency' principle of nervous representation, as found in the telephone theories of Rutherford and others. And finally there was a compromise position, taken in the theories of Meyer and Wrightson, in which this frequency principle was combined with a form of place representation that permitted at least a degree of peripheral analysis.

According to these divergences, as the accompanying outline shows, the theories fall into four groups, two in each of two

THE CLASSICAL THEORIES SINCE HELMHOLTZ

I. Place Theories

    A. Resonance theories

        1. Tuned-element theories
            Helmholtz, 1857, 1869

        2. Membrane-resonance theories
            Hasse, 1867
            Ewald, 1898
            Shambaugh, 1907

        3. Tube-resonance theories
            Ranke, 1931
            Reboul, 1937

    B. Non-resonance or wave theories
        Hurst, 1895
        ter Kuile, 1900
        Watt, 1914
        Békésy, 1928

II. Frequency Theories

    A. Telephone or non-analytic theories
        Rutherford, 1886
        Ayers, 1892
        Bonnier, 1895
        Hardesty, 1908

    B. Frequency-analytic theories
        Meyer, 1898
        Wrightson, 1918

general classes. The two classes are the place theories and the frequency theories, distinguished by the manner of accounting for the perception and discrimination of pitch. The place theories depend upon the spatial distribution of response in the cochlea, so that every tone has its proper location and therefore its specific nervous representation. These theories subdivide further according to whether they accept or reject the resonance principle, and hence we have both resonance and non-resonance types of place theory. The frequency theories are characterized by the assumption that the frequency of the mechanical vibrations is communicated to the auditory nerve and thence to the higher nervous centers, and that this frequency as centrally represented provides the basis for pitch perception. These theories separate into two groups accordingly as they accept or reject the principle of peripheral analysis, thereby giving the telephone or non-analytic theories and the frequency-analytic theories. In the following pages these several forms of auditory theory will be treated in detail.

CHAPTER 3

THE PLACE THEORIES AFTER HELMHOLTZ

As we have seen, the objections found to Helmholtz's particular hypothesis led at once to two types of theory in which the place concept was retained: the membrane-resonance theories and the non-resonance place theories. Ultimately, in more recent times, there appeared a third type, the tube-resonance theories. As the outline shows, this last belongs logically with the other resonance theories. In the treatment to follow, however, these theories will be taken up in the order mentioned; the historical order is preferred to the logical because in many respects each type builds upon the foundations of its predecessors.

THE MEMBRANE-RESONANCE THEORIES

Only through two special assumptions was Helmholtz able to formulate a stretched-string theory while accepting the basilar membrane as the responding structure. These assumptions were that the membrane is subjected to great transverse tension but is lax in the longitudinal direction and that cross connections impose only negligible restraint on the independent movement of the fibers. If these assumptions are denied, but the principle of resonance is retained, the result is a form of membrane-resonance theory. The earliest example of this type of theory was the theory of Hasse, formulated in 1867 on the basis of his study of the cochlea of birds.

HASSE'S TECTORIAL MEMBRANE THEORY

Carl Hasse was a comparative anatomist, at first at the University of Würzburg and later at Breslau. In his work of 1867 he opposed Helmholtz's view that the rods of Corti were the resonators because in the avian cochlea these elements are absent. At the same time he rejected Hensen's suggestion about the basilar membrane fibers and argued instead in favor of the tectorial membrane as the responsive structure.   By then it was known that the auditory nerve fibers have their endings on the hair cells, and Hasse accepted these cells as the ultimate points of excitation.   Yet he considered them to be too loosely suspended on the surface of the basilar membrane to be stimulated readily by it.   On the other hand, the tectorial membrane lies in close proximity to these cells, and in its movements ought to excite them easily.

Though Hasse did not elaborate upon his theory, it evidently belongs to the membrane-resonance type, for he put forward no special assumptions that would lead to a response of isolated fibers.   A little later he grew doubtful about his hypothesis and went over to Hensen's view, then raised in prestige by Helmholtz's adoption of it, to the extent of accepting the basilar membrane as at least the primary resonator.   In later years others, including Siebenmann, von Ebner, Kishi, and Shambaugh, pursued the tectorial membrane theory further, and in their hands the contrast of membrane resonance as against stretched-string resonance was made explicit.

SHAMBAUGH'S MEMBRANE THEORY

In 1907, G. E. Shambaugh, an anatomist and otologist connected with the University of Chicago and the Presbyterian Hospital, made the latest and most extensive formulation of this theory.   His arguments include first of all his reasons for rejecting Helmholtz's simple resonance theory.   The transverse fibers of the basilar membrane, he pointed out, are not independent but are united in a close meshwork.   Moreover, the cells lying on the membrane are in contact and must affect one another. He argued, too, that a simple 'tone to a fiber' relationship ought to give a high stability of action, with relatively fixed powers of pitch discrimination, whereas actually there are great differences in the powers of discrimination among individuals and variations in any given person as a result of training.   As arguments against the choice of the basilar membrane as the resonator, Shambaugh observed that near the base of the cochlea this membrane is thick and rigid and apparently ill-adapted to movement.   Sometimes, he said, the basilar membrane is missing at the extreme basal end, yet the organ of Corti is present, resting on the solid bony lamina. On the other hand, the tectorial membrane is found here and, indeed, is everywhere associated with the organ of Corti; and this close relationship provides what he considered to be 'strong presumptive evidence' for the tectorial membrane as the resonator. This structure is exceedingly delicate, semifluid in nature, and of the same specific gravity as the endolymph. Therefore it could be set into vibration with great readiness. It lies over the hair cells, and, he believed, the hairs are embedded in its lower surface, hence its movements will excite these cells.

This theory conceives of resonance only of a general sort, with any particular tone involving a considerable area of the membrane and hence exciting a rather extensive group of hair cells. Discrimination of pitch is possible, according to Shambaugh, because a higher or lower tone will excite a few more cells above or below the previously excited region.

The tectorial membrane theory as sketched here has two important features. One, treated in a rather incidental manner by the proponents of the theory but actually of great significance, is the emphasis on a broad form of response of the membrane rather than an action of isolated elements; this feature will appear again in bolder outline in the modern developments of the resonance theory.

The other feature and the one that was uppermost in the minds of Hasse and his successors was their choice of the tectorial membrane as the locus of the cochlear resonators. Most of the arguments advanced in support of this choice have now been mentioned. It is fair to say that they are not taken very seriously at the present time.

EWALD'S PRESSURE-PATTERN THEORY

A different form of membrane theory was elaborated in 1898 by J. R. Ewald, Professor of Physiology in the University of Strassburg. He rejected the idea of a resonance of specific elements and also that of a broad local response as conceived in the theories of Hasse and others. Instead, he proposed a theory in which the basilar membrane is thrown into general and extensive vibratory patterns, something like the patterns demonstrated long before by Chladni in vibrating plates. These patterns, or 'acoustic images,' as Ewald called them, were regarded as distinctive for every discriminable sound.

The manner in which the 'acoustic images' arise is through the establishment of standing waves upon the membrane. Ewald was not altogether explicit on this point, but he evidently conceived of waves traveling over the basilar membrane from base to apex and then after reflection passing backward toward the base. Such an action will give rise to standing waves, as is

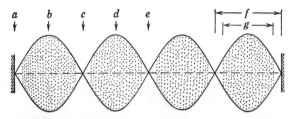

Fig. 8. Ewald's theory. Shown here is the standing wave pattern conceived for the basilar membrane when stimulated by a tone of 40 ∽. Points *a, c, e* are nodes; *b, d* are loops. A loop covers half a wave length, *f*, and is effective over only part of its length, *g*.

easily demonstrated with a cord when one end is secured and the other end is moved rapidly up and down. Certain segments of the cord will be observed in vigorous up-and-down movements while others remain at rest; these segments are called loops and nodes, respectively (see Fig. 8).

It may be observed also in this demonstration that the number of loops and nodes increases with the frequency of the vibration, and at the same time the distance between nodes decreases. The distance from one node to the next is one-half the wave length of the vibration. The basilar membrane is thought of as acting like the cord in this example, except that it is anchored at both ends and is moved by energy communicated to its mid-portion.

In this situation, two cues are available for the perception and discrimination of pitch. One is the spatial separation of the loops, which is great for low tones and progressively less as the frequency increases. The other is the width of the band in the region of each loop where the amplitude of movement is sufficient to give nerve excitation.

The limits of the tonal scale will depend on the practical limits of spatial separation of the loops. One of these limits is reached, according to Ewald, for the simple pattern of two loops and three nodes, which gives an internodal distance of half the length of the basilar membrane; this pattern he took to represent 20 $\sim$, the lowest perceptible pitch. The other limit, presented by the highest perceptible pitch, he set out to calculate. The highest pitch he accepted as 32,000 $\sim$, and as this frequency is 1600 times that of the lowest tone, it should have 1600 times as many loops, or 3200 loops. If the basilar membrane is 32 mm long, the highest tone will be represented by an acoustic pattern containing 100 loops to the millimeter, and discrimination of this tone from others will require a distinction of elements only 0.01 mm apart. Such fine discrimination Ewald regarded as anatomically reasonable.

According to this theory, the analysis of complex sounds involves the ability to recognize different tonal patterns when they are present simultaneously, superimposed on one another in the response of the membrane. We should expect such ability to vary among individuals and to be improved greatly by practice. Here is one of Ewald's chief arguments for his theory, for analytic abilities indeed are variable and are noticeably subject to training.

The specific arguments that Ewald set forth in favor of his theory as opposed to the simple resonance hypothesis are itemized as follows:

1. The theory avoids the physical and anatomical difficulties of the assumption of specific independent resonators. The basilar membrane is regarded as a true membrane, and critical assumptions do not have to be made regarding its physical characteristics.

2. The theory possesses a desirable flexibility. In the simple resonance theory, the loss of a single element must be immediately obvious in the inability to hear a particular pitch. In this theory a local injury would not be serious, for the pattern could still be represented satisfactorily on the remaining regions of the membrane. The theory is even able to embrace a limited

kind of regional differentiation. It is likely, Ewald agreed, that the highest tones do not spread over the entire extent of the membrane but are restricted to its narrower portions. Hence the high tones are found in the basal region, and the low tones are distributed over the whole membrane.

3. The facts of pitch discrimination are satisfactorily explained. On a resonance theory there is no good reason that a given tone should be any more difficult to distinguish from a neighboring tone than from one more remote, for every tone is represented by a separate element. In this theory, on the contrary, discrimination is in a measure a matter of spatial differentiation, and the separation of the patterns increases with the frequency difference.

4. Consonance and dissonance are simply accounted for as the degree to which two patterns coincide. Two tones that form the interval of an octave give the maximum consonance because there is a high degree of overlapping of their patterns: the loops of the lower tone coincide with alternate loops of the higher tone. Other simple intervals give lesser degrees of coincidence. On the other hand, tones with incommensurable ratios show no coincidences and are heard as dissonant.

5. Noises are accounted for by the absence of fixed patterns and the formation instead of moving, ever-changing patterns.

6. Difference tones and interruption tones are easily explained as the result of a periodic interruption of sound patterns. The periodic gaps in a pattern are appreciated because they form a pattern of their own. Any periodicity whatever can thereby be perceived.

In support of his theory Ewald carried out extensive tests on a model, his 'camera acustica,' which consisted of a thin rubber membrane stretched over a wedge-shaped opening in a block. When the membrane was excited by bringing a vibrating tuning fork near it, a pattern was formed that varied with the frequency of the sound but was constant for any given sound. Ewald considered that the forms of these patterns provided the basis for pitch discrimination in the manner already described.

Ewald's theory has received relatively little attention and support from other investigators. Lehmann criticized it, saying that the patterns were largely 'optical illusions' determined by the particular way in which the membrane was illuminated during its vibration. He constructed models of his own and usually, on exposing them to vibrations, observed complicated patterns that spread over nearly the entire surface of the membrane. Under some conditions, however, he was able to obtain simple cross striations, largely restricted to one region. He suggested that in the actual cochlea the damping may be great enough that only two or three of these striations are effective; and by this means his theory is reduced to one of general localities in the representation of pitch.

For the high tones, according to Lehmann, the patterns of action are near the base of the cochlea and fairly restricted, whereas for the low tones they are farther toward the apex and more extensive. Because the effective areas are larger for the low tones than for the high tones the quality of 'expansiveness' possessed by the low tones is accounted for.

Lehmann thought of his theory as a variant of Helmholtz's, and there is indeed a resemblance at many points, especially in the means proposed for cochlear differentiation. Without going into details Lehmann suggested that the breadth, tension, and stiffness of the basilar membrane, and possibly its thickness also, determine the regions of movement in response to particular frequencies. The theory departs from that of Helmholtz in a denial of the principle of specific energies. The areas of action are broad, and perhaps there are two or three of them that are effective for any given tone. At this point the theory comes close to Ewald's.

Much later, Zoth adopted Ewald's theory, but he substituted Reissner's membrane as the resonating structure. His argument was that a thin membrane is required and that this membrane fills the requirement better than the basilar membrane.

Koch developed Ewald's theory (with the basilar membrane as the resonator) from a mathematical standpoint. He advanced two chief arguments in addition to those made by Ewald. He considered the natural frequency of the membrane to be about $16,000 \sim$ and thus well above the greater part of the auditory range, but he did not think this a handicap to the Ewald theory, though obviously it must preclude a Helmholtz form of theory.

Further, he sought to show that damping is far from negligible, as it is assumed to be on a specific resonance theory.

One significant feature of Koch's theory is that he regarded damping as operating in a progressive fashion, increasing toward the apex. A result is that the amplitude of the loops formed on the membrane is greatest near the basal end and less toward the apex. In fact he inclined to the view that the rate of the decline in amplitude is so great that only the first and second loops are effective. This condition would restrict the response of the higher tones rather sharply to the basal end, and a kind of localization would be established that in some respects resembles the one assumed by the Helmholtz theory.

Gildemeister (2), who worked with Koch in developing this theory further, suggested that for two reasons, because the sound energy has its principal access to the cochlea at the basal end and because the damping increases rapidly from there toward the apex, only the first loop of the response will have appreciable amplitude. These assumptions increase the agreement with the Helmholtz theory of localization. The remaining difference is that the low tones, with their long wave lengths, affect large regions of the membrane, basal and apical alike, whereas in the Helmholtz theory they affect only narrow bands in the apical region.

It should be added that this concept of the progressive damping of a wave that begins at the base of the cochlea and moves upward is a very significant variation from Ewald's theory. It will not harmonize with the standing wave principle through which Ewald supposed the acoustic pattern to be established. If the primary wave is severely damped out there will be no reflected wave, and hence no standing waves can arise. Thus on scrutiny Koch's theory appears to be a form of traveling wave theory, like those to be considered later in this chapter.

The outstanding advantage of the membrane-resonance type of theory is the relative simplicity of its assumptions about the physical properties of the membrane. The Helmholtz theory, as we have seen, is forced to make assumptions of a specific (and it can be argued a rather improbable) character, so that the membrane will act like a set of independent stretched strings and not at all like a membrane. This theory, on the contrary, does not demand any particular mode of response of the cochlear structures, except that the response shall vary significantly for different sounds.

As far as pitch perception and pitch discrimination are concerned, the theory compares favorably with the Helmholtz hypothesis. At first glance it seems to suffer in that the cue for pitch is a more complex affair: it is a pattern involving many areas of stimulation rather than the excitation of a single fiber or small group of fibers; yet this feature seems not very serious if we accept Ewald's suggestion that the cue to pitch is the spatial separation of stimulated areas, and perhaps at the same time it depends upon the breadth of these areas. The difficulty is even less if we consider Koch's idea that somewhat as in the Helmholtz theory itself it is the general locus of the excitation that acts as the cue to pitch.

One obstacle for the theory arises in the matter of the analysis of complex sounds. When several patterns are simultaneously present it is difficult to conceive how they may be separated. The service rendered by the peripheral mechanism in the interest of analysis is certainly less under this hypothesis than in the Helmholtzian 'pitch to a fiber' theory. There are two answers, or partial answers, in the face of this difficulty. One is that auditory analysis is not nearly so general and well developed a capacity as Helmholtz made out, that it depends upon long practice, and that it is possessed in high degree by only a few. The other is that analysis is not a peripheral activity and that its burden must be cast upon the higher brain centers. This last was Koch's position.

A serious objection to Ewald's hypothesis follows from the assumption that in its action the membrane is divided into an integral number of loops: two or three or four and so on up to the limit of perhaps 3200. If this kind of response occurs there is a significant consequence for pitch discrimination. If two loops represent 20 $\sim$, three must represent 30 $\sim$, and so on; and hence at the low end of the scale the steps are large—only two in the first octave. Then as the scale is followed upward the steps continue in linear progression until finally a point is reached where the spatial separation of the loops is too small to be appreciated and discrimination fails. Before this point is reached the discrimination should be extraordinarily keen as reckoned by tonal interval: 16,000 ~, represented by 1600 loops, ought to be distinguishable from 16,010 ~, represented by 1601 loops. In general, the difference limen for pitch ought to have the constant value of 10 ~ regardless of the region of the frequency scale. We are certain that discrimination at the low end of the scale is better than indicated by the theory and that it is poorer at the high end; and that though it is roughly constant in terms of frequency difference at the low end it is not so at the high end.

The objection just outlined does not apply, at least not in any simple manner, to the form of theory held by Koch, for apparently in his theory the patterns do not arise through standing waves.

Other criticisms might be made of the Ewald theory in regard to various details, but they will not be developed here. Presently it will be shown that a similar theory arises in another way, as a development of the Helmholtz theory when a high degree of damping is admitted, and in this connection a further evaluation of the pattern hypothesis will be attempted.

The Non-Resonance Place Theories

In this class of place theories the principle of resonance is rejected, but a spatial distribution of pitches in the cochlea is attained by a different process. These are sometimes called 'wave theories,' or 'traveling bulge theories,' since they depend upon a progressively moving wave of displacement on the basilar membrane. Theories of this class were proposed by Hurst, ter Kuile, and Watt.

HURST'S TRAVELING BULGE THEORY

C. H. Hurst's theory, presented at a meeting of the Liverpool Biological Society in 1894, was the first of the traveling bulge theories. It is a remarkable theory in many respects. Its basic assumption is that sounds set up waves that move up and down the cochlea and in their travels meet with one another at positions that are a function of their wave lengths.

The conception in detail is as follows. A wave of displacement of the basilar membrane is formed during the period when the stapes is moving inward with positive acceleration. This wave is a narrow bulge that retains its restricted form as it moves. It begins at the basal end of the membrane and rapidly moves upward toward the apex. When it reaches the apex it runs around the terminal wall to Reissner's membrane and then continues down Reissner's membrane to the base of the cochlea.

If the stapes moves inward once more before this circuit of the first wave is completed, the second wave will meet the first at some point in the cochlea. At the place of meeting of the upgoing and downgoing waves the cochlear fluid will be concentrated, since one wave produces pressure in one direction and the other in the contrary direction, and at the point where this concentration is great—so it is said—the tectorial membrane will be thrust down upon the hairs of the hair cells and stimulation will occur.

The region of the basilar membrane so stimulated will depend simply on the time interval between the two waves. If the time interval is great, the first wave will have covered most of its path before the second wave begins, and their meeting point will be near the basal end. If the time interval is short, one wave will follow closely behind the other, and they will meet soon after the first has made the turn at the apex. Therefore the excitation for low tones will be localized in the base of the cochlea and that for high tones will be localized in the apex.

For the very low tones, the meeting of the two waves can occur at only one point. For higher tones, however, there may be several points of meeting when there is a continuous series of waves. If, say, ten waves are moving down the cochlear pathway at any one instant, a new upgoing wave will meet with every one of them in its course from base to apex. Hurst made certain special assumptions to reduce the complexity that would result if all these meetings were effective in stimulation.

The first assumption is that the amplitude of the displacement increases as the wave moves from base to apex. This increase of amplitude takes place because the membrane becomes broader toward the apex and resistance to displacement grows correspondingly less. He then assumed that after the apex is reached, and the wave moves downward again over Reissner's membrane, the amplitude decreases rapidly on account of damping. Therefore, on both membranes, the amplitude is greatest in the apical region. Consequently, when there are multiple meeting points, the one nearest the apex will be the most effective. For weak intensities it must follow that only the most apical meeting will give rise to a perception of pitch.

A further assumption is that the middle ear introduces a marked compression of amplitude, so that the range of variation of amplitudes from the smallest to the largest will be much reduced at the stapes from what it is as the sounds enter the ear. For tones ordinarily encountered the amplitudes at the stapes will vary over a narrower range than the variations introduced within the cochlea itself by the two conditions mentioned: the width of basilar membrane and the damping. In consequence, at the primary or most apical meeting point the stimulating effect of a tone of moderate intensity will be only a little larger than that for a barely perceptible tone, and at secondary and more basal points the amplitude will be insufficient to stimulate. For all tones ordinarily encountered, therefore, only one meeting point will be effective.

For tones of extraordinarily great intensity there will be a second and possibly a third meeting point where stimulation will occur, but the 'spurious' pitches resulting from these excitations will be faint and therefore not very noticeable in comparison with the principal pitch.

The first objection to Hurst's theory arises from the form of cochlear localization that it involves: low tones in the base of the cochlea and high tones in the apex. The available evidence points to the contrary relation. Hurst discussed some of this evidence. He mentioned the reported observation that injuries to the apex of the cochlea caused a loss of hearing for low tones. His explanation was that the injury to the apex allowed the transmitted wave to pass from the basilar membrane to Reissner's membrane at the site of the injury and thereby reduced the usual path of travel so that a given wave would reach the basal end sooner than usual. If it arrived there before its successor had started upward, no stimulation could occur. The tones at the low end of the frequency scale would therefore be lost.

As will be shown later, the selective loss of low tones does not occur. The well-authenticated observation of the isolated loss of high tones as a result of basal injury will not permit of ready explanation on Hurst's theory.

Hurst's theory suffers also from the improbable nature of its special assumptions. The theory assumes a very low velocity of conduction, around 1 meter per second for the lowest tones in order for two waves to be present in the cochlea at the same time. Though a case might be made for velocity of this order by assuming a very great viscosity, it is not at all probable.

If damping operates for the wave going down Reissner's membrane, it should be present also, in moderate degree at least, during the upward passage along the basilar membrane. If there is damping, then it is difficult to conceive of a progressive rise in amplitude during the transmission apicalward.

The idea that the middle ear in some unexplained fashion produces a compression of amplitude is a weak point in the theory. Such a compression would make it difficult for us to distinguish variations of loudness. From evidence available to us now, though not to Hurst at the time, it is certain that no such compression takes place.

Finally, this theory supposes that when the intensity of a tone is raised to a very high level we hear additional tones whose frequencies are simple fractions of the fundamental frequency, whereas what we actually hear are overtones—multiples of the fundamental frequency.

TER KUILE'S THEORY

Emile ter Kuile was a physician specializing in otology, who shortly after presenting his theory in 1900 was located in the city of Amsterdam. His theory was developed in connection with a general treatment of the form of movement of the basilar membrane. Like Hurst's it is based upon the idea of wave motion in the cochlea, but for ter Kuile the motion occurs in only one direction, from base to apex, and Reissner's membrane has no important role. The pitch depends on how far up the cochlea this wave motion extends.

When, according to this theory, the stapes starts from its most outward position and moves inward it displaces a quantity of fluid which causes the basilar membrane to bulge downward. The bulge begins at the extreme basal end of the membrane

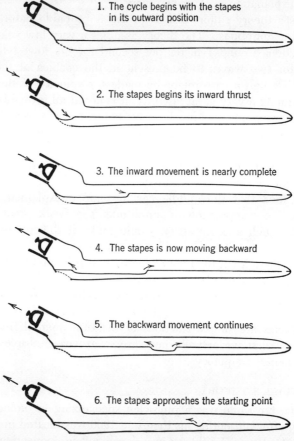

1. The cycle begins with the stapes in its outward position

2. The stapes begins its inward thrust

3. The inward movement is nearly complete

4. The stapes is now moving backward

5. The backward movement continues

6. The stapes approaches the starting point

FIG. 9. Ter Kuile's theory. The progression of a wave along the basilar membrane is represented in six successive views. The cochlea is shown as unrolled, and the stapes is pictured as though it were a piston working in a cylinder. The arrows on the left indicate the stapedial motions. Other arrows represent the fluid pressures as exerted on the basilar membrane.

but at once is propagated apicalward along the membrane. This propagation of the bulge takes place both on account of the elastic properties of the membrane and because as the stapes continues to move forward the amount of fluid displaced is greater than can be accommodated by the bulging of the basal portions of the membrane.

When the stapes reaches its most forward position the bulge attains its greatest length. It continues to travel apicalward at constant velocity, but from now on it suffers a curtailment of its length. As the stapes has reversed its direction and is pulling away, the fluid is sucked backward. The effect is to erase the bulge in a progressive fashion, beginning at its most basal end and continuing until at the moment the stapes has returned to its most external position the bulge vanishes.

During the first half-period of the vibration, when the stapes moves from its most external to its most forward position, the bulge travels one-half a wave length along the membrane. During the second half-period, when the stapes moves backward, the bulge continues to travel up the membrane but suffers a progressive diminution in length at its lower end. At the close of the period the most advanced portion of the bulge will approach a position along the membrane which is one wave length from the base—but it reaches this position only just as it ceases to exist.

The significant feature for pitch perception is the extent of basilar membrane excited, measured from the basal end to the farthest point reached at the moment the bulge disappears. The length of this excited portion of the membrane depends simply upon the period of the wave, which varies inversely as the frequency; the low tones, with their long periods, will have a more extended path of travel than the high tones. The result is a distribution of response along the basilar membrane according to frequency, much as in the resonance theory except that here it is the whole extent of the stimulated portion of the membrane that affords the cue to pitch rather than an isolated point of stimulation.

It is to be noted that the backward movement of the stapes only erases the depression that has just previously been formed, and does not produce a displacement in the upward direction. This condition arises, ter Kuile said, because the movement of the stapes itself is asymmetrical: forward movement is relatively free, but backward movement encounters a heavy resistance from the drum and other middle ear structures. As a result the stapedial system is shifted as a whole in the forward direction, so that true negative movements do not occur. As has been described, positive stimulation takes place only for the inward thrust of the stapes.

Because in general the high tones have small amplitudes relative to the low tones a problem arises as to their effectiveness in the process of excitation. It is assumed that the feature of the inward thrust of the stapes that is important in producing displacement of the basilar membrane is the velocity * of the movement, not simply the amplitude. This condition gives the high tones a more favorable status than if amplitude alone were the determinant, for the velocity of the movement varies with the frequency as well as with the amplitude.

Frequency operates in still another way to enhance the effectiveness of the high tones. The excitation of hair cells occurs once during every cycle, and therefore the high tones are favored in proportion to their frequency. This feature of the excitation process balances that of the spread of effect along the membrane. The low tones involve relatively great lengths of membrane and thus large numbers of hair cells, but excite them only at moderate rates, whereas the high tones excite few of the sensory elements, but do so at rapid rates. What may be called the 'intrinsic intensity' of tones thus depends upon the frequency.

There is in addition a variable intensity that depends upon the energy of the sound wave and is included in the velocity of the stapedial movement and therefore is represented in the degree of displacement of the basilar membrane. However—and here the theory really gets complicated and resorts to assumptions somewhat similar to Hurst's—the variation of stapedial

* Ter Kuile here is referring to the velocity of the reciprocating motion, often called the particle velocity, and not to the propagation velocity, which is the rate at which a wave moves forward through a medium. Incidentally, the spreading of the bulge over the basilar membrane is akin to this second kind of velocity but is not really to be identified with it, because in ter Kuile's view the bulge does not represent a freely propagated wave. The stapes itself, and the particles of fluid beyond it, may have considerable motions about some point in space without going forward in a progressive wave.

movement and of membrane displacement can occur only within narrow limits. The peculiar properties of the middle ear and of the basilar membrane provide the limitations. In the first place, the stapedial movements undergo only rather restricted changes of velocity, despite the changes in the external stimulus. When the intensity of the external sound is carried beyond a moderate level it brings in overtone frequencies, and the excess intensity is carried by these additional tones rather than by the fundamental. Secondly, when the stapes displaces a quantity of fluid the membrane in its immediate vicinity yields almost to the whole extent that it is capable of doing, and further room for the fluid can be found mainly by the yielding of portions of the membrane farther up the cochlea. Therefore the more intensive sounds, despite their greater particle velocities, can cause only slightly greater displacements in a given region than the weaker sounds do.

An important accompaniment of the larger displacements for intense sounds is an alteration of pitch. When the stapedial thrust is great and the membrane displacement is large, the rate of propagation of the bulge is increased beyond the normal. As a result the bulge reaches a point somewhat farther along the membrane than it would have done for the same tone at a weaker level of intensity. Therefore, ter Kuile concluded, a strong tone is heard as lower in pitch than a weak tone of the same frequency. This change of pitch with intensity is small, because as just indicated the variations of stapedial velocity and membrane displacement with stimulus intensity are limited.

A given tone stimulates its own segment of the basilar membrane at a rate equal to the tonal frequency. The question arises whether the frequency of stimulation of hair cells operates as a cue to pitch. Ter Kuile decided against such a possibility, for three reasons. In the first place, such a cue would be out of harmony with the relation between pitch and stimulus intensity just mentioned. If frequency operated as a cue the pitch ought not to vary with intensity in the manner described. Also he thought that a frequency cue would be confusing whenever several tones were sounded at once. Finally he argued that if every cell could respond to any tone there would be no point to the long evolutionary development of the ear: the simplest form of ear would show as good musical ability as the most complex.

Noises are accounted for as the result of a stimulation of the entire basilar membrane, usually in an irregular manner.

Ter Kuile pointed out that his theory accounts for the reported observation of a loss of hearing for low frequencies after injury to the apex of the cochlea. He considered his theory to be on a level with the resonance theory in this regard.

Likewise, the theory can account for our arrangement of pitches in a continuous series from high to low, and for tonal analysis. Analysis depends simply on the ability to discriminate quanta of lymph and membrane displacements that correspond to the components of the compound wave. At the same time, combination tones are said to arise from the superposition curve.

A thoroughgoing criticism of ter Kuile's theory was made by Max F. Meyer, whose own theory, formulated a little earlier, has many points of resemblance to this one but differs in important details. He objected to ter Kuile's assumption that the basilar membrane is elastic and that a bulge formed on it is propagated forward by virtue of this characteristic of the membrane itself.

Apart from these fundamental drawbacks, Meyer continued, an obvious difficulty of the theory is brought out by a consideration of what would happen in response to a combination of two frequencies. The compound wave form may be such as to give the wrong tones, as the components in the wave are no longer operating independently. A bulge that ought to go to a given place to correspond to one of the components is erased too soon, or fails to be erased completely and so extends too far. In a compound curve the ups and downs vary markedly with the phase relations of the components, and according to the theory different sets of tones ought to be heard when the phase relations of the components are made to vary. Further difficulty is presented by non-sinusoidal pulses of sound such as are produced by a siren when the holes are widely spaced. If the in-and-out movement of the stapes is completed in the early part of every cycle, the period during which the bulge can travel is extraordinarily small, and a very high tone ought to be heard. On the contrary, we hear a noisy tone whose fundamental frequency corresponds to the number of pulses per second—and which may be one or two octaves below what the theory would require.

Meyer objected to the explanation given for the reported loss of low tones after injury to the apex of the cochlea. If the cue to pitch is the length of the stimulated path, the loss of the apical elements ought not to cause a disappearance of all response to these tones. The low tones still should stimulate all the elements remaining, and therefore all frequencies below some point should sound alike.

Ter Kuile's theory gives a picture of a generalized kind of spatial distribution of response as a function of frequency. In this it is in a favorable position with respect to the available evidence. The theory suffers, however, as Meyer's critique brought out, from the dubious character of some of its assumptions. Two of these that still need to be mentioned have to do with the form of the stapedial motion. A reciprocal movement in which the return phase is essentially suppressed is hardly in the bounds of comprehension. Also the idea of a compression of the range of intensity, as we have already seen in Hurst's theory, is not only weak in itself but must encounter the indisputable fact that we are able to make discriminations of loudness over a broad range.

WATT'S THEORY

Henry J. Watt, who was Lecturer on Psychology at the University of Glasgow, in 1914 developed a 'psychological' theory of hearing. That is to say, he attempted to deal with the problem of hearing primarily by the interrelation of aspects of auditory experience. On its physiological side the theory is based upon ter Kuile's. It differs in its emphasis upon a certain resilience of the basilar membrane, from which arise important variations from ter Kuile's notions of the form and persistence of the bulge.

In Watt's theory, as in ter Kuile's, the bulge develops during the forward motion of the stapes and then is further extended during the recession of the stapes. However, according to Watt, its basal end is not erased. The elastic properties of the membrane are such as to sustain the pressures that have been developed in the cochlear fluid, though not at their original levels because the backward movement of the stapes has its effect. A balance is established between the elastic force of the membrane and the force represented by the position of the stapes, but this balance is a changing one since the stapes is continually retreating, and the communication of pressures through the cochlear fluids is not instantaneous but takes a little time. When the stapes has gone back to its initial position the bulge attains its greatest length, and extends all the way from the basal end of the cochlea to a point that is determined by the period of the wave—the same point as in ter Kuile's theory. The bulge has its greatest amplitude at its midpoint, which is the point reached at the moment of the most forward thrust of the stapes, when the exerted pressure is the greatest. From this midpoint toward the apex the amplitude diminishes, until it becomes zero at a distance of one wave length; this diminution represents the continual falling off of pressure as the bulge is conducted along the membrane. From the midpoint toward the basal end likewise the amplitude diminishes because the negative pressure exerted by the retreating stapes is increasingly felt. During the backward movement of the stapes the amplitudes are everywhere diminishing along this basal half of the path, so that at the close of the period they are well below their original levels. The distribution of pressures is such that at the end of the period the bulge is symmetrical about the midpoint, where a moderately sharp maximum lies.

The bulge does not vanish as the period ends, though it continually decreases as time goes on. Its rate of recession is slow enough that some effect persists over several periods of the sound wave. The result is to accumulate a certain positive displacement that mounts during successive periods to an equilibrium level.

The cue to pitch is the location along the membrane of the maximum at the midpoint of the bulge. When several tones are present simultaneously there will be several such maxima. The analysis of complex sounds depends upon the ability to perceive these persisting maximal points.

Distinct advantages are claimed for the persisting effect on the membrane. It explains the 'action time' of the ear—the time during which a prolongation of stimulation gives an apparent rise in the loudness of a tone. It explains also the 'expiration time' or after-effect of stimulation. More important still, it avoids any difficulty of phase relations in a compound tone, for every component will exert its own effect regardless of its phase position relative to the others.

Watt's theory places much emphasis upon the attribute of volume in auditory experience, and this characteristic is referred to the bulge as a whole, while the pitch is represented by the point of maximum. This theory accounts for the alteration of pitch with stimulus intensity in the same manner as ter Kuile's theory. The effect of experimental injury to the cochlea with loud tones is said to be compatible with the theory, but the evidence is not deemed sufficient for a full account of the matter. No attempt was made to explain the combination tones, for Watt, in company with Helmholtz, regarded these as arising outside the cochlea.

As far as excitatory effect is concerned, Watt's theory bears a remarkable resemblance to a resonance type of theory in which the resonance is very broad. It therefore has many of the advantages and limitations of such a theory. Its weakness, like ter Kuile's, lies in its basic assumptions, which are largely of an improbable character.

BÉKÉSY'S THEORY

In a series of papers beginning in 1928 and running over a number of years Georg von Békésy, then a communications engineer in Budapest, developed a theory that initially took the form of a traveling wave theory, but without any commitment then as to details of the process by which the wave arises and is propagated.

Békésy worked at first with mechanical models of the cochlea, constructed much after the fashion of Ewald's by covering a slot in a metal plate with a rubber film. He observed, as Ewald had, that such a membrane responds to a tone at several places. Then he discovered that by thickening the rubber film suitably the response could be restricted to a narrow region or even to a sharply defined spot.

This membrane when acted upon by sound is thrown into wave motion of a peculiar kind. An undulating wave is seen to travel from one end of the membrane to the other, varying continually in amplitude with its position at any one moment and also varying its pattern from moment to moment. As the wave proceeds its amplitude rises steadily to a maximum somewhere along the membrane, and then it rather rapidly falls toward zero. Figure 10 illustrates this conception. Consider first only

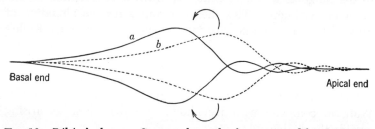

FIG. 10. Békésy's theory. Curve *a* shows the form assumed by the basilar membrane at one instant, during the outward movement of the stapes. Curve *b* shows the form a little later, when the wave has moved farther apically. The other curves, mirror images of these two, show the corresponding forms when the stapes is moving inward. The curved arrows represent local eddies in the surrounding fluid. Modified from Békésy (1) and (6).

the two uppermost curves, marked *a* and *b*. These represent the forms assumed by the membrane as a result of negative pressure on the fluid bounding the upper surface of the membrane, a pressure that in the actual cochlea would be caused by an outward thrust of the stapes. Curve *a* shows the form at a certain instant and curve *b* the form a bit later, after the wave has proceeded a little way up the cochlea. The lower two curves show correspondingly the forms of the membrane as a result of an inward thrust of the stapes. For the particular waves represented here the maximum displacement will occur somewhere near the middle of the membrane.

Békésy (1, 9–14) pursued this problem further by the observation of wave motion in fresh or preserved specimens of human and animal cochleas. Preparation of these specimens consisted usually of first decalcifying part of the bone of the cochlear capsule, opening the apical end (under fluid to avoid ripping the delicate parts) and replacing the lymph with a solution containing solid particles of carbon or fine metals. Movements of these particles during stimulation with sounds then were observed under moderate magnification with stroboscopic illumination. The principal observations were made near the apical end of the cochlea, at a point about 30 mm from the base. Observations were made at other positions also but were hampered by the greater difficulty of making suitable exposures. The forms of movement as revealed here agreed with those that had been found in the mechanical models.

From these results Békésy inferred the forms of the waves throughout the cochlea. He outlined, as seen in the mechanical models, a systematic variation in the location of the maximum, with the high tones in the basal part and the low tones toward the apex, just as in the Helmholtz theory. However, this localization is only gross, as Fig. 11 shows. This is so because the damping is great.

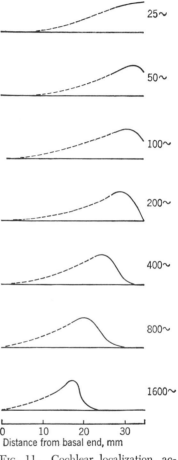

Fig. 11. Cochlear localization, according to Békésy (13). The relative amplitude of motion along the basilar membrane is shown for seven different stimulating frequencies. [From the *Acta Oto-Laryngologica*.]

Békésy observed also the phase relations among the cochlear structures. He found first of all that for the low tones there is complete phase agreement in all the moving parts at the exposed position; the tectorial membrane, the organ of Corti, the basilar membrane, and usually Reissner's membrane also undergo vibratory movements as a whole. Then he measured the phase relations between the movements of these parts and the movements of the stapes and found systematic variations with frequency over the range up to 300 ~. For the lowest tones these apical structures move in phase with the stapes, or nearly so, and then as the frequency is raised, beginning noticeably as the tuned frequency is approached, the phase of the apical structures progressively lags behind the stapes. The phase lag becomes π radians (180°) at the frequency giving the maximum displacement and thereafter continues to increase up to an amount as great as 3π radians (540°).

Because this sort of phase variation is different from what we expect in a series of resonators Békésy argued that we are dealing not with a Helmholtzian system of tuned elements but with traveling waves whose wave lengths grow shorter as the frequency rises.

This investigator was convinced that the differentiation of cochlear action with frequency is due to properties of the dividing partition. To determine which ones among the various parts making up this partition possess the differential properties he made measurements of their stiffness. To Reissner's membrane, the tectorial membrane, the organ of Corti, and the basilar membrane in the different regions he applied known pressures by means of fine hairs and observed the resulting depressions. Only for the basilar membrane did he observe systematic variations along the cochlea. For it he found the stiffness to vary about 50-fold between the 10 mm and the 30 mm positions. By a different procedure, in which he observed the displacement of the membrane resulting from a steady pressure applied to the fluid of the cochlear duct, he obtained a 100-fold variation over the entire membrane. Though its resistance to displacement varies, this membrane is not under tension, but rather is "an unstressed, gelatinous, elastic plate."

In his model experiments Békésy (1) reported along with the traveling waves some curious vortex movements in the cochlear fluid. These appeared in both 'scalae' above and below the place where the amplitude of vibration was a maximum. Their nature is indicated by the arrows in Fig. 10. Békésy's belief was that these eddies in the fluid established steady pressures on the partition near by and constituted the actual excitation of the hair cells. Thereby he supposed the action to be considerably restricted compared to what it would be if the whole wave were effective along the membrane in proportion to its amplitude. Even with this restrictive condition the action as pictured is still a broad one, and Békésy sought further limitations of it. He resorted to what he called a 'law of contrast, described in more detail later on, in which any demarcation in a sensory function is supposed to be emphasized. He considered that by these two means, one peripheral and the other central, the broad action of the stimulus may be converted into a narrow one. Specificity, though lost at first, is finally regained.

In the later discussions of this theory a surprising feature emerged: the cochlear action is regarded as relatively independent of various mechanical disturbances. Békésy reported that the nature and locations of the vortex movements remained unaffected by many kinds of manipulations that ordinarily would be considered drastic. In the actual cochlea, drilling through the cochlear wall and pushing a probe through the hole so as to displace and crush the basilar membrane had not the slightest effect upon the response pattern. Also, Békésy claimed, preserved specimens behaved in the same way as fresh ones. In the models, adding an extra membrane, varying the lengths and diameters of the fluid columns, or even eliminating one scala altogether had only minor effects. Moreover, altering the place of application of the stimulus from the basal to the apical end, or to the middle, had no effect either. From these considerations it grows doubtful whether this ought really to be classed among the traveling wave theories. Evidently the response patterns are a function merely of properties of the basilar membrane itself, as in the conventional resonance theories, and indeed are even less dependent upon the surrounding structures than is envisaged in most of these.

Zwislocki in 1946 outlined a theory that differs from Békésy's mainly in the assertion that the analytic action of the cochlea depends upon only two variables, the elasticity and damping of the basilar membrane. From a consideration of hydrodynamic principles he concluded that every tone produces a wave that travels up the cochlea, reaches a maximum amplitude at some position, and then rapidly falls away. The location of the maximum varies with frequency in the usual manner: it is near the basal end for the high tones and toward the apex for the low tones. Zwislocki adduced evidence in support of his views from the study of a model of about the same construction as the ones described by Ewald, Békésy, and others: a rubber membrane stretched over a triangular opening in an elongated, fluid-filled chamber.

The wave theories in general encounter a difficulty because of the specific nature of the assumptions that they make about the action of the stapes in initiating the cochlear waves and about the paths of travel of these waves. The difficulty grows particularly serious in a consideration of stimulation other than by the usual aerial route.

When the stimulation is by bone conduction the energy is no longer applied only at the stapes, but presumably it may enter the cochlea from any one of various directions. The ingress of energy must be further complicated in otosclerosis, a disease of the bone in the region of the oval window whereby the stapes becomes firmly embedded and finally immobilized. And though in this disease the hearing is impaired to aerial sounds it is not seriously affected (in simple cases) for vibrations communicated to the bones of the skull. Further problems of conduction arise when this condition is relieved and the serviceable reception of aerial sounds is restored by means of the fenestration operation, in which a new opening is made into the lateral semicircular canal or into the vestibule (see Lempert).

Further evidence on this matter comes from animal experiments (Wever, Lawrence, and Smith). It has been found that sounds are quite as effective in producing electrical potentials of the cochlea when applied to the round window as when applied to the oval window. Plainly a specific path of travel for the acoustic energy is not necessary for cochlear stimulation. Here is a difficulty that the wave theories will have to face.

THE TUBE-RESONANCE THEORIES

A comparatively late development is a type of theory that resembles both the wave theories and the resonance theories;

essentially it is a wave theory in which the wave motion is ascribed to physical conditions of much the same kind as those assumed in the resonance theories for the differentiation of individual elements. In this type of theory the cochlea is treated as a tube with partially elastic walls.

RANKE'S RECTIFIER-RESONANCE THEORY

The first of these theories was elaborated by Otto F. Ranke in 1931, then an assistant in the Physiological Institute of the University of Heidelberg. He called it a 'rectifier-resonance theory.'

The starting point for Ranke's theory was a mathematical treatment worked out by Frank on the transmission of pulse waves through the blood vessels. Ranke conceived that the general principles developed for the pulse waves can be applied to the cochlea if it is regarded as a tube bent back upon itself, with the basilar membrane as a common elastic wall. A number of modifications of Frank's treatment are found necessary, however, to handle the special conditions. The scala vestibuli plus the cochlear duct form one canal and the scala tympani forms a second canal parallel to it. The wave motions are probably similar in these two, but not identical.

According to the theory, the movements of the stapes set up waves of pressure that travel along the two scalae from base to apex at a rather moderate velocity, varying with the frequency. These waves cause complex movements of the basilar membrane as shown in Fig. 12. There are two important zones of action, one called the initial zone and the other the transition zone. The initial zone shows a gradual rise of amplitude from zero at the basal end to a maximum somewhere up the cochlea, and then a sharp fall to zero. The transition zone begins at this zero point and extends a little farther up the cochlea and is distinguished by relatively rapid changes of amplitude, with two maxima or loops and possibly more. These patterns of action are similar in form for all tones, but their locations vary systematically with frequency. Those for the low tones spread far toward the apex, and those for the high tones extend only short distances.

The location of the transition zone depends upon the relation between the wave length of the traveling wave and the breadth of the canal. In the initial zone the wave length is large with respect to the size of the canal, which in Frank's development of the problem is one of the necessary conditions for the continued systematic propagation of the pressure wave. In the transition zone, however, these two become of the same order of magnitude; in fact, this zone is defined as lying beyond the point where the wave length equals π times the diameter of the

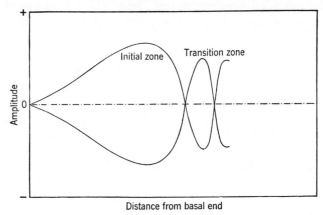

FIG. 12.   Ranke's theory.   Shown is the pattern of basilar membrane movement as conceived for a low tone.

canal and accordingly the wave movements in the canal become transverse as well as longitudinal.

To obtain a suitable distribution of the wave patterns over the cochlea for the whole gamut of audible tones it is necessary not only that the velocity of propagation be low but that it vary rapidly as the wave proceeds up the cochlea. Ranke estimated that this velocity ought to be 5.02 cm per second for a 20 $\sim$ tone and 63 meters per second for a 10,000 $\sim$ tone, which is a variation of 1235-fold.

Now the propagation velocity, according to his derivations, depends upon the cross-sectional area of the canal and the mechanical properties of the basilar membrane. It remains to be seen whether their variations are sufficient to make the theory tenable.

The cross-sectional area, according to data that he used, varies about 6.2-fold. Therefore from Frank's formula, in which the velocity of propagation varies as the square root of the tube cross section, this dimension gives a variation of $\sqrt{6.2}$ or 2.5-fold. At the same time the basilar membrane (according to Hensen's data) widens by 12-fold; and since the velocity varies as the square root of the width cubed ($v \propto \sqrt{w^3}$) we have a further variation of 41.6-fold. Besides, it can be supposed, Ranke said, that the transverse tension on the fibers of the basilar membrane diminishes about 4-fold from base to apex, giving a variation of velocity of $\sqrt{4}$ or 2-fold. Altogether, then, for these three conditions, we have a variation of 208-fold.

This amount is well below the total variation needed (1235-fold), and Ranke sought to meet the situation by supposing that tonal discrimination is diminished or fails at the upper and lower ends of the auditory scale. Below about 30 $\sim$ and above 4000 or 5000 $\sim$, he averred, the estimation of pitch is only crude. If differentiation is limited to about 8 octaves the required variation in velocity becomes only about 256-fold. This variation is approached by the figure of 208-fold given above; and he thought that the small amount still needed might be obtained through variations in the viscosity and mass of the basilar membrane. Accordingly, he considered that his basic assumptions were fully justified by the anatomical conditions.

Thus far we have a picture of rather extensive fluid movements through the cochlea. Now we learn how a simplification is worked out in the stimulation of the sensory cells. The vibratory patterns are supposed to cause lines of flow in the fluid of the two canals, lines that are roughly symmetrical on the two sides of the membrane. In the initial zone these lines of flow are well spread out in the canal, but in the transition zone they change rapidly to become dense in the close vicinity of the membrane. The effect of the flow lines is to produce a continuous negative pressure on the membrane in the initial zone and a continuous positive pressure of much greater magnitude at the beginning of the transition zone. It is the large positive pressure, in Ranke's view, that probably constitutes the local stimulus for the organ of Corti. It is because the lines of flow set up pressures that are continuous, not following the undulations of the waves, that this becomes a 'rectifier' theory. Watt, we recall, made a somewhat similar assumption regarding the action of sound on the basilar membrane.

The positive and negative pressures, Ranke went on to say, have a curved form, so that the fluid in the region of the transition zone is given a rotary motion. An eddy therefore appears on each side of the membrane. Békésy's observations made on his cochlear model indicated the general form of movement conceived in this theory, and he saw the eddies as well.

According to Ranke, the position of the transition zone depends simply on the velocity gradient, and not at all on the setting up of standing waves as in the usual form of wave theory. However, he admitted the presence of standing waves, produced as a result of a reflection of the progressive wave back from the transition zone. These waves reinforce the local movements and to this extent determine the amplitude of the displacements of the membrane. In this aspect of the action it is proper to speak of resonance, and so Ranke justified his designation of the theory as a 'rectifier-resonance theory.'

On this theory the pitch depends upon the locus of the transition zone, or rather the beginning of it, where the rectified pressure undergoes a change from negative to positive. Low tones have a transition zone near the apex, whereas high tones have one near the base. The analysis of complex sounds depends upon the formation of transition zones corresponding to every component present. However, this analysis is not strictly of the Fourier type. The partials are not so loud as Fourier's principle predicts, on account of mutual disturbances within the responsive areas. Also, combination tones arise when parts of the membrane are affected by two or more components at the same time.

Noises are heard when the rectified pressures appear at several places along the membrane and at irregular rates.

The time of onset and also the persistence time of tones depend upon the damping. Damping does not have any important effect, however, upon the sharpness of the tuning. The time required to recognize the pitch of a tone is explained as the time during which the rectified pressure is being built up to an appreciable level.

REBOUL'S HYDRODYNAMIC THEORY

A more recent form of tube-resonance theory was worked out by J. A. Reboul and presented in 1937 as a thesis to the medical faculty of the University of Montpellier. Like Ranke he regarded the cochlea as a tube with elastic walls and sought to treat its behavior as a problem in fluid mechanics. The result is a wave theory like the foregoing, and also like Ranke's it bears certain points of resemblance to the more traditional resonance hypothesis. On the other hand, because he differed in some of his basic assumptions and in his conception of the relations among the variables, Reboul's theory departs widely from the others in many respects.

The general conception is as follows. The compressions and rarefactions of the perilymph of the scala vestibuli set up by the stapedial movements pass up the cochlea, and if they are rapid enough they discharge through the flexible partition, the basilar membrane, to the scala tympani. The place at which the discharge occurs depends upon the frequency of the wave and its velocity of propagation. This velocity depends upon a number of conditions: the density and compressibility of the fluid, the diameter of the scala, and the thickness and elasticity of the basilar membrane. As most of these conditions vary along the cochlea, the velocity does also. Most important here are the changes in the diameter of the scala vestibuli and in the elasticity of the membrane on account of its variation in width; both these changes are such as to increase the propagation velocity as the wave moves toward the apex of the cochlea. Reboul estimated the velocity near the oval window as 38 meters per second and that near the apex as 415 meters per second, an increase of nearly 11-fold. We note in passing that this is both a smaller variation than the one worked out by Ranke and, even more important, it is in the opposite direction.

The cochlear patterns depend on both the varying wave velocity and the locally varying compressibility, which latter largely reflects the properties of the basilar membrane. Reboul considered the patterns both of displacement and of pressure, which in general are contrary in form: at the place where the displacement of the membrane is a maximum the pressure is a minimum, and conversely.

To present a realistic picture of these patterns Reboul was forced to make a number of assumptions of somewhat arbitrary nature, since so many of the variables are not quantitatively known. He concluded that tones below some limiting frequency, which he took to be about 750 ∼, do not have any clear maximum of displacement amplitude but spread over the entire membrane, rising progressively toward the apical end. For tones above this frequency the amplitude rises to a maximum and then falls, and for the higher tones (above perhaps 4000 ∼) there are multiple maxima. For 4000 ∼, for example, the calculations indicate two maxima, and for 10,000 ∼ four. The maximum nearest the basal end is the largest, and the others fall off rapidly.

Corresponding to the principle already laid down, the patterns of pressure show a phase difference from the displacements described above. For all the low tones, below 750 ∼, the pressure is zero in the middle of the cochlea and it rises positively toward the base and grows increasingly negative toward the apex. For the higher tones there are broad maxima of negative pressure that move toward the base of the cochlea as the frequency increases. For tones above 4000 ∼ there are undulations of the pressure curves which are larger toward the apex and smaller toward the base.

What we are to picture here is a movement that for the low tones is like that of a reed or flexible strip, and for the high tones is similar to the waves moving along an extended rope. For the high tones the resulting excitation corresponds closely to what has been predicated on the more traditional resonance theory.

Reboul developed his discussion further to show the consistency of his conceptions with new data obtained in the study of the electrical responses of the ear, and their consistency also with the volley theory; but these relations are more conveniently treated later on.

What can be claimed for this theory, as for Ranke's, is that it achieves something like the differentiation of specific resonators by a different approach and, superficially at least, a different set of assumptions. The traditional difficulty about the question of damping, that Wien labored against Helmholtz's theory with so telling effect, seems here to be avoided.

It is hardly possible with our present information to make a meaningful comparison of these two forms of tube-resonance theory or to weigh their individual merits. Their development is largely mathematical, but the assumptions that are made are not always clearly indicated, and at best the variables are imperfectly known. The latter defect is inescapable, because we know too little even of the simple anatomy of the structures and hardly anything about the magnitudes of such variables as the elasticity and tension of the tissues.

CHAPTER 4

THE FREQUENCY THEORIES

According to the frequency theories the auditory nerve receives and transmits a pattern that corresponds in all essential details to the pattern of the external sounds. The ear therefore serves as a kind of relay mechanism for the characteristics of the stimulus. The analogy with a telephone transmitter is obvious, and the simpler forms of frequency theories are often called 'telephone theories.'

THE SIMPLE FREQUENCY THEORIES

The first suggestions for a frequency theory were made by Rinne in 1865, soon after Helmholtz had advanced his resonance hypothesis. Rinne did not develop a formal theory but was chiefly concerned with criticisms of the ideas of resonance and peripheral analysis. He contended that the problem of analysis is not solved by a spatial distribution over the cochlea of the components of a complex wave. If each component is represented in the action of a separate nerve fiber, he pointed out, there still remains the matter of our appreciating and relating these several processes by means of some integrating mechanism in the higher centers. In other words, peripheral analysis simply raises a new problem, that of a synthesis later on. Therefore, he concluded, it is quite superfluous to set up an artificial mechanism for the purpose of an analysis of sounds in the ear. It is simpler to suppose that the acoustic pattern maintains its unity and conveys the whole complex of movements to the mind simply as intensive states, without any spatial separation.

Voltolini in 1885 presented a simple frequency theory and compared the ear with the telephone and the phonograph. He vigorously opposed Helmholtz's theory, which then was held in wide esteem, and went so far as to hold it up to ridicule as "the product of a great mind in an hour of weakness." He insisted that every hair cell responds to every sound, rather than some one cell to each discriminable sound. The advantage of a large number of cells is simply to increase the acuity of hearing. He argued that in general the auditory process is similar in all animal forms from fish to mammals, and the arch of Corti is not a resonator but only a special device developed in mammals for increasing the delicacy of reception.

RUTHERFORD'S TELEPHONE THEORY

The most famous and influential of the telephone theories is that of William Rutherford, Professor of Physiology at the University of Edinburgh. He conceived the theory in 1880, but first presented it publicly in a lecture delivered in Birmingham in 1886. He made a more detailed discussion without any substantial changes in a second lecture in 1898, twelve years later.

Rutherford's theory supposes, like Voltolini's, that all the hair cells can be stimulated by every sound, whether simple or complex, and that through these cells "sound waves [are] translated into nerve vibrations of corresponding frequency, amplitude, and wave form." Theoretically, a single hair cell could give all the different auditory sensations. He suggested, however, that a large number of cells is advantageous in providing a high sensitivity to slight differences of quality. The character of a sound is appreciated directly on the basis of the vibratory pattern that is presented to the higher centers.

Rutherford recognized that his theory makes severe demands upon the auditory nerve fibers. These fibers must be capable of transmitting frequencies throughout the auditory range. At the time that the theory was developed this requirement appeared even more extreme than now, for owing to the faulty calibration of test instruments the upper limit of hearing was generally accepted as around 40,000 to 60,000 vibrations per second, which is two or three times too high. Nevertheless, Rutherford did not consider the demand for so high a rate of action on the part of the nerve fibers any serious obstacle to his theory.

Not much was known then about the characteristics of nerve fibers, and Rutherford himself set out to determine their maximum rates of activity. He worked on a nerve and its muscle in the rabbit and found that the currents set up in the muscle by stimulating the nerve gave an audible tone if run into a telephone receiver. He obtained impulses up to 352 per second, but not higher. He cited an observation made by Helmholtz's assistant, Bernstein, that the action current in the frog's sciatic nerve lasts only 0.0007 sec, and inferred on this basis that a frequency of about 1400 per second was possible. As (perhaps unjustly) he considered these experiments rather crude, he believed that the limits of frequency of the nerves had not been approached. Hence it seemed to him that frequencies 10 times as high or even higher, as demanded by the theory, were entirely reasonable.

Rutherford attacked the concept of selective resonance of the fibers of the basilar membrane on the basis of the anatomical evidence. He pointed out that the transverse fibers are not isolated and free, and he stressed especially the fact that in certain animals, like the rabbit, birds, and reptiles, there are two layers of fibers, sometimes with connective tissue binding the whole together.

He cited Hermann's evidence on 'beat tones' as contrary to the resonance hypothesis. Hermann had reported that two tones when sounded together will not affect a resonator tuned to the frequency of their 'beat tone,' though this tone is easily audible to the ear. It then could be argued that, if an external resonator will not respond to a frequency difference, a resonator within the ear cannot be assumed to do so either. (Helmholtz adroitly got around this difficulty by postulating a distortion process in the middle ear through which a new tone was produced at the frequency of the beat tone.)

According to Rutherford, the analysis of complex sounds is not a peripheral process but is a function of the brain. It is not a native capacity but must be acquired through meticulous practice, and in only a few persons does it reach a high level of development.

Rutherford examined carefully the evidence then available on the effects of experimental destruction of portions of the cochlea in animals. Baginsky had reported that destruction of the apex and part of the middle turn of the cochlea of dogs left the animals with hearing only for high tones. However, his attempts to perform similar destructions in the region of the basal turn were unsatisfactory; some of the animals were able to hear both high and low tones after the operation. Corradi, in work on the guinea pig, obtained results similar to those of Baginsky. On the other hand, Stepanow, working also with guinea pigs, obtained contrary evidence: responses remained to low as well as to high tones after destructions in the apical region of the cochlea. Somewhat similar evidence was derived from clinical observations of local damage to the cochlea in human subjects. Moos and Steinbrügge reported a reduction of the upper limit of hearing as a consequence of atrophy of the nerve in the basal region. Bezold likewise observed deafness to high tones associated with basal atrophy.

Though this experimental and clinical evidence was generally accepted as favoring the Helmholtz theory, Rutherford pointed out that it was by no means consistent or conclusive. He conceded the possibility that high tones are dependent upon the basal portion of the cochlea but perceived no evidence that the low tones were correspondingly restricted to the apical region. He suggested that there was no incompatibility with the telephone theory in the restriction of the actions aroused by certain tones to particular regions of the cochlea, but he did not develop this idea as a feature of his theory.

Other theories that evidently are variants of Rutherford's were put forward by Waller and Ayers. Waller's statements, however, were too brief to convey his ideas clearly, and some have included his among the wave theories.

AYERS' 'AUDITORY HAIR' THEORY

Howard Ayers was a morphologist in charge of the Lake Laboratory of Zoology at Milwaukee. His theory, developed in 1892 on a background of study of the evolutionary history of the ear, contains a number of peculiar features. Ayers took the position that the ear has developed out of the lateral-line organ of fishes and as such must operate everywhere in an essentially simple manner. Auditory stimulation, he said, always consists in the setting in motion of sensory hairs floating freely in the fluid of an auditory sac.

The tectorial membrane of the higher vertebrates as ordinarily represented is an artifact, he claimed, and actually is merely a 'hair band,' a field of long slender hairs growing out of the ends of the hair cells. These hairs respond with great delicacy to vibrations in the endolymph and communicate their movements to the nerve fibers associated with their cells.

This action was compared with the waves of motion in a field of standing grain blown by a fitful wind. All the hairs may be affected by any tone, and there is no peripheral analysis.

This theory received a good deal of attention a few years later from W. S. Bryant, but generally it has been passed over without comment because its anatomical claims can not be justified.

BONNIER'S REGISTRATION THEORY

Another form of frequency theory with a number of distinctive features was developed by Pierre Bonnier, who began his career as a comparative anatomist and then became an otologist, associated with the Rothschild Polyclinique in Paris. According to his views, first expressed briefly in 1895, the function of the cochlea is a 'registration' of the form of the stimulating waves. An analogy is drawn with recording apparatus, like the early phonograph, which inscribes a wave by means of a stylus on an impressionable surface.

The process is conceived of as follows. The vibrations of the stapes produce to-and-fro movements of the basal part of the basilar membrane. The epithelial structure comprising the basilar membrane and associated elements is in the form of a spiral ribbon and is lightly suspended, so that it has extraordinary freedom of movement, especially in the transverse direction. This freedom is progressively greater toward the apex, so that when the basal portion is thrown into vibration the movements are readily conducted up the spiral. The process is similar to the conduction of waves in a rope when one end is vibrated back and forth.

This process results in a spreading of the excitation over a large sensory area. The larger the area, the greater is the number of sensory cells involved and the greater is the sensitivity.

Moreover, this spreading of the excitation facilitates our analysis of the wave, for the wave form is presented to every sensory element. The analysis is not peripheral, but central; but the peripheral 'recording' of the wave facilitates the central analysis of it, just as the accurate picturing of a wave in the form of a curve will aid in its graphic treatment.

The pitch of the sound corresponds to the periodicity of the sensory irritation and of the nerve excitation; here the theory agrees with the other telephone hypotheses. The intensity of the sensory irritation is reflected in the intensity of the central nervous effects. The timbre depends upon a perception of the details of the wave form.

Bonnier worked out a curious hypothesis to account for Broca's evidence that a tone is perceived as lower in pitch when its intensity is raised. He supposed that a powerful wave would be propagated along the basilar membrane at a faster rate than normal and that therefore the wave form would be represented on a larger segment of the membrane. He further supposed that any given sensory element when displaced more than usual from its equilibrium position would return to that position relatively slowly and hence would suffer a retardation of phase. Consequently, Bonnier thought, the frequency of vibration of such an element would be decreased, and the impulses relayed to the higher centers would represent a lower pitch. This hypothesis hardly needs comment, as it violates principles of physics and logic; the first part of the argument regarding speed of propagation and wave length is irrelevant; and a phase retardation, if it occurred as a result of an increased amplitude of vibration, would hold for each successive vibration and hence would not alter the frequency.

HARDESTY'S THEORY

In 1908, Irving Hardesty, an anatomist at the University of California, formulated a type of telephone theory in which the tectorial membrane rather than the basilar membrane is regarded as the responding mechanism. As an anatomist he appreciated the weight of the objection to Helmholtz's theory on the ground that the fibers of the basilar membrane are not free but compose a feltwork of fibers many of which run in a crosswise direction. At the same time he rejected the concept of selective resonance for the tectorial membrane as well, on a basis of its observable structure and from tests that he made on a large model.

According to Hardesty, the tectorial membrane is much more free to move than the basilar membrane, because it is more flexible and is anchored on only one edge. Hence he regarded it as receiving the waves from the endolymph and in turn exciting the hair cells.

Though he did not conceive of this membrane as a resonator, Hardesty suggested that tones of high pitch affect it near the base where it is thin and narrow, and those of low pitch affect it in a more general way, traveling farther toward the apex. He perceived this difference in the locus of excitation for different frequencies and also a difference in the extent of excitation according to the intensity of stimulation; but beyond these conditions he regarded the finer analysis of sounds as "almost wholly cerebral."

The various formulations of the telephone theory that have now been described hardly deserve consideration as separate theories, because all are characterized by the single hypothesis of a representation of sound frequency in the auditory nerve response, and in their development they go little beyond an expression of this idea. The most serious fault of these formulations is their limited scope: their concentration upon a single aspect of audition, that of pitch perception. This fault of course arises from their appearance as opposition hypotheses; they reflect this preoccupation with pitch from the resonance theory that they are seeking to supplant. Rutherford went somewhat farther than most in his concern with the neural implications of the theory, and also in his weighing of the available evidence on the effects of local cochlear destruction, and deservedly his formulation has had more prominence and consideration than the others.

A second form of frequency theory is still to be considered. In this form of theory the concept of resonance is rejected, as it is in the simple telephone theory, but peripheral analysis based on a spatial distribution of response in the cochlea according to the sound frequency is accepted. Theories of this form, therefore, are known as the frequency-analytic theories.

THE FREQUENCY-ANALYTIC THEORIES

Like the wave theories treated earlier, the frequency-analytic theories include a special means apart from resonance for the allocation of different frequencies to different parts of the basilar membrane. They differ from these theories in the particular mechanism that is conceived for bringing about this spatial distribution and also in their inclusion of the principle of pitch representation in terms of the frequency of nerve impulses.

There are two formulations of this type of theory, one by Meyer and another by Wrightson.

MEYER'S HYDRAULIC THEORY

Max F. Meyer when he launched his theory was a research assistant in the psychological laboratory at the University of Berlin. He continued its development and defense during more than three decades of teaching and research in psychology at the University of Missouri. He based the theory on a geometrical analysis of compound waves, an analysis not of the Fourier type. This form of analysis he first outlined in 1896 in an attempt to account for the formation of combination tones, and two years later after considerable modification he incorporated it into a general theory of hearing.

Meyer's theory rests upon the assumption of rather simple physical properties of the basilar membrane. He regarded this membrane as leather-like in nature and as laxly suspended between the vestibular and tympanic scalae. When a movement of the stapes occurs and the pressure becomes different in the two scalae, the membrane must bulge until the pressures are equalized. As the membrane is lax it imposes almost no resistance to lateral displacement so long as the displacement is small, but after its slack is taken up its resistance rapidly rises and further movement practically ceases. An analogy is the action of a leather chair seat, which at first yields easily to one's weight and then offers nearly maximum resistance.

Meyer conceived the action as follows. When the stapes moves inward and exerts a positive pressure on the cochlear fluid, the response of the basilar membrane is at first restricted to its most basal portion. This part of the membrane is bulged downward, and the bulging continues until the limit of free motion is reached, and then it begins to spread to the more remote portions. The bulge extends in the apical direction only as far as necessary to give room to the fluid displaced by the stapes.

When the stapes reaches its most inward position and starts backward it causes a second displacement of fluid, but in a direction contrary to the first. Consequently the membrane is drawn upward. This reversed motion of the membrane, like the other, begins at the basal end of the cochlea and spreads toward the apex. If the backward movement of the stapes has the same amplitude and velocity as the preceding forward movement, this second movement of the membrane extends the same distance as the first and exactly erases the original bulge; the membrane then is in its initial position. If the reverse stapedial movement is somewhat less in amplitude, the second displacement of the membrane will erase the first only in the basal region, and the most apical part of the original bulge will remain undisturbed.

It should be noted that the membrane is conceived as nearly inelastic and under great frictional resistance; it is almost completely damped or 'dead beat.' Indeed, the natural frequency of the membrane is so low that if left to itself after a primary displacement it would take several seconds to return to its equilibrium position. Hence, for all practical purposes, it moves only in response to some positive force. It does not transmit motion along its own length to any appreciable extent. The spreading is brought about through the fluid and not by a wave motion of the membrane as such. It is primarily in this feature that the theory differs from the wave theories mentioned earlier, in which a bulge travels on the basilar membrane.

The distance of spread of a displacement depends not only on the amplitude of the stapedial movement but also, to a degree, on its velocity. The reason is that the fluid has a high viscosity, and imposes a resistance to movement that increases with the velocity. If the velocity is very low, the fluid is able to flow from one scala to the other through the helicotrema, and no depression of the membrane occurs. If the velocity is great, the fluid moves a shorter distance and the membrane is displaced. It follows that high-pitched tones (which have relatively high stapedial velocities) have a more limited spread than equally strong tones of low pitch.

Excitation of the hair cells probably occurs on the upward phase of every up-and-down cycle of displacement, though this point is not finally determined. At any rate, one excitation occurs for every cycle, and hence the nerve response has a frequency equal to the frequency of the stimulating sounds.

The loudness of the sound is determined by the extent of the spreading over the membrane and hence the number of hair cells involved.

The analysis of a compound wave follows the principles already laid down. However complex the form of the stapedial movement, a bulge always starts at the basal end of the cochlea and continues to be extended until there is a change in the direction of the stapedial movement. The number of bulges formed, therefore, corresponds to the number of maximum and minimum points in the compound wave; and the length of each bulge depends upon the amplitude as measured from one of these points to the next. Since the amplitudes between successive maximum and minimum points always vary in a compound wave, the different bulges will spread for different distances. This process may be made clear in an example.

The upper part of Fig. 13 shows a curve formed by compounding two tones with a vibration ratio of 2:3; to be definite, let us say that the tones have frequencies of 200 and 300 ~. The successive maxima and minima in this compound wave are lettered for ease of reference.

The lower part of this figure indicates the basilar membrane movements corresponding to the changes in this compound wave. A number of views are given to represent successive positions taken by the membrane to one side or the other of the resting position (which is indicated by the dot-dash line). If we think of a rising amplitude in the wave as representing an inward thrust of the stapes, then the resulting membrane displacement will be toward the tympanic scala and is shown here as a displacement to the right; and correspondingly an outward movement of the stapes will result in a displacement to the left.

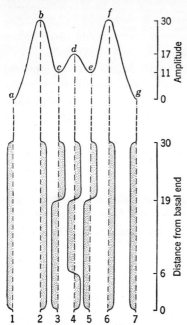

FIG. 13. Max F. Meyer's theory of cochlear analysis. Shown above is a compound wave, and below are shown a number of views of the forms taken by the basal portion of the basilar membrane. The views are oriented vertically so as to represent the motion at selected points within the wave cycle. The scale units are arbitrary for both wave amplitude and distance along the membrane, but they are made to correspond one to the other. For further explanation, see the text.

The amplitude of the wave is scaled as shown, and so is the portion of basilar membrane concerned.

Let us follow the sequence of action in detail. When the wave is at a, which is a minimum from which the amplitude rises, the first 30 units of the membrane have the position shown at 1, displaced to the left of the dot-dash line. As the amplitude rises from a to b, a bulge is formed on the membrane and extends a distance of 30 units from the basal end, erasing the initial displacement and substituting another in the contrary direction, as shown at 2. Now the wave amplitude falls from b to c, an amount equal to 19 units, and a second bulge forms, carrying the membrane this number of units to the left and leaving it as shown at 3. Next, as the wave rises from c to d, a distance of 6 units, a smaller portion of the membrane is displaced to the right, as at 4. So the process continues, until 6 bulges are formed in the course of a single period of the compound wave.

Now let us examine these bulges in a little more detail. It will be noted that the part of the basilar membrane nearest the basal end is involved in all these movements, and, since the direction of the movement changes successively, this part, 6 units in length, will be moved back and forth (or up and down, as more conventionally pictured) three times in one period of $\frac{1}{100}$ sec, or 300 times a second. The next portion of the membrane, which extends from the farther end of this 6-unit portion to the 19-unit position, and is thus 13 units long, will be moved back and forth twice during the period, or 200 times a second. Finally, a third portion, 11 units long, will be moved back and forth only once per period, or 100 times a second. If excitation occurs once for each reciprocal movement, as already assumed, there should be 300, 200, and 100 excitations per second for the three different portions of the basilar membrane. Three tones should be heard, the two original components of 200 and 300 $\sim$ and a new tone of 100 $\sim$ that represents their frequency difference. Our ability to perceive these separate components, that is, our analysis of the complex sound, is made possible, according to the theory, by the distinctive action of separate regions of the basilar membrane. The theory thus accounts at the same time for analysis and the production of combination tones. Moreover, it derives the relative intensities of these components as a function of the lengths of the portions of basilar membrane involved in the movements.

One feature of this analysis deserves particular attention. It may already have been noted in this example that whereas the middle portion of the basilar membrane undergoes two up-and-down displacements per cycle, these displacements are not evenly spaced within the cycle. One is at the beginning of the cycle and the other at the end. The resulting nerve excitations, therefore, assuming that they occur only for movements from a maximum to a minimum, should give a pattern of two impulses separated by a space. Moreover, as a little consideration will show, this pattern varies somewhat for different strips of the membrane within the area under consideration, so that we must conceive of groups of nerve impulses that are somewhat spread out in time.

When other examples are considered, in which tones with less simple frequency ratios are compounded, the irregularities just mentioned are even more prominent. However, it was Meyer's belief that this is not a fatal obstacle to the theory and that perceptually we may be able to tolerate such variations from true synchronism.

The loudness of any component of a complex stimulus, just as of a simple tone, depends upon the length of the particular portion of the basilar membrane involved. It is necessary to add that in the example just given the functional relation between the stapedial movements and the lengths of basilar membrane has been oversimplified. Though the amplitudes of stapedial movements for the components 300, 200, and 100 ∼ have ratios of 6:13:11, the lengths of the portions of basilar membrane do not bear these same ratios. The function, Meyer indicated, is a complex one; it includes the varying width of the basilar membrane, and especially the velocity of the stapedial movement. Since the membrane widens from base to apex, the amount of spread for any given increment of stapedial movement must vary as a function of the length of the bulge at the moment. Near the basal end, where the membrane is narrow, a unit of stapedial movement will cause a larger spread than it will farther up the spiral where the membrane is wider. Meyer did not specify the exact form of this variation for lack of information on the form of the variation in width of the membrane. He pointed out, however, that it is an advantage to have the larger variations of length at the smaller amplitude levels, for faint tones thereby are relatively favored in representation and the upper end of the intensity scale is compressed.

The intensity relations for the components of a complex sound are further complicated by the fact that a general increase in the magnitude of the complex wave moves all the response areas apicalward, and since the width of the membrane is changing the several components are affected differently. Their intensity ratios thus vary with the level of stimulation. Generally speaking, a combination tone will be relatively louder for strong primary tones than for weak ones.

The intensity relations vary also according to the phase relations of the primary tones, though this effect is considered only a minor one.

Meyer's theory has had far less consideration than it deserves. It is a difficult theory: difficult in conception and perhaps more so in its presentation; and herein may lie part of the reason for its continued neglect.

The theory has a number of outstanding merits. Foremost is the simplicity of its assumptions about the basilar membrane. This structure is treated merely as a membrane, with only the orthodox properties of one that is both lax and strong, acting under heavy damping. There are no rigid specifications of shapes, sizes, tensions, masses, or the like, as are found in most other theories.

A signal contribution is the relation of loudness to the areal extent of the cochlear action and thus to the number of neural elements. Most subsequent theories have incorporated this idea.

Meyer's theory accounts for the masking of high tones in terms of overlapping: the low tones spread farther along the basilar membrane than the high tones do. But it does not explain so well the masking of low tones by high tones, which also occurs in some degree.

It is a virtue of the theory that it accounts for combination tones as a feature of the action in the cochlea in response to two or more tones presented at the same time. It is a disadvantage, however, that the periodicities of these tones as well as of others resulting from the analysis of complex sounds are not entirely regular. A still greater drawback is that some periodicities are theoretically derived that are of doubtful existence in the ear. The theory is indeed ingenious in its conception of a mode of analysis without recourse to resonance.

WRIGHTSON'S THEORY

The second form of frequency-analytic theory is that of Thomas Wrightson, a British engineer and industrialist. He outlined it first in an address before a group of engineers in 1876 and then developed it more fully some years later, in 1918. Like Meyer's theory, it was elaborated on the basis of a graphic kind of wave analysis. However, Wrightson's conception of the physical characteristics and mode of operation of the cochlea as well as the precise method of analysis differs from that of Meyer in many respects.

According to Wrightson, the cochlear fluid is entirely incompressible, and therefore the pressures set up by the movements of the stapes are communicated instantaneously to all parts of the cochlea. All particles of fluid and likewise all the membranes move simultaneously; there is no time lag for the more remote parts. Thus there is no spatial differentiation according to the frequency of tones, but every ending is subject to stimulation by any sound.

The sensory cells are stimulated whenever their hairs are bent as the result of relative movement between the basilar mem-

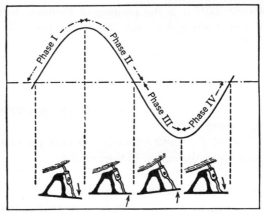

Fig. 14. Wrightson's theory of the 'phases' of excitation of the hair cells. Above is a sine wave, and below are the four positions taken by a portion of the organ of Corti as a result of the wave action. Shown schematically are Corti's arch and a single hair cell with its cilia impinging upon the lower surface of the tectorial membrane.

brane and the tectorial membrane. Ter Kuile's conception of the cochlear mechanics is followed closely here. When the basilar membrane is made to bulge, the arch turns as on a pivot formed by the foot of its inner pillar, which rests solidly on the edge of the spiral lamina. The hair cells, because they are securely linked to the arch by means of the reticular membrane and other parts, are carried along in this movement. These cells, therefore, are moved somewhat sidewise as well as vertically. Now, the tectorial membrane, though it is free to move up and down, is anchored to the limbus so that lateral movement is prevented. While the roots of the hairs are moved laterally their ends remain practically fixed, since they rest on the lower surface of the tectorial membrane or possibly are embedded in it. Hence the hairs are bent toward the limbus when the basilar membrane bulges downward, and are bent in the contrary direction when the membrane bulges upward.

Wrightson conceived that a flexure of a hair occurs every time the hair cell is moved either away from or back toward its equilibrium position. Therefore there are four flexures per cycle: one when the membrane moves downward from its equilibrium point, another when it moves back to this point, a third when it bulges upward, and a fourth when again it moves back to the equilibrium point. Figure 14 illustrates these four 'phases' of a single cycle of movement. These phases correspond in the aerial wave to the points of maximum pressure, zero pressure, minimum pressure, and zero pressure again, as shown in the figure.

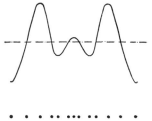

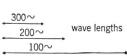

300~
200~ wave lengths
100~

FIG. 15. Wrightson's theory of wave analysis. Above is a compound wave, containing two components of 200 and 300 ~. The line of dots represents the pattern of nerve impulses produced: one impulse for every crest, trough, and 'crossing point' of the wave. Below are indicated the wave lengths of the two components and their difference tone.

According to Wrightson, there is excitation of the hair cell and its nerve fiber at every flexure of the hairs. Hence there are four nerve impulses for every cycle of the stimulus. This frequency theory therefore differs from the others mentioned in that sound frequencies are not directly reproduced in the nerve action but are quadrupled. A tone of 1000 ~, for example, would excite a series of nerve impulses with a frequency of 4000 per second.

When the wave form is complex, just as when it is simple, nerve excitation occurs at every crest, trough, and 'crossing point' of the wave. A curve like that of Fig. 15, which represents a compound wave formed by two tones whose frequencies are 200 and 300 ~, will set up a pattern of nerve impulses indicated by the dots below.

A fundamental feature of Wrightson's theory is his contention that this nerve pattern actually contains two rhythmic series, one corresponding to one component (the 200 ~ tone) and another corresponding to the other component (the 300 ~ tone). The wave lengths corresponding to these two tones are to be found in the distances separating various pairs of the dots.

Wrightson's method of analysis makes use of either the wave pattern or the equivalent dot pattern. He sets a pair of compasses to the wave length of one component and then applies them at various regions of the curve until separations are found that match their span. It is not required that the agreement be exact, and the degree of variation that is allowable seems to be a matter of personal judgment. Moreover, the series representing a given component is not a continuous one: pulses are often missing. The argument was made that the ear will tolerate a considerable amount of variation from perfect synchronism. This point was supported with evidence from siren experiments that used a siren disc in which the holes were not all equally spaced, but some were shifted slightly from their regular positions. It was found that despite these variations a tone was heard, though it steadily grew more noisy in character as the variations from true synchronism became numerous. Similarly, the omission of holes left the original pitch unchanged, though this measure too introduced noisiness.

The theory goes further. Not only are there rhythms corresponding to the primary components of the compound wave (200 and 300 ~ in the example), but also there are rhythms representative of combination tones. In the example, a difference tone of 100 ~ is said to be present. Curiously enough, however, this component does not have four pulses per cycle, but only one.

There are usually some pulses that belong neither to the primary rhythms nor to the combination tones; they are inharmonic, and are said, like the variations from perfect synchronism, to add a noise quality to the sound. In certain compounds of more complicated character, which Wrightson analyzed in this fashion, as many as 20 per cent of the pulses are classed as inharmonic.

The compound wave illustrated in Fig. 15 is the one obtained for a particular intensity relation and a particular phase relation of the primary components. If either the intensity or phase relation is altered, the form of the compound wave will change. Correspondingly there will be a variation in the nerve pattern produced. These variations, like the others mentioned, Wrightson regarded as not very serious. He suggested also that by reason of certain distortions introduced in the middle ear by the operation of the tympanic muscles, and by further distortions in the inner ear, the aperiodicities referred to tend to be minimized. The argument here is not easy to follow.

In Wrightson's theory, little is said about sound intensity. The point is made that the spread-out character of the end organ gives room for a large number of sensory cells and thereby affords higher sensitivity, and that it provides also a factor of safety in case of functional failure of some of the elements. Further it is claimed that since the scalae are narrowest at the apical end the velocity of fluid motion must be maximal there, and hence this region is the most sensitive one. A very faint sound will affect only the apical hair cells, and as the intensity is raised the effect will spread toward the base. In a minor degree, therefore, loudness varies with the number of hair cells stimulated; this aspect of loudness is minor because it is effective only for sounds near the threshold, or at the moment of expiration of a sound. Principally, loudness depends upon the acoustic power communicated to each of the sensory cells, but how this is converted into nerve action is not specified in the theory.

Wrightson's theory contains a number of weaknesses for which it has been severely criticized. Certainly dubious are the assumptions that the cochlear fluid is inelastic and incompressible and that the pressure within the cochlea caused by a sound wave is everywhere the same. Boring and Titchener pointed out these difficulties and objected to the peculiar conception of excitation at four 'critical points' within each cycle. Especially curious is the assertion that motion or momentum falls to zero at the crossing points as well as at the peaks and troughs of a wave. They pointed out the inconsistency of having four excitations per cycle, yet in the graphical analysis looking for whole wave lengths rather than quarter wave lengths. They commented favorably, however, on Wrightson's 'discovery' that critical points in a compound wave may represent its periodicities.

This 'discovery' is the focal point of the objections to the theory made by Morton, and more emphatically by Hartridge. Hartridge carried out the graphical analysis as described on several samples of waves and found that purely arbitrary distances would give just as many coincidences as the constituent wave lengths themselves. He concluded that the analysis was unreal and that Wrightson's seeming success grew out of his selection of certain chance relations and the neglect of others.

This chapter and the others preceding have dealt with a long array of theories that may properly be regarded as the classical ones. These for the most part sprang up early, in the latter part of the past century, in the wave of interest in sensory activity stimulated by Müller's doctrine of specific energies. A few other theories came later, but still deserve the classical designation, as they have served to round out the possibilities of explanation of the auditory phenomena. These theories have shared among them the responsibility for stimulating and guiding the subsequent thought and research in this field.

Still, this list of theories is by no means complete. There have been others, indeed a good many others, that have been put forward by their inventors, either tentatively or with vigor, but always hopefully, and yet have had only slight effect upon the main stream of development. For this and other reasons they have not been treated here. Some such theories that come to mind are those of Tominaga, Dunlap, Lucae, Goebel, Mygind, and Leiri; and there must be others still. Also, and too numerous for even this passing reference, are the many modified versions and individualized presentations of the classical theories, and Helmholtz's in particular. Their peculiarities, and sometimes perhaps involuntary departures from the original forms, are not of any serious concern to our present problems.

Part II
The Modern Developments

MODERN DEVELOPMENTS OF THE CLASSICAL THEORIES

THE MODERN RESONANCE THEORY

As seen in the perspective of recent times there have been three principal problems to be faced by the resonance theory. These are (1) the conditions determining the differentiation of the resonant elements, (2) the specificity and independence of these elements, and (3) the manner of representation of stimulus intensity in the auditory nerve action. The first two problems were treated by Helmholtz, as we have seen, but the third could arise only after the development of our modern knowledge of the nature of sensory nerve activity.

THE FACTORS OF DIFFERENTIATION

If the transverse fibers of the basilar membrane act as simple stretched strings, like the strings of the piano and violin, their natural frequencies of vibration will be determined by three factors: the length, tension, and mass of the fibers. A low natural frequency is produced by increasing the length of the string, or reducing its tension, or increasing its mass. On the other hand, a high natural frequency results from reducing the length, increasing the tension, or reducing the mass. Precisely, these three conditions act jointly to determine the tuned frequency in a manner expressed by the formula

$$f = \frac{1}{2l}\sqrt{\frac{T}{m}}$$

where f = natural frequency, l = length of the string in centimeters, T = tension in dynes, and m = mass in grams per centimeter of length. It must be added at once, however, that the laws of vibrating strings of which this formula is an expression are founded upon certain assumptions, chiefly the following: that the string is of negligible rigidity, its mass is uniformly distributed along its length, its end supports are immobile, and it is subjected to only negligible friction. If these conditions are not met, then rather drastic modifications of the formula must be made.

The Factor of Length. Helmholtz in his treatment of the tuning of the basilar membrane fibers considered explicitly only the factor of length. He cited Hensen's observation that the width of the basilar membrane (*i.e.*, the length of its transverse fibers) increases from 0.041 mm at the basal end to 0.495 mm at the apical end, which is a 12-fold variation. He pointed out further, following Henle, that most of this increase takes place in the outer zone of the membrane, beyond the arches of Corti, so that if only this outermost and presumably more mobile portion of the membrane is considered the variation in Hensen's measurements comes to nearly 20-fold. This expansion of the range of variation is quite specious, however. There is no advantage in the resonance of just the outermost, free portion of the basilar membrane, for this part alone cannot have any excitatory effect. It must carry with it the remainder that bears the sensory structures. It is remarkable that this kind of suggestion was ever taken seriously.

Hensen's measurements had been made on only one specimen, and it remained to be seen how representative they were of ears in general. Unfortunately, the succeeding decades brought more confusion than clarification to this matter. Retzius in 1884 made measurements in a single ear at three positions, one each in the basal, middle, and apical turns, and obtained widths of 0.210, 0.340, and 0.360 mm, respectively; and these measurements have been the most extensively quoted since that time. Keith in 1918 made measurements in three ears and reported averages of 0.160 mm near the basal end and 0.520 mm near the apex. Held in 1926, in measurements on two specimens, obtained values of about the same order as Keith's.

The trouble with these results is that they do not include sufficient information about the positions along the cochlear spiral at which the measurements were made. Expressions like 'in the basal turn' and 'near the apex' are too indefinite. What was wanting was a procedure for dealing precisely with a structure of this complicated form. Guild (1) supplied it in his method of graphic reconstruction. This method yields an accurate scale projection of the cochlear spiral, on which any part of the structures may be located and the distance found from either end of the spiral. This method is now the basis of all our quantitative dealings with the cochlear anatomy.

Guild (2) applied his method to the guinea pig ear. He made graphic reconstructions of 3 ears to locate 9 positions along the spiral where the membrane had been cut 'radially,' *i.e.*, along its radius of curvature, and from these data he estimated the positions in 32 other ears. He then made measurements of the width of the basilar membrane in the 35 ears at these 9 positions. He found rather large individual differences, but on the average a variation in width of a little over threefold. A curious feature was revealed: the membrane in the guinea pig does not taper continuously from one end to the other but attains its maximum width near the beginning of the apical coil and then declines rapidly.

I have made use of Guild's method in a series of measurements of the width of the basilar membrane in man (Wever, 4). The study was made on 25 cochleas that had been prepared for histological examination by serial sectioning. An extension of the method made it possible to include positions at which the plane of section was oblique as well as the simpler radial sections, so that altogether the measurements were made at 17 to 19 positions along the membrane, depending upon the number of cochlear turns.

The results showed that in man, as Guild found for the guinea pig, the basilar membrane is not uniformly tapered. The width increases from the basal end upward at first slowly and then more rapidly. Individual differences are large, especially in the apical region. In most cochleas the maximum width is found about one half-turn before the apical end is reached, after which the width decreases sharply. In a few cochleas, and more commonly in those in which the total length of the membrane is below average, the width continues to increase almost to the very end.

Because the most basal part of the membrane fails to continue the spiral form of the main portion but curls around into a terminal hook, any attempt to treat it by simple projection is unsatisfactory. The measurements are likely to be too large because a full correction is not made for the obliquity of the section. The results obtained by the regular graphic method gave widths for this portion that varied from 0.100 mm upward

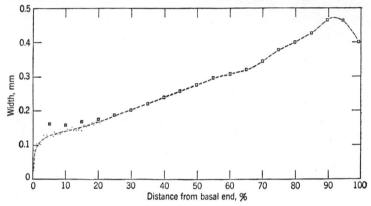

FIG. 16.   Width of the human basilar membrane. The square points represent averages of measurements on 25 cochleas, and the small dots represent results obtained on a single ear by a special method. To obtain abscissa distances in millimeters for the average ear, multiply the percentage numbers by 0.3152.

to more than 0.200 mm. Two series of sections that were cut in the frontal plane, that is, perpendicular to the axis of the cochlear spiral, were more satisfactory for this purpose and showed a gradual taper to a lower value of about 0.100 mm near the basal end. The most satisfactory results were obtained by a special method of sectioning. The block of tissue was observed with a microscope during the sectioning and was continually reoriented so as to keep the basilar membrane at right angles to the knife. This procedure was laborious and was carried out on only one ear. It proved that the membrane tapers gradually and then ends bluntly and that close to the end it has a width of 0.080 mm.

In Fig. 16 the square points show averages of the measurements on the 25 ears, and the dots indicate the results obtained at the basal end by the special method just described. The average figures are significant for the middle portion of the cochlea where the different ears are in fairly good agreement,

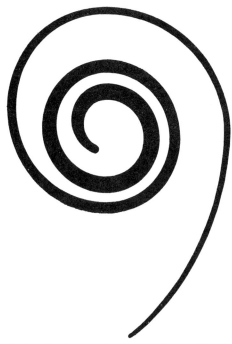

FIG. 17.   Spiral plot of a human basilar membrane, 10 times natural size. From Wever (4) [*Annals of Otology, Rhinology, and Laryngology*].

but are much less so for the apical end where there are large variations of form.   Figure 17 is a diagrammatic representation, to scale, of a basilar membrane of rather more than average length.

The maximum width of the membrane varied in different specimens from 0.423 to 0.651 mm, with an average value of 0.498 mm.   Hence the variation in width was a little over 5-fold at one extreme and about 8-fold at the other, with a $6\frac{1}{4}$-fold variation as the average.

It is evident that if the width of the basilar membrane is accepted as one of the factors of tuning in the ear, the theory must be flexible enough to allow for these large individual differences. In any case the factor of length can account for only a rather small amount of the frequency differentiation required. The vibratory frequencies to which the ear is responsive and which it can discriminate extend (in young persons) from 15 to 24,000 ~, a variation of 1600-fold or $10\frac{1}{2}$ octaves. If the length of the transverse fibers varies on the average by $6\frac{1}{4}$-fold then we can by this factor account for somewhat less than $2\frac{1}{2}$ octaves of the frequency range.

The greater share of the frequency differentiation, amounting to 256-fold or 8 octaves, is left to the variables of tension and mass. Moreover, since in the formula these two variables appear under the square-root sign, they must undergo jointly a variation of 256^2 or 65,536-fold if the theory is to be substantiated.

The Factor of Tension. The first material support of the view that tension enters into the differential tuning of the basilar membrane fibers was obtained by Gray (1) in a study of the form of the spiral ligament. This structure, a ribbon of fibrous connective tissue, connects the basilar membrane with the external bony wall of the cochlea. Gray pointed out that it presents a continuous graduation in size throughout the cochlea. At the basal end it is dense and bulky, but at the apical end it is reduced greatly in size and fiber content. It is inferred that the spiral ligament exerts transverse tension on the basilar membrane, a tension that is greatest in the basal region and progressively less toward the apex. This variation of tension, Gray pointed out, operates for differential tuning in the same sense as the variation in breadth of the membrane; the transverse fibers in the base are short and strongly stretched, and therefore tuned for high tones, whereas those in the apex are long and lax, and tuned for low tones.

Gray made no estimate of the amount of tension or its range of variation. Later, Wilkinson offered some suggestions as to what is left for tension after suitable shares of the differentiation have been assigned to the other factors of length and mass. He accorded length a $3\frac{1}{4}$-fold variation and mass a 20-fold variation; and on his assumption of an auditory range of 30 to 30,000 ~

this left tension with a variation of 4734-fold, which is much the largest share. (If we use the range cited above of 15 to 24,000 ~ this figure becomes 12,119-fold.) More specifically, Wilkinson determined from the formula for vibrating strings that a segment of the membrane 0.1 mm long in the extreme basal region must sustain a tension of 1843 dynes, and a segment of the same length in the apical region a tension of 0.39 dynes. He carried out tests on silkworm gut and other fibers to show that they could bear the maximum tension here required. The minimum tension of 0.39 dynes he conceded to be "fairly low, but not infinitesimal."

Berendes sought to decide this question experimentally. He worked with fresh human material, and determined the tension of the basilar membrane by ascertaining the distance that it was depressed by the exertion of a known force upon it. He was able to expose the membrane suitably only in the first half-turn of the basal end of the cochlea so that his measurements were restricted to this one place. The tensions observed varied from 4.59 to 10.7 dynes per cm of length; let us take 7.6 dynes per cm as a middle value.

It might be argued that Berendes' measurements do not indicate the maximum tension of the basilar membrane, as they were made a little distance, perhaps about 7 mm, from the basal end. If we assume that tension varies uniformly from base to apex, we can estimate that Berendes' measurements represent about $\frac{4}{5}$ the maximum tension, as 7 mm is $\frac{1}{5}$ of the way from base to apex. On this basis we have 9.5 dynes per cm as the maximum tension, or 0.095 dynes for a strip of the membrane 0.1 mm long. This value of 0.095 dynes is quite out of the range of Wilkinson's calculation of 1843 dynes for this size of strip at the basal end of the membrane—the discrepancy is more than 19,000 times. If we calculate a minimum tension by dividing the figure of 0.095 dynes per 0.1 mm by 4734, we obtain the ridiculously small figure of 0.00002 dynes per 0.1 mm.

Measurements of the size of the spiral ligament indicate far less variation than Wilkinson supposed. The cross-sectional area indeed varies progressively from base to apex, as Gray described. However, as Fig. 18 shows, its range of variation is only about 15-fold. It is reasonable to suppose that if the ligament exerts tension it does so in simple proportion to its bulk, and hence a 15-fold variation of tension is the most that can properly be assigned to it.

Békésy (11) in a recent experiment was unable to observe any tension at all in the basilar membrane, which is reminiscent of

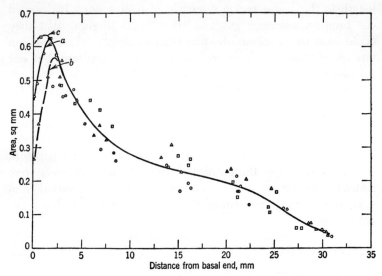

Fig. 18.   The size of the spiral ligament in the human cochlea.   The cross-sectional area is shown for three different ears, as represented by the three kinds of points.   Over most of the range—all except the basal end—a single curve represents the data reasonably well.   See Fig. 2 for orientation. (The measurements were made on serially sectioned ears made available by Dr. Stacy R. Guild.)

Helmholtz's own result which he would not accept.   What we seem to have in this membrane is not an active tension but rather a resistance to displacement, or a stiffness.   Békésy, as we have already seen, measured such a stiffness by two methods and reported its variation along the cochlea as about 100-fold.

The Factor of Mass.   Helmholtz offered no detailed explanation of the factor of mass, yet he considered it an important variable and called upon it for scaling down the responses of the cochlear resonators to the extent required at the lower end of the frequency range.   He wrote: "That such short strings should be capable of corresponding with such deep tones, must be explained by their being loaded in the basilar membrane with all kinds of solid formations; the fluid of both galleries in the cochlea must also be considered as weighting the membrane, because it cannot move without a kind of wave motion in that fluid."

Two or three distinguishable conditions are suggested here: (1) the inertia afforded by the cellular structures attached to the basilar membrane, (2) the frictional damping to which the movements are subjected, and perhaps (3) loading by fluid columns.

1. Inertia Effects. Several writers since Helmholtz have referred to the loading of the basilar membrane by the organ of Corti. Gray pointed out that such loading operates in the same direction as the variation in breadth of the membrane and as the assumed variation of tension, for the cellular masses are greatest in the apex and progressively smaller toward the base of the cochlea. Hartridge and Banister estimated this variation as having a range of 12-fold.

This estimate of Hartridge and Banister is much too large. My own measurements of the area of the cellular structures made in three cochleas show a variation of about threefold in two of them and fivefold in the other. Figure 19 gives some of the data. The rise in bulk of the structures is fairly uniform from the basal end upward to within a few millimeters of the apex, and then there is a leveling off and finally a rapid decline. The central mass of the organ, which loads the middle of the membrane, shows somewhat smaller variations than the entire basilar structure.

2. Damping. The movements of the basilar membrane encounter frictional resistances that must be considerable. The membrane itself is fibrous in composition, and in its action friction must appear in the sliding of the fiber layers on one another. The cellular structures that are attached to the membrane form a somewhat consistent mass, and at some places these parts have connections with relatively immobile bodies, as in the internal and external sulcus regions, so that the parts are not perfectly free but undergo deformations when the membrane moves; these deformations create internal friction in the parts concerned.

Finally, the movements are executed in a fluid medium and are damped by that medium in so far as there is relative movement between the fluid and its confining walls.

Damping has effects of great importance, some of which have already been referred to. For the present problem we have the principle that the greater the degree of damping the lower the

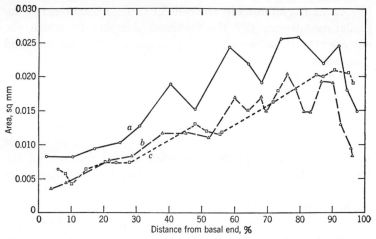

FIG. 19. The size of the sensory structures borne by the basilar membrane. Included in the measurements are all parts between the two anchorages of the membrane at the spiral ligament and the limbus: the organ of Corti proper and the tympanic lamella below. See Fig. 5 for orientation. To obtain the abscissa distances in millimeters, multiply the percentage figures by 0.315 for curve *a*, by 0.317 for curve *b*, and by 0.288 for curve *c*. These ears are the same as were used for Fig. 18.

natural frequency. Now there are two main considerations for a variation in damping. On the one hand we may expect the damping to depend upon the bulk and surface area of the cellular structures, because these structures in moving undergo internal deformations and also present a frictional surface to the surrounding fluid. Because the cellular structures grow more massive toward the apex the damping so produced will increase in this direction. This condition, therefore, may aid in differential tuning.

A further consideration is that the surface and internal friction may increase with the velocity of motion, and so it must increase

with the frequency. However, this variation is a function of
the stimulation and not a local characteristic of the tissues themselves; and though its effects are to be seen in the degree and
spread of activity it is not to be regarded as a factor in differentiation in a strict sense.

3. Fluid Columns. A hypothesis of differentiation by means
of fluid columns was first put forth by F. Lux, according to an
account by Budde. This hypothesis was further developed by
Wilkinson. It is supposed that every segment of the basilar
membrane is associated in its movements with a double column
of fluid, namely, the fluid that extends from the oval window
to the segment on the one hand and from the segment to the
round window on the other hand. (See Fig. 72.) As the lengths
of these columns are greater for segments farther toward the
apex, the fluid loading is progressive.

The fluid is not assumed to move in the form of a narrow band
or column, yet it is supposed that the mass moved is equivalent
to such a column. The moving mass has a cross-sectional area
equal to the area of the basilar membrane segment and a length
determined by the distance of the segment from the base of
the cochlea.

Since the cochlear fluids have a specific gravity approximately
equal to 1, the mass in grams, and of course the degree of variation, can be computed from the dimensions. Wilkinson estimated that for the highest audible pitch the length of the double
column was 0.2 cm, and for the lowest pitch 4 cm, which is a
variation of 20-fold for a constant element of cross section.
Fletcher (1) in a later estimate gave 30-fold as the possible
variation.

This claim for loading of the membrane by fluid columns is
enticing but not quite convincing. It is somehow reminiscent of
the fabulous feat of lifting yourself by your bootstraps. A column of a given length is determined by the fact that the membrane yields only at a particular place; how then does the
column's length determine that place? If this part of the membrane had its own separate column the matter would be different,
but the liquid is common to all parts and when a given tone is
sounded will reinforce the movement of any part as readily as
this particular one.

Let us now review this differentiation of the basilar membrane in terms of the length, tension, and mass of its transverse fibers. The factor of length varies $6\frac{1}{4}$-fold and can account for $2\frac{1}{2}$ octaves. The factor of tension is doubtful altogether, for neither the older observations of Helmholtz nor the modern ones of Berendes and Békésy indicate any active tension at all. But if we grant the argument, the variation in bulk of the spiral ligament can justify a variation in tension of but 15-fold, which can account for about 2 octaves. The remaining 6 octaves must depend upon the factor of mass.

For mass proper we have a variation of, let us say, 4-fold on the average; this will account for one octave. What contribution to the mass factor a variation in damping can make is quite speculative; shall we say another octave? Remaining are a little over 4 octaves, which now must be assigned to fluid loading. This calls for a variation of 273-fold, far more than either Wilkinson or Fletcher was willing to credit to this factor. If we take Fletcher's estimate of 30-fold as an outside figure, we shall still have nearly 2 octaves unaccounted for.

At the best—granting every claim—we can work out a total differentiation of about $8\frac{1}{2}$ octaves; and at a more realistic level, denying the claims for tension and fluid loading, we have a differentiation of perhaps $4\frac{1}{2}$ octaves. Obviously the stretched-string theory does not do well in the face of the modern evidence.

THE SPECIFICITY AND INDEPENDENCE OF THE COCHLEAR RESONATORS

The resonance theory in its simplest form rests upon the assumption that the ear contains a large number of specific, independent resonators—one for every discriminable pitch. The Helmholtz theory is often presented as such a simple theory, and, indeed, Helmholtz introduced his theory in a way that emphasized the specificity of the resonant and nervous elements. Thus he said, "The sensations of simple tones of different pitch would under the supposed conditions fall to the lot of different nervous fibres, and hence be produced quite separately, and independently of each other."

It has been easy to overlook the fact that in this passage Helmholtz referred to 'supposed conditions' and that later on in the development of his theory he found it necessary to complicate these conditions materially. Because damping in the cochlea must be considerable and because his observations on 'musical shakes' demanded it, he postulated a moderate degree of spread of resonance in the cochlea. His specific assumption was that any given resonator may be set in motion by all frequencies within a band extending about a semitone above and an equal distance below the tuned frequency. In a figure he indicated that within this band the amplitude of vibration ought to fall off rapidly as the frequency departs from the tuned frequency. Stated differently, Helmholtz's assumption was that when any given tone stimulates the ear it sets into vibration to an appreciable extent all the resonators—a score or more, he thought—whose tuned frequencies lie within the range of a whole tone. The problem is, why then do we perceive only one pitch, rather than all the pitches proper to the resonators in action? Helmholtz did not treat this problem and perhaps did not have any clear perception of it as a problem, but the matter was one of concern to many who followed after him.

The first presentation of the problem is due to Hostinsky, who in 1879 brought out an elucidation of Helmholtz's principles for the benefit of musicians. He interpreted Helmholtz's discussion of the spread of resonance to mean that a single tone arouses not one sensation but a whole group of sensations. Then to reduce the complexity he applied a principle that had become widely known from its use in Herbart's psychological system, the principle of the interaction of sensations in the unconscious. The several sensations aroused by a single tone do not appear in consciousness as a group, he said, because they first compete with one another in the unconscious, and only the strongest survives to pass the conscious threshold. This he called a 'focusing' process.

Little attention was paid to Hostinsky's treatment of this matter, in some measure perhaps because the notion of unconscious sensations was not attractive, but mainly because Helmholtz's remarks about the spread of resonance were generally ignored and his theory was thought of in a very simple way, as involving specific, independent resonators. Because it was regarded in this way, the theory came to face an ever-mounting clamor of criticism.

The most trenchant of these criticisms, and the one that had the most influence among physicists, was made by Wien in 1905. He pointed out that in the presence of damping no resonator can be altogether inactive toward any vibratory frequency that is brought to bear upon it. Hence every cochlear element responds in some degree to every tone. How then, he asked, can we perceive a single pitch? In his opinion the resonance theory could give no suitable answer to this question.

The theory was most often attacked by anatomists and physiologists on the ground that the fibers of the basilar membrane are not free to vibrate separately. Later was added the argument that the nerve supply to the hair cells is not specific either, so that even if an element could resonate alone it could have no distinct neural representation. At the beginning of the present century these criticisms had become so general and compelling that many were ready to cast the theory away altogether. Thereupon appeared Gray's principle of maximum stimulation to give the theory a new significance.

THE PRINCIPLE OF MAXIMUM STIMULATION

Gray formulated his principle, it would seem, quite independently of Hostinsky, yet it is essentially an assertion of the same focusing principle. Gray's formulation met with more ready acceptance in part just because he made no specific commitment as to the process by which the focusing is achieved. He stated simply that we react by a perception of pitch only to the particular nerve fiber that corresponds to the point on the basilar membrane where the stimulation is a maximum. Impulses from other nerve fibers that are excited at the same time are either suppressed or are integrated with those from the one representing the maximum.

Gray took his main evidence from the field of touch. He observed that when any blunt object is pressed upon the skin we feel the contact at only one point, though the skin is depressed over a considerable area. If the object is applied more strongly the intensity of the pressure sensation is increased, but still (he thought) we perceive only one locus of stimulation, namely, that at which the excitation is a maximum.

In this connection the term 'maximum' is used in its mathematical sense, as a point on the basilar membrane where the amplitude of movement is greater than it is immediately above and below, regardless of what the amplitude may be elsewhere along the membrane. Thus there may be any number of maximum points at different regions of the membrane at any one time. Figure 20 gives a schematic representation of the maxima that might be formed by three different tones acting independently; and if we should sum up the amplitudes for all three curves we should have their composite pattern. Such a pattern might be the result of stimulating with a musical note made up of a fundamental tone and two overtones. The pitches heard are those proper to the positions at *a, b,* and *c.*

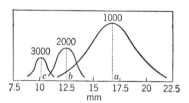

FIG. 20.   Gray's principle of maximum stimulation. The horizontal scale represents the position along the cochlea and the vertical scale the amplitude of basilar membrane movement.

According to Gray, the limits of pitch discrimination are determined simply by the ability to differentiate adjoining maxima. If two maxima are far enough apart to be distinguished, two pitches are heard. If they are very close together the result is a single tone, which, however, will exhibit beats because at that part of the membrane affected by two stimuli in common the vibratory movements combine at some moments and oppose one another at others.

Gray (2) used his principle to explain certain abnormalities of hearing. The condition known as disharmonic paracusis is one in which a simple tone is heard as a tone in one ear and as a buzzing noise in the other ear. Gray supposed that the noise is heard because in that ear a few resonators or nerve fibers in the region of the maximum have been impaired, yet the elements above and below this region are functioning normally. The result is that there are two regions of stimulation so close together as to be indistinguishable. If the impairment is broader, so that the two normally acting regions are rather distant from one another, the rarer disorder known as monaural diplacusis appears, in which a single tone is heard as double. The more common binaural diplacusis, in which a single tone is heard as of different pitch in the two ears, is accounted for as a shift of the maximum point away from its normal position in one of the ears.

Gray's principle saved the day for the resonance theory. It made it possible—or so it was believed—to admit a high degree of spread in the action of sounds in the cochlea without loss of the specificity that is the heart of the theory. For though specificity was given up in the initial action of the stimulus it was recovered later on through this principle of the maximum.

One point of theory remained. As we have seen, Gray only asserted his principle; he did not explain the process underlying it. This mystery could not long be ignored, and two types of hypothesis were offered.

Fischer made an effort to locate the process in the periphery. He conceived it in a peculiar mode of excitation of the hair cells. He supposed that in the resting position, when no tone is acting, the hairs of the hair cells stand a little distance away from the tectorial membrane. When a tone appears and vibrates the basilar membrane it forces the hairs into contact with the tectorial membrane but it does so only at one place, where the tuning is best and the movement is strongest. Elsewhere no contact is made, both because the amplitude of vibration is smaller and because to some extent the tectorial membrane moves along with the basilar membrane.

Another peripheral hypothesis was advanced by Békésy (1). According to his theory of cochlear action, described earlier, the movements of the stapes set up waves that travel down the basilar membrane to the helicotrema. They vary in amplitude as they travel and reach a maximum at some place where the tuning is most favorable. There they produce an eddy in the endolymph. It is likely, he thought, that excitation occurs only in the region of the eddy, not over the full course of the disturbance.

The second type of explanation looks to the higher centers for the means of emphasizing the point of the maximum and of neglecting the remaining areas of movement. We have already met one such hypothesis in Hostinsky's early treatment of the problem. Békésy presented another which he called a 'law of contrast.' According to this conception the nerve excitation is particularly great in a region of the basilar membrane that forms a boundary between relatively little movement and relatively great movement. He drew an analogy with visual contrast, by means of which the brightness difference between two adjoining surfaces is emphasized. This emphasizing will be the greatest in the region of a maximum, for here are two transitions, from weak to strong and from strong to weak, and the two contrast effects are added. According to Békésy, this narrowing of response is superimposed upon that already afforded by the local eddy, and so specificity of tone perception appears even in the face of heavy damping in the cochlea.

Objections can easily be raised against all these hypotheses. Those based upon peripheral processes may seem to ease the difficulty, but they do not solve it, because the intensity range to which the ear responds is much wider than any conceivable restriction of excitation by the means suggested. For many tones the amplitude from threshold to the largest bearable magnitude varies more than a million-fold. If, in Fischer's theory, the hair cells in the best-tuned region just make contact at threshold, then certainly when the intensity becomes a million times greater other hair cells must make contact as well. It does no good to space the hair cells away from the tectorial membrane as he suggested, for this only makes excitation more difficult in general and does not change the problem. Békésy's local eddy theory suffers from the same limitation, as evidently he was well aware when he sought to supplement it by his contrast hypothesis.

The central hypotheses, like Hostinsky's competition of sensations and Békésy's law of contrast, are not really explanations but assertions of the principle of the maximum in other terms. If competition and contrast are general characteristics of the nervous system—and they may well be—we still need to know how they are displayed, by what processes, and under what conditions.

Even if we admit the physiological basis of the principle, or pass over the problem as Gray did, there are many inherent difficulties. Let us first consider some particular ones.

Frequencies at the upper and lower ends of the scale, according to a resonance theory in which even a small amount of damping is admitted, ought to produce patterns (as shown in Fig. 21) in which the terminal resonator is always at the maximum. Hence all tones below the natural frequency of the lowest resonator ought to have the same pitch, as also should all tones above the natural frequency of the highest resonator. Helmholtz and others did indeed assert a dullness of pitch perception in these regions, yet modern observations show no lack of discrimination at the lower end of the scale, and even at the upper end though discrimination is poor it continues all the way.

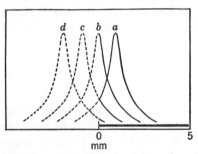

FIG. 21. Patterns of stimulus action at the basal extremity of the basilar membrane (hypothetical). According to the principle of maximum stimulation, the curves *b, c, d,* all of which involve the terminal resonator more strongly than any other, ought to have the same pitch.

Another difficulty comes in the raising of a tone to a high intensity. At some level the resonators in the middle of the stimulated area ought to reach their limits of action, and the curve of the response then should have a flat top and no point of maximum. A further increase of intensity would extend the flat area. Such tones, it would seem, ought to be poorly defined in pitch, perhaps noisy, and not readily discriminable. Gray asserted as much. The evidence indicates quite the contrary: strong tones acquire harmonics but do not grow noisy, and discrimination is at its best at the highest intensities.

A more serious difficulty appears when two or more tones are applied simultaneously. If their stimulated areas overlap, the combined pattern will have maximum points whose locations depend not only on the frequencies but also, in a complicated way, on the intensities and phase relations.

The most serious issue for the Helmholtz type of theory will now be evident. Once the elementary and complete form of specificity has been given up the theory is in difficulty. The principle of maximum stimulation does not eliminate this difficulty but only adds further complications. A burden is thrown upon the higher centers in the perception of even the simplest tones. For the complex tones this burden is greater still. A distinction in this respect between the resonance theory and the other theories that deliberately depend upon the higher centers for discrimination and analysis has largely disappeared.

THE REPRESENTATION OF STIMULUS INTENSITY

In the early development of the resonance theory the representation of stimulus intensity was not thought of as presenting any special problem. Helmholtz referred to the matter only briefly and dismissed it with the suggestion that "for each individual fibre of the nerve there remains only the quantitative differences in the amount of excitement." He took it for granted that the size of the nerve impulse could vary in such a way as to represent the amplitude of response of the cochlear resonators and hence the gradations of the external sound. This simple and seemingly obvious explanation of intensity was set at naught by the discovery of the all-or-nothing principle of nerve action.

The All-or-Nothing Principle. Gotch in 1902 first suggested that a nerve fiber when stimulated always responds to the utmost degree permitted by its condition at the moment, regardless of the intensity of the excitation. His evidence was slender, so much so that it is fair to regard his conclusion as essentially a bit of brilliant insight, but in the ensuing years many experiments established the validity of the principle. The impulse of a nerve fiber varies, but only according to the physiological condition of the fiber, particularly its degree of recovery from a preceding excitation. The magnitude of the impulse does not vary according to the intensity of the stimulus, and hence it cannot represent that intensity except in one detail, namely, to the effect that the stimulus is over threshold strength.

Adrian (1–3) was responsible for much of the final experimental support of the principle, and he provided also a simple explanation why the principle holds. Any stimulus, he pointed out, will necessarily spread through some appreciable length of the nerve fiber on which it acts, and an excitatory effect will be established at every point along the fiber where this influence exceeds the threshold value. At some advanced point, where the excitation is barely above threshold, a nerve impulse will arise and will be propagated forward. At all more adjacent points, though the stimulus influence is stronger, the action will be strictly local: propagation cannot occur because ahead are regions where the fiber is already undergoing changes and is left in a refractory condition. Accordingly, all nerve excitation effectually is threshold excitation. Raising the intensity of the stimulus merely extends a little farther along the fiber the point at which the propagated impulse arises, and does not alter the size of the impulse.

This explanation needs a little modification in the light of more recent ideas of nerve excitation. It now appears that a propagated impulse does not arise at a point in a fiber independently of the rest of the fiber. Rather it requires the mutual reinforcement of activity over a segment of the fiber. However, the essential argument still stands, that the effective place from which propagation proceeds will be one most advanced where the excitation level is just at threshold.

The Theoretical Implications. For the simple resonance theory, which restricts the response aroused by a given tone to a single resonator or at most a small group of resonators, the limitations on intensity representation imposed by the all-or-nothing principle are particularly severe. One suggested solution is that each resonator might operate in association with a group of nerve fibers, so that several steps of intensity could appear by stimulation of the fibers in varying numbers. This solution, however, calls for an abundance of nerve fibers that is not to be found. Forbes and Gregg pointed out that the apportionment of only 10 fibers to each resonator—an all too niggardly quota—and the assumption in agreement with Helmholtz that there are 4500 resonators would call for a total of 45,000 nerve fibers, far more than there are in the cochlear nerve. A similar calculation based on more modern knowledge of our capacities for pitch and intensity discrimination yields the enormous figure of 540,000 fibers, which is something like 18 times the available number.

Evidently, if the framework of the resonance theory is to be retained, some further dimension of variation of the nerve fiber must be found for intensity representation. Forbes and Gregg proposed for this purpose the frequency of nerve impulses. They suggested that the intensity of excitation of a given fiber might be reflected in its rate of firing.

This suggestion was raised to the status of a principle of sensory nerve action in the work of Adrian and his associates, who in a notable series of experiments proved that in various sensory nerves—those serving muscular, tendinous, pressure, pain, and tactual endings, among others—the rate of impulses is a regular function of the intensity of stimulation. This we call the intensity-frequency principle.

The representation of stimulus strength by the frequency of nerve impulses is now understood as a consequence of the varying excitability of a fiber in its relative refractory period. During the early part of this period only the strongest stimuli are effective; later those more moderate in strength will suffice. It follows that a continuing stimulus will set up a train of impulses whose rate increases as a function of the stimulus intensity.

In this modification enjoined by the discovery of the all-or-nothing principle the resonance theory may be said to have attained its modern form. All recent formulations of the theory, as for example that of Wilkinson and Gray, embody the principle that intensity is represented by the frequency of nerve impulses.

The Modern Frequency Theories

The simple frequency or telephone theories now as throughout their history have met with two major obstacles, one the problem of analysis and the other the limitation in the frequency of impulses carried by nerve fibers.

THE PROBLEM OF ANALYSIS

Ohm's law of auditory analysis, by which a complex sound is resolved perceptually into a series of simple components, is the starting point of the resonance theories and their most distinctive feature; as is well known, they refer this ability to a spatial distribution of action according to the principle of resonance. The telephone theories, on the contrary, can offer no peripheral explanation of analysis, but refer it instead to the brain where it remains shrouded in the mysteries of the higher intellectual processes. How serious a matter this is we shall come to see.

FREQUENCY REPRESENTATION IN THE AUDITORY NERVE

Although the frequency theories may dispose of the problem of analysis by relegating it to the higher centers, they must face directly the problem of frequency representation in the auditory nerve. The assertion that sound frequencies themselves, over the extensive range to which the ear responds, are relayed by the auditory nerve must be measured against our knowledge of the limitations of nerve transmission.

The absolute refractory period of a nerve fiber is the interval of time after one impulse that the fiber requires before it again is capable of being excited. The individual firings cannot crowd one another more closely than the interval thus defined. Thereby an absolute limit is set upon the frequency of impulses that a fiber is able to transmit.

We have seen how in the early development of the frequency theory this problem arose, and how Rutherford set out to solve it by experiments of his own. He failed to observe nerve frequencies even approaching the upper limit of hearing, but he felt certain that such frequencies were possible; and considering the little that was known about nerve fibers in his time his conviction was a reasonable one to cherish.

Boring in 1926, after a review of the evidence on frequency theories and especially of that on the refractory properties of nerves, was led to reassert Rutherford's position. He found that the figures on the refractory periods of various nerves exhibited a range of 4.46 to 0.43 milliseconds, which if steadily maintained would permit the transmission of frequencies from 224 per second for the slowest up to 2325 per second for the fastest. Here is a range of frequencies of more than tenfold in different kinds of fibers. There were no determinations for the auditory nerve itself. Boring felt that it was only necessary to extend the present ratio and to suppose that the auditory fibers stood as much above the fastest fibers so far measured as these are above the slowest. The frequency theory has never enjoyed wide popularity. Boring's presentation of it is the most favorable of recent times. It was his contention that the rival theories based upon resonance put an undue emphasis on pitch and auditory analysis to the neglect of other phenomena. Such things as loudness and the localization of sounds in space deserve a weightier consideration; and these, he thought, lend themselves more readily to explanation on the basis of a frequency theory.

We have seen how embarrassing is the problem of intensity for the resonance theories, and how Forbes and Gregg gave a solution in terms of nerve impulse frequency. The frequency theories on their part were able to handle the problem more simply. They correlated intensity with the spread of the stimulus in the cochlea and consequently with the number of active nerve fibers.

As regards the problem of sound localization the frequency theories are in a favorable position. One cue to our perception of the direction of a sound is the difference in the time of arrival at right and left ears. Another is the phase relation of the binaural stimuli. The differences in time or phase required for this localization are extraordinarily small: under appropriate conditions of the order of a few millionths of a second. It seems obvious that the temporal patterns of the stimuli must be transmitted with great accuracy to permit the definiteness and regularity with which we appreciate these cues. The problem gives no difficulty to the frequency theories, for they assume the whole temporal pattern to be transmitted by the nerve fibers. On the other hand, the resonance theories can provide no ready solution; and they have usually resorted weakly to a denial of the facts of time and phase localization themselves.

Both place and frequency theories deal with other phenomena like beats, combination tones, and aberrations of hearing through special hypotheses with about equal success.

A recapitulation of the basic assumptions of the simple frequency and place theories in their most modern forms will show up these theories as essentially alternative in character. In the place theories, pitch depends upon the vibration of particular portions of the basilar membrane, and hence the excitation of particular nerve fibers, whereas loudness depends upon the amplitude of the basilar membrane movement and the frequency of impulses conducted by the nerve fibers. In the frequency theories, on the other hand, pitch is not referred to any specific locus on the basilar membrane but depends upon the frequency of impulses transmitted by the nerve fibers; and loudness depends upon the areal spread of the action along the basilar membrane and hence the number of nerve fibers set in operation.

As Boring pointed out in his discussion, the contrasting character of the two theories in their assumptions as to how the nerve represents intensity and pitch sets the stage for a crucial experimental test. A definite choice between these two directions that auditory theorizing has taken ought to come, he said prophetically, from experiments in a suitable animal on the nature of the auditory nerve impulses during stimulation with sound. It was a consideration of this situation in which auditory theory found itself that led to the modern series of investigations of auditory nerve action.

CHAPTER 6

AUDITORY NERVE RESPONSES

The use of the electrical responses of the auditory nerve in the search for evidence on the questions of theory just outlined rests upon two closely related developments of nerve physiology. One of these is the growth of understanding of the principles of nerve action, with an appreciation of the significance of the electrical manifestations of nerves. The other is the achievement of suitable technical procedures for handling nerves and recording their potentials.

THE ELECTROPHYSIOLOGY OF NERVES

A nerve fiber, like other living cells, is the seat of electrochemical processes, one notable result of which is the establishment of a state of polarization between the outer membrane of the fiber and its plasmic core. To demonstrate this polarization a nerve trunk, made up of many fibers, is cut across at one place, and two electrodes are placed, one on the cut ends of the fibers and the other on the intact surface a little distance away. When the electrodes are connected to a sensitive galvanometer a deflection is observed. The current in the galvanometer not only proves the presence of polarization, but also reveals its character: the exterior surface of a fiber is electrically positive with respect to the interior.

If both electrodes are located a little distance apart on the outer surface of the nerve the galvanometer shows no deflection, for the positive charge is the same at the two places. If now the nerve is stimulated in some manner the galvanometer needle gives a brief flick in one direction, returns to zero, then gives a flick in the other direction, and once more returns to zero. This experiment is especially revealing when a motor nerve is used and its muscle is left attached to serve as an indicator of the conduction of a functional impulse. Then, if careful time records are made of the instant of stimulation, of the appearance of the two galvanometer deflections, and of the twitch of the muscle, it will be found that the deflections occur precisely at the moments when the conducted impulse passes under first the one and then the other electrode. At the time that the im-

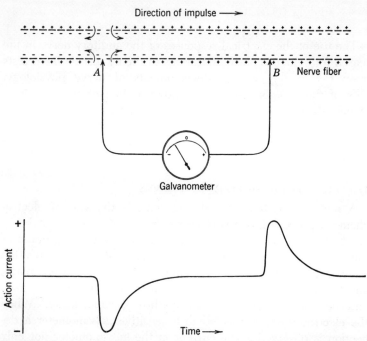

FIG. 22. Action currents of nerves. Above, a polarized nerve fiber, contacted by two electrodes, *A, B*, which lead to a galvanometer. An impulse is now at *A*, represented by ionic movements suggested by the arrows. A point on the graph immediately below *A* shows the action current measured at this moment. Later as the impulse proceeds along the fiber the measured potentials change, and at *B* the current through the galvanometer is reversed. This is a diphasic form of action current.

pulse reaches a given electrode, that point on the nerve becomes negative with respect to the inactive portion of the nerve at the other electrode.

Many variations of the above experiment have been carried out, with all sorts of nerves, and the results consistently demonstrate that the electrical change is everywhere coincident with the functional impulse—with the impulse that is represented by the capacity of the fiber to set in action another fiber or a muscle with which it makes connection.

The electrical change is referred to variously as an 'action current' or 'spike potential,' or in view of its polarity as a 'negative variation' or a 'wave of negativity.' Considered strictly, according to the best interpretation, what we have here is not an increase of negative charge, as the latter expressions might imply, but a decrease in positivity, a breakdown of the normal condition of positive potential of the fiber membrane.* A clear picture of the action is afforded by the membrane hypothesis, which represents the nerve fiber as a semi-permeable membrane enclosing a solution of electrolytes. The ions formed by the dissociation of the electrolytes encounter in the membrane a barrier of a special sort. It is a selective barrier: the membrane has the power of determining what ions shall pass through it. It allows certain ions with positive charges to pass freely, but is largely impervious to the negative ions. Hence the exterior surface of the membrane acquires a positive charge and the interior a negative charge. The polarization potential that is established in this way depends for its magnitude upon the electrolytes that are present and the selective capacities of the membrane. From a study of the electrolytes found inside and immediately outside nerve fibers, it is calculated that the maximum possible polarization is in the region of 118 millivolts. This figure is based on the assumption of perfect selectivity on the part of the membrane, and we should hardly expect this maximum to obtain in fact, but it is significant that in nerves studied under particularly favorable conditions it has been possible to record potentials as high as 30 millivolts (Erlanger and Gasser).

It has already been mentioned that after a nerve fiber has once been caused to respond there is an interval of time during which it cannot again be excited however strong a stimulus be applied; this is the *absolute refractory period*. During this period there are processes of restoration through which a new polarization is formed to replace that which has been broken down. The absolute refractory period bears a close relation to the course of the negative variation; specifically it extends from the mo-

---

* We now know that the nerve impulse is not merely a breakdown of the existing polarity but includes also a momentary reversal of polarity.

ment of appearance of the spike potential and its abrupt rise to a maximum negative value through its somewhat less rapid fall to a level close to the base line, where it merges with other, secondary potentials.

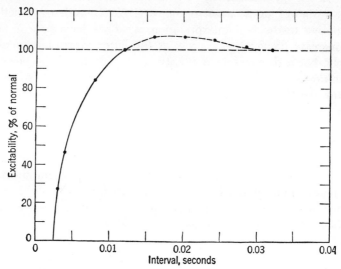

Fig. 23. The recovery process in nerves. A frog's nerve was stimulated once, and then a second time after varying intervals as indicated on the abscissa. The excitability was actually measured as the reciprocal of the current required to excite the nerve this second time, but here is referred to as the percentage of normal excitability. The time up to the first appearance of excitability (0.0025 sec) is the absolute refractory period, and the added time required to reach normal excitability (0.0095 sec) is the relative refractory period. The further course of the curve, above the 100 per cent line, represents the supernormal phase, which is sometimes absent. Data from Adrian and Lucas [*Journal of Physiology*].

Then follows the *relative refractory period* during which the fiber is excitable but only by a stimulus of more than the normal threshold strength. At the beginning of this period the restoration processes have proceeded only far enough to make an impulse possible; the polarization is low and the spike potential correspondingly small. As time goes on and the restoration processes continue, the excitability increases and so does the magnitude of the spike potential. Finally, as the period ends, both excitability and spike magnitude have returned to their resting values.

From all these intimate relations between action potentials and functional changes in the nerve fiber it is clear that the electrical variations form an essential part of the fiber's activity and can safely be regarded as indicative of the propagation of a functional impulse.

The Recording of Nerve Potentials. The natural indicator of nerve action is the muscle, which by its visible contraction signalizes the passage of an impulse. This indicator, obviously, limits the observation to motor nerves and to the end result only of the process. By use of the electrical signs the study is extended to the sensory nerves and in more detail to the entire course of the action.

The study of action potentials in nerves is complicated because these potentials not only are small, but also they exhibit extraordinarily rapid changes in magnitude. A recording instrument must be both sensitive and capable of following these changes with reasonable faithfulness. Either of these physical characteristics is easy to achieve by itself, but because they are in some sense contradictory it is difficult to obtain them both at the same time.

In view of the rather large polarization potentials of many millivolts that theoretically are established in nerve fibers, and that sometimes are measurable, it is necessary to explain why under the usual conditions a high sensitivity is required in the recording instruments. There are two reasons. The electrodes are not often in the most favorable locations, but are some distance away from the place of production of the potentials. The resistance of the intervening tissues then causes a serious falling off in the potentials that are actually picked up. At the same time there is a large shunting effect of other fibers, fluids, and tissues in the vicinity. These limiting conditions are particularly severe when the nerve is left in its normal position in the body, for the nerve then is more difficult to approach with electrodes and is closely surrounded by other tissues. For these reasons the size of nerve potentials as measured at the electrodes is often only a few microvolts.

The spike potential rises and falls in so short a time—in rapid-acting fibers in less than half a millisecond—that no ordinary electrical measuring instrument can keep pace with it. To be altogether suitable a recording instrument must have a natural frequency that is high with respect to the changes to be observed. A practical rule is that the natural frequency should be at least 5 and preferably 10 times the frequency of the phenomena. For a half-millisecond spike this means a natural frequency of 10,000 to 20,000 vibrations per second, which is difficult to achieve in an instrument without unduly impairing its sensitivity.

Throughout the history of the electrophysiology of nerves the pace of progress has been set by the development of instruments that would satisfy these technical requirements. The early investigators had available only the moving-coil galvanometer, an instrument of great sensitivity but distressingly sluggish action. It fails to record the true height of the spike and irons out all minor variations, so that it serves for little more than a qualitative indication of nerve action.

Then came the development of two new instruments, the capillary electrometer and the string galvanometer. These represented a compromise of qualities: they were reasonably sensitive and moderately rapid in action, but not wholly satisfactory in either respect.

Finally, within recent years, the development of the vacuum tube and of circuits for its use brought a revolution in this technical field. Vacuum tube amplification, by which minute potentials may be raised to almost any level of magnitude, freed the electrophysiologist from primary concern with the sensitivity of his recording apparatus. Instruments that are rapid acting but inherently insensitive now became usable. Also important was the development of the cathode-ray oscillograph, the heart of which is a special type of vacuum tube in which a beam of electrons is played upon a fluorescent screen so as to form a visible trace. The action here is as free of inertia as the electron itself, and action potentials are portrayed with complete fidelity.

Along with the development of apparatus has come the equally necessary elaboration of knowledge and skill in the handling of nerve tissues. The result has been a remarkable enlargement of our understanding of nerve action in general, and particularly of the sensory nerve processes.

The Study of Sensory Nerves. With the refinement of technical methods, active attention returned to the old problem raised by Johannes Müller's doctrine of the specific energies of nerves, and new efforts were made to bring to light the nature of the messages sent along the sensory channels. Here our particular problem, the representation of auditory stimuli, lagged far behind because the interest at first was in sensory nerve action in general rather than in points of special theory, and there was an undercurrent of belief (amply justified in general) that all sensory messages would turn out to be alike. A choice of nerve for study therefore was pretty much a matter of convenience, and the auditory nerve, of all the most inaccessible and difficult to deal with, was passed over in favor of others more fortunately placed. The earliest studies of sensory nerves were carried out on the cutaneous and kinesthetic nerves easily approachable in the peripheral regions of the body.

The study of these various sensory nerves established certain general principles. The two most important, the all-or-nothing principle and the intensity-frequency principle, have already been referred to in Chapter 5. Evidence for their validity has been found in every sensory nerve in which a specific inquiry has been made.

As already brought out, the all-or-nothing character of the nerve impulses becomes understandable on the basis of the membrane hypothesis. The propagated disturbance consists in the progressive breakdown of a state of polarization, and hence the magnitude of the effect produced at the far termination of a fiber depends simply upon the condition existing there, and not on the magnitude of the stimulus that initiated the action, or even upon the size of the impulse that has passed along the fiber to that place. The stimulus must of course be above threshold strength to cause a propagated impulse; but any strength above that level makes no difference so far as this particular impulse is concerned.

Because a misapprehension is common here, it is necessary to add and emphasize that 'all or nothing' does not signify a constancy in the magnitude of nerve potentials; the potentials vary widely according to the condition of the fiber at the moment it is called upon to act. Especially in the relative refractory period the condition of a fiber changes greatly, and consequently the size of the spike varies all the way from its normal maximum to practically zero.

As mentioned earlier, the intensity-frequency principle grows out of the special nature of the excitability of a fiber during the relative refractory period. If a stimulus is steadily maintained at barely the threshold strength, one excitation of the fiber can follow another only after the full refractory period is past; but if the stimulus is above the threshold it can excite the fiber within the relative refractory period, and the stronger the stimulus the earlier in this period will it be effective. Hence the intensity of a continuing stimulus becomes translated into frequency of impulses in the nerve message.

The nerve impulse seems to be everywhere the same, regardless of the type of nerve in which it appears. The modes of variation of nerve transmission therefore are strictly limited. The following dimensions are generally regarded as exhausting the possibilities of representation by nerves of the physical characteristics of the stimulus: (a) the particular fiber or fibers set in operation, (b) the number of fibers excited at any one time, (c) the frequency of impulses in each fiber, (d) the duration of the train of impulses, and (e) the time relations of the separate impulses passing through different fibers. The problem of auditory theory is to show how these variables represent the properties of the stimulus and determine the nuances of auditory experience.

DISCOVERY OF THE AUDITORY IMPULSES

The earliest observations of electrical potentials as a result of stimulation by sounds were made with electrodes placed on the surface of the brain and led to a sensitive galvanometer. After Caton in 1875 had obtained potentials in an animal as a result of stimulating its eye with light, first Beck and then Danilewsky in 1890 and 1891 obtained similar results on stimulating with loud sounds.

The first study of the electrical responses of the auditory nerve itself was made by Beauregard and Dupuy in 1896. They conceived the plan of utilizing the action currents of this nerve as a measure of the range of sound reception. In experiments on frogs and guinea pigs they exposed the eighth nerve, cut it across, and placed an electrode on the cut surface. They connected another electrode to the drum membrane and led the two electrodes to a galvanometer. On stimulating with sounds they obtained small deflections, which seemingly were true action currents because they disappeared on disturbance of the electrodes and death of the animal. The original purpose of the experiment of ascertaining the auditory range evidently was defeated by the small size of the deflections.

Piper in 1906 began a series of experiments to study the operation of the acoustic mechanism in the fish. The observations were concerned with the sensory apparatus rather than the nerve. He placed electrodes on the exposed otolith of the saccule and obtained galvanometer deflections on stimulation with sounds. Notes from pipes of low frequency produced in the water in which the preparation was submerged and sounds from beating on the sides of the tank gave positive results, which were interpreted to mean that in the fish, or at least in the species investigated, the saccule is an auditory receptor.

Buytendijk in 1910 obtained results from the auditory nerve similar to those reported previously by Beauregard and Dupuy. Electrodes on the auditory nerve of rabbits and guinea pigs showed galvanometer deflections when the ear was exposed to intense sounds of various kinds, like the shot of a pistol and the note of a flute.

In 1927 Forbes, Miller, and O'Connor reported an experiment that was stimulated by Boring's suggestions on auditory theory. Their problem was to ascertain the maximum frequency of operation of the auditory nerve in response to an acoustic stimulus. They used a string galvanometer, sometimes with a single stage of vacuum tube amplification, and recorded photographically the potentials from the medulla oblongata or the brain stem of cats during stimulation with sounds. Results were obtained readily with brief clicking sounds, like those of two metal objects struck together or the snapping of a 'watchman's rattle.' Such sounds produced a sharp spike, evidently representing the nearly simultaneous operation of a good many auditory fibers.

Continuous sounds were less satisfactory. The 'watchman's rattle' rotated rapidly, or a spinning cog wheel against whose teeth a card was held, gave a series of spikes whose frequency followed that of the clicks continuously at the low rates and for brief intervals as high as about 220 per second. Tones from a tuning fork gave deflections so small as to be uncertain, but upon examination of the record with a lens the authors considered the responses to have the frequency of the waves at 104 ~ and possibly at 200 ~, though not continuously or perfectly represented. These authors considered the results to be inconclusive as regards the questions of theory originally raised, and they suspected that the degree of synchronism found between sound waves and nerve responses was a matter of a following of the bursts of sound intensity rather than a frequency representation as such.

In 1930 Foà and Peroni, using a string galvanometer, recorded impulses from the auditory nerve of the giant sea turtle. They obtained discharges of 50 to 60 per second, irrespective of the sounds used in stimulating the ear.

All these early studies suffered from severe limitations of method. As has already been brought out, the moving-coil galvanometer is capable of showing only the slowest changes of potential, and even the string galvanometer, employed in the last two experiments mentioned, is too sluggish to reproduce high frequencies of nerve current. The development of high-gain vacuum tube amplifiers altered this situation. In 1930 Wever and Bray reported experiments on the auditory nerve that made use of these new technical developments.

In these experiments an electrode was placed on the auditory nerve of the cat, with an inactive electrode in other tissues near by, and the nerve currents were led through a vacuum tube amplifier to a telephone receiver where they became audible as sound. The responses reproduced the frequency of the stimuli applied to the animal's ear, over a wide range. A number of tests were carried out to insure that this effect was not an artifact but was a true physiological response.

These experiments were promptly repeated and confirmed by other investigators, and various refinements of technique were worked out. The following account will deal in a general way with the technical methods that have proved of greatest value in these investigations.

TECHNICAL PROCEDURES IN AUDITORY NERVE EXPERIMENTS

Apparatus. The instrumental requirements include sources of sound, amplifiers, and recording equipment. An electrical oscillator operating into a loudspeaker is the most practical sound source, as such an apparatus will deliver relatively pure tones over any desired ranges of frequency and intensity. The oscillator is usually followed by electric filters which remove any harmonics present in the generated currents, and by attenuators which control the voltages applied to the speaker and hence the sound intensity.

The amount of amplification required depends upon the recording apparatus, but generally speaking the available gain should be as large as possible within the limits imposed by technical conditions. There is a practical limit to amplification on account of inherent irregularities in the operation of the vacuum tube itself, and there is no advantage in raising the amplification beyond the point where these irregularities become prominent in the recorded picture. If the response to be observed is smaller than these irregularities it is not made any more discriminable by a continued raising of the level.

Even more important as a limitation in this situation is physiological noise of two sorts. One is noise in a literal sense: the slight but nonetheless significant sounds of respiration, heart beat, and blood flow, and in all but the most deeply anesthetized animal of other motor activity as well—sounds that stimulate the ear and produce unwanted responses. The second sort, usually more disturbing, consists of stray electrical effects from muscles and other tissues in the region of the electrodes. It is not possible to escape these stray potentials altogether, but careful technique can minimize them: we keep the animal quiet by deep anesthesia and curarization, include between the electrodes as little extraneous active tissue as possible, and make as good a contact with the nerve fibers as we can.

If the amplifier operates into a telephone receiver, where the signals become audible as sound, observations are possible with as little as 50 db of amplification, but 75 db is more satisfactory.

With the cathode-ray oscillograph as the recording instrument a gain of 100 db or more is required.

For exploratory work the telephone receiver is a valuable instrument, as the observer, utilizing the analytical capacities of his own ear, can differentiate the response from its background more successfully than is possible by any other means. This method of observation was employed in most of the early work, and it is still useful in inquiring into any new phenomena. For quantitative measurements, however, it is not sufficiently exact,

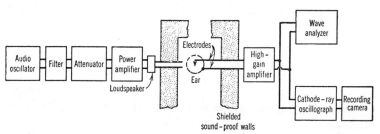

FIG. 24. Apparatus for the investigation of the electrical potentials of the ear.

and a method must be employed that yields a visible trace. Here the cathode-ray oscillograph is the most serviceable instrument. Its deflections may be observed visually or may be photographed to give a permanent record.

Besides these instruments a practical necessity is a room that is both electrically shielded and soundproofed. Within it the animal is isolated from external electrical and acoustical disturbances, including those incidental to the experiment itself. It is desirable to have the sound-generating apparatus outside this specially treated room. The amplifying and recording apparatus likewise are best located outside the room, and at a distance from the stimulating equipment. Figure 24 shows a suitable arrangement.

Procedure. The animal may be prepared by anesthetizing with an injected anesthetic, like one of the barbituric acid derivatives, whose effects last throughout the experiment. An alternative method is to anesthetize the animal with ether and then decerebrate, after which the ether is discontinued; this method is usually preferable when impulses from middle levels of the acoustic nervous system are to be studied, because an anesthetic depresses the action of central neurons.

A skull opening is made posterior to the occipital ridge on one side of the midline, and the exposed portion of the cerebellum is displaced medially, or sometimes removed in part. The eighth nerve is exposed deep in the crevice between the petrous bone and the medulla oblongata. This nerve is a composite of two trunks, cochlear and vestibular. The cochlear division is formed within the cochlear spiral by the gathering in a close bundle of a good many small twigs issuing from the bony spaces of the modiolus. It takes a short course through the petrous bone and is joined by the vestibular division from the endings of the saccule, utricle, and semicircular canals. The nerve emerges into the cranial cavity through the internal auditory meatus and immediately expands conically as it enters the medulla. In most cats the available length of nerve is only 2 or 3 mm. A minute artery and vein accompany the nerve and must not be damaged, as they form the principal, perhaps the sole, vascular supply of the cochlea proper.

One electrode is placed on the nerve and another on some other tissue near by; the location of this second, indifferent electrode matters little so long as the tissue is inactive and affords a good contact. Special pains are necessary to place the active electrode on the cochlear fibers, which in the cat run in the forward and ventral portion of the nerve.

Precautions. In an experiment of this kind, where a high degree of amplification is used, it is necessary to exercise all care to avoid the introduction of artifacts. Artifacts are of two kinds, induction effects and microphonics.

Induction effects appear when a sound source like an oscillator produces an electrical field, either magnetic or capacitative, which extends to the electrode wires and sets up currents in them. These effects sometimes appear in most unexpected ways; in the early experiments, for example, it was found that steel tuning forks when struck and held near the cat's ear often set up induced currents because they are almost invariably magnetized.

Microphonics include any means by which sound waves produce electrical effects independently of the animal's ear, and are of several kinds. Most common is vibration of parts of the amplifier, especially the elements of the vacuum tubes. Microphonics arise also from the electrodes in the tissues, if the wires or the tissues themselves are free to move under the influence of the sound, for such movements produce either a periodic variation of resistance or a varying potential. It is easy to demonstrate such an effect by placing two electrodes in a vessel of water and then exposing the fluid surface to intense sounds.

Induction effects are eliminated by drastic shielding of all electrical apparatus and by maintaining the animal as well in a metal shield with only a small opening for the introduction of sounds. Or, since the experimenter usually must have free access to the animal during the tests, the shield is made to enclose the entire operating room.

The avoidance of microphonics involves the careful handling of the sounds and the use of soundproofing. It is preferable to produce the sounds within a closed chamber and to introduce them into the ear through a tube, rather than to permit them to be scattered about the experimental room. It is further necessary to insulate the amplifier, especially its earlier stages, against the entrance of sound both as aerial waves and as vibrations of the surface on which the apparatus rests; in this treatment we use massive, air-tight cases and suspend the parts within by means of rubber or spring mountings.

Fortunately, these extraneous effects are usually slight, and become noticeable only with the loudest sounds and the highest degrees of amplification. They may be tested for in a number of ways, all of which involve measures that impair nerve action but may be expected to have little if any effect upon electrical and mechanical phenomena. These measures include placing the electrodes on tissues away from the head, restricting the blood supply to the ear, destroying the cochlea, or killing the animal. All these measures eliminate the nerve response; hence if a signal remains after they are carried out an artifact is indicated.

Forms of Audioelectric Response

Electrical potentials in response to sounds are not restricted to the auditory nerve but arise at every level of the acoustic receptor system from the cochlea itself to the final nervous projections at the cerebral cortex. Of the various forms of audioelectric effect, the cochlear response deserves special consideration, both because it is primary in the action of the stimulus and because it is a sensory as opposed to a nervous activity.

The Cochlear Response. Potentials that have their origin within the sense organ have a magnitude that within limits is a linear function of the stimulus, and for strong sounds they reach high levels. They may be picked up from any point in the immediate vicinity of the cochlea, but more readily the closer the approach to the interior. A convenient and at the same time a particularly favorable location for the electrode is the membrane of the round window, for this membrane bounds the fluid of the inner ear and itself presents a moist surface of low resistance.

The response from the cochlea is a true sensory effect and is independent of the presence of nervous elements within the organ. The evidence that this is so is both direct and indirect. A direct approach to the problem is made possible by the fact, first reported by Wittmaack (3), that after the eighth nerve is cut near its connection with the medulla the whole nerve degenerates, and all nervous elements within the cochlea disappear. Guttman and Barrera cut the nerve in cats, and after time had been allowed for the nerve degeneration to become complete they found that the cochlear response remained unimpaired. Three other experiments of this kind have been reported by Hallpike and Rawdon-Smith and their collaborators, but with somewhat inconsistent results. The first experiment of the series (Hallpike and Rawdon-Smith, 3) contradicted the results just stated. The second (Ashcroft, Hallpike, and Rawdon-Smith), which included several animals, showed various degrees of change of histological elements and cochlear responses, and no consistent dependence of the one upon the other. The third (Rawdon-Smith and Hawkins), on one animal, agreed with Guttman and Barrera's findings. Responsibility for these uncertainties may perhaps be charged to technical inadequacies; there is little doubt that Guttman and Barrera's original observations are the proper ones. They have recently been confirmed by Neff and me, in experiments in which the condition of the sensory and nervous elements was mapped out by Guild's graphic reconstruction method (Neff; Wever and Neff). In certain ears in which conditioning tests showed complete deafness, a histological examination revealed only a trace of nerve fibers and ganglion cells, whereas the hair cells and other sensory structures were completely normal. So also were the cochlear potentials, as Fig. 57 will show.

A complementary line of evidence comes from observations on animals in which the nerve is intact but the sensory cells are absent. Opportune for the purpose here is the occurrence in certain animals of a form of congenital sensory defect in which the organ of Corti along with other cochlear structures suffers from maldevelopment or atrophy. The albino cat is the most notable case of this kind, known since Alexander's description in 1900 of a female and her three kittens. Howe and Guild first observed that in this animal the cochlear response fails to appear, and a histological examination showed that there was a sensory defect of the type that Alexander had described: nearly complete absence of the organ of Corti with its hair cells, collapse of the cochlear duct, and shrinkage of the stria vascularis. Similar observations have since been made on waltzing guinea pigs, dancing mice, and a strain of Dalmatian dogs, all of which, like the albino cats, appear to be completely deaf (see Hughson, Thompson, and Witting; Grüneberg, Hallpike, and Ledoux; and Lurie). Invariably in the animals in which the cochlear response is lacking the organ of Corti is absent or only partially differentiated; and in some of these animals, though not in all, the auditory nerve is normal or approximately so.

Further evidence like that from the albinotic animals comes from experiments on stimulation deafness (Lurie, Davis, and Hawkins; K. R. Smith, 2). A sound of great intensity impressed upon an animal's ear for a minute or so will produce an impairment of the cochlear response, and in the cases in which the loss amounts to 30 db or more a subsequent histological examination reveals an injury to the sensory structures. In the milder grades of histological damage, the changes are limited to the hair cells, and in the more severe grades it includes the whole organ of Corti, whose cells are loosened from their anchorages on the basilar membrane and sometimes thrown off altogether. In acute experiments there is no apparent damage to the nervous elements except for the ends of the dendritic processes that run out into the organ of Corti and which necessarily are torn away in the disruption of that structure.

The above evidence supports the view that the cochlear response is a result of the primary action of sound upon the ear and is independent of the nerve excitation that follows. A study of the two forms of electrical activity reveals further distinctive characteristics.

DISTINCTIVE FEATURES OF COCHLEAR AND NERVE RESPONSES

Wave Form. The cochlear response (under usual conditions) reproduces faithfully the form of the sound wave, or, more

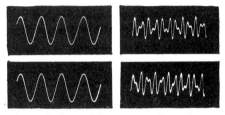

Fig. 25. Wave form of the cochlear potentials. The wave at the upper left represents a stimulus tone of 1000 ∼ as recorded with a condenser microphone, and the wave immediately below represents the cochlear potentials recorded in a guinea pig. The wave on the upper right represents a stimulus made up of two tones, 1000 and 1500 ∼ (which form a musical fifth), and the curve below represents the resulting cochlear potentials. (The variations of wave form in both these curves are due to a slight drifting of frequency in one of the oscillators.)

strictly, the form of the wave as represented at the inner ear. When the stimulus wave becomes complex the response does so likewise. Figure 25 gives some examples.

The nerve response, on the other hand, has its own distinctive form, which may sometimes approach the form of the stimulus but does not always do so. See Fig. 26.

Magnitude. The cochlear response varies in size according to the strength of the stimulus, over a range from the weakest signal that it is possible to observe with present instruments to a maximum that varies characteristically with the ear studied.

The lowest level of reliable measurements so far attained is 1 or 2 ten-millionths of a volt, but there is every reason to believe that an improvement in recording equipment would extend this range farther toward zero. Thus no threshold appears for this response. The maximum level may reach 1 millivolt in the cat and guinea pig, for very loud sounds.

The nerve response has a threshold: stimuli below a particular level are without effect. As later will be described in more detail, the magnitude varies according to the number of fibers in action and their physiological states, and hence this response only imperfectly reflects the intensity of the stimulus.

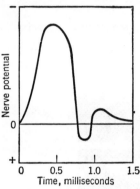

FIG. 26. Wave form of the nerve potentials. The nerve spike shown was obtained by recording both cochlear and nerve potentials with an electrode on the round window membrane of a guinea pig and by then subtracting the cochlear potential wave. The stimulus was 300 ∼, and a spike of this kind appeared once in every cycle.

Frequency Limits. The cochlear response reproduces the frequency of sounds over a wide range, which varies with the species of animal concerned. Nerve responses follow the stimulus frequency faithfully at slow rates, but cease to do so at the highest rates where the cochlear potentials are still present.

Animal Species. The cochlear potentials have been observed in numerous species among the higher vertebrates: in a few reptiles, in birds (the pigeon), and in all the mammals so far tried, including opossums, mice, rats, rabbits, guinea pigs, cats, dogs, monkeys, and man. The human observations are only fragmentary, because they are carried out in the face of special difficulties: they have to be made on pathological ears in the course of a surgical operation, or on other defective ears that have suffered a perforation of the drum membrane large enough to permit the insertion of an electrode (Lempert, Wever, and Lawrence). These observations are of interest, however, in showing that everywhere, in man as in the lower animals, the electrical activity of the cochlea is of the same general character.

The nerve potentials have been studied less extensively, but as far as the evidence goes they too seem to be similar in form in the different animals. Yet for both these types of electrical response there are characteristic differences among species in the range of effective frequencies. Generally speaking, this range is extended on the high-frequency end as we go upward in the evolutionary scale.

Physiological Conditions. Both cochlear and nerve responses reflect the physiological state of the animal, and more particularly the conditions existing at the ear itself. In general, the cochlear response is the more resistant to adverse conditions.

Restriction or failure of the blood supply to the head affects both types of response, but the nerve response fails the sooner. If the stoppage of the blood supply is carried out judiciously, for a few moments only, these responses can be reduced and then returned to normal when the circulation is re-established.

A restriction of the respiration has no noticeable effect until it becomes extreme, and then it reduces both types of response just as a circulatory impairment does. A restriction of oxygen intake that is severe but still is not carried so far as to be fatal to the animal will cause a slow, progressive deterioration of the cochlear potentials over a period of a few hours, ending sometimes in their complete disappearance (Wever and Lawrence, 3).

On the death of the animal the nerve response ceases at once, while the cochlear response, though suffering a marked decrease in magnitude, lingers on for a matter of hours. Considerable attention has been given to the course of these changes in the cochlear potentials (Wever, Bray, and Lawrence, 6). The abrupt loss that follows immediately after cardiac failure (which is taken as indicative of the moment of death) varies in amount depending upon the cause of death; a violent form of death, such as that produced by a stoppage of circulation, gives an initial loss of the order of 15 to 20 db, whereas a milder form of death, as that produced by curare poisoning, gives an initial loss of about 10 db. The reason for this difference is uncertain, but it may be the pressure changes in the cochlea produced by strong muscular contractions. After the initial stage, the further decline is gradual, and feeble potentials can still be observed after as much as five hours have passed.

The course of decline of the potentials after death is affected little if at all by stimulation of the ear by sounds (provided that the sounds are within normal limits of intensity). This observation was made in a cat in which both round windows were exposed and an electrode placed on the membrane of each. One ear was stimulated continuously with a rather strong tone of 1000 ~ and the other with the same tone at an intensity 20 db lower. Measurements of the cochlear potentials were made over a period of two and a half hours after death, and gave practically parallel curves of change in the two ears. This observation evidently signifies that in the stimulation there is no exhaustion of a sensitizing substance or other reserve of material on which the potentials depend.

A study of the effects of temperature upon the electrical responses is difficult to make in the living animal because of its ability of temperature regulation. Bray and I placed a decerebrate cat in an ice pack, but observed no change in the responses up to the point where the cat died. Adrian (6) likewise found no change in potentials from the cat on packing ice about the auditory bulla, but in a continuation of this experiment (by Adrian, Bronk, and Phillips) by use of the guinea pig, in which the bone about the cochlea is thinner, the ice was found to cause a definite weakening of the responses. When the ice was removed the responses returned to normal, provided that the circulation was intact. If the circulation had ceased, the cooling depressed the responses irreversibly: a restoration of normal temperature failed to restore them to their former level. These experiments included both cochlear and nervous potentials, without any clear distinction.

The effects of temperature on the cochlear potentials were considered further by Wever, Bray, and Lawrence (6) in the course of their study of the death function. The slow subsidence of the responses after death was strikingly interrupted on the application of gentle heat to the auditory bulla, and then the curve resumed its former course when the heat was removed. Larger amounts of heat caused a marked rise and then a serious fall in the level of response, a fall from which there was only a partial recovery after the heating was stopped.

General anesthesia does not directly affect the cochlear response, and apparently it has little effect either upon the nerve response.

Localization. As indicated in the earlier discussion, the cochlear response has its focus of intensity at the cochlea itself, whereas the nerve response is most readily picked up from the nerve trunk. In the process of recording, however, these two effects usually are incompletely separated. Nerve potentials arise from all portions of the cochlear neurons, including the ganglion cells and the dendritic processes. An electrode in the vicinity of the cochlea picks up these potentials along with those from the sensory cells. Fortunately this contamination of the cochlear potentials is not usually serious, as the nervous component is relatively small under most conditions. Only for tones in the medium low range of frequencies, and at faint levels of intensity, do the nerve effects loom large with respect to the cochlear effects.

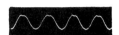

FIG. 27. Cochlear and nerve potentials, as recorded at the round window membrane (guinea pig). A nerve spike appears at the peak of each wave. The stimulus was 150 ~.

Correspondingly, both effects are recorded from an electrode on the nerve trunk. Here the overlapping is more of a nuisance; though the nerve response does not change much with intensity, the cochlear response reaches high magnitudes when the stimulus intensity is great. At low stimulus levels the nerve response can be obtained in reasonably free form. For the stronger stimuli it is more practical to record from neurons of secondary and higher levels beyond the auditory nerve proper, for at these levels the electrode is far enough away from the cochlea to make negligible the spread of its sensory effects.

THE SOURCE OF COCHLEAR POTENTIALS

The albinotic and other deaf animals already referred to, in which the cochlear potentials are lacking, exhibit two invariable histological features: the organ of Corti is malformed to a degree that is always serious and sometimes complete, and the stria vascularis is shrunken and partially atrophied. The animals made deaf by overstimulation show on their part a grave loss of cochlear potentials and a disruption of the organ of Corti, including the tympanic lamella (the layer of cells covering the lower surface of the basilar membrane), but the stria vascularis is unaffected. In the milder cases of stimulation deafness only the hair cells and the tympanic lamella are involved, as indicated in Fig. 28. These results therefore point to the organ of Corti, and more particularly to the hair cells, as the source of cochlear potentials. What we observe is no doubt a summation of effects produced in all the hair cells exposed to the stimulus action. There remain to be considered the specific operations through which these potentials are generated.

The Mechanics of Hair-Cell Stimulation. As described earlier and illustrated in Figs. 5 and 6, the hair cells are supported in a kind of trusswork, formed by cuticular struts joining the basilar membrane to the reticular plate above. The most prominent of these supporting members are the pillars or rods of Corti, rising from the basilar membrane and running obliquely to a common junction at the inner edge of the reticular membrane. Also rising from the basilar membrane are numerous smaller pillars which are the processes of the Deiters cells. They are found in several rows, three or more corresponding to the rows of outer hair cells. They run upward and then send off a branch; the main part expands to form a little cup that supports the lower end of a hair cell, and the branch (called a phalangeal process) runs on to the reticular membrane.

The course of the phalangeal processes is oblique: they do not join the reticular plate immediately overhead but first run a little way in an apical direction. They swing outward around the hair cells and usually pass by two of these cells and form the reticular collar for the third. The effect is to provide a certain amount of cross bracing to the structure. Additional bracing of this kind is afforded by Corti's arches, which are not isolated arches but are all firmly united at their headpieces. The inner and outer pillars are not even present in equal numbers, and they

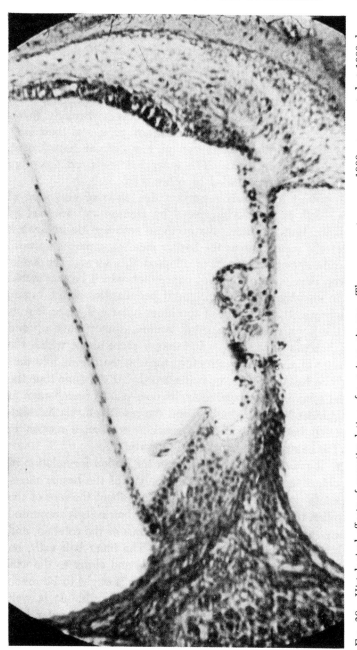

FIG. 28. Histological effects of overstimulation of a guinea pig ear. The exposure tone was 1000 ~, presented at 1000 dynes per sq cm for 4 min. From K. R. Smith (2) [*Journal of Experimental Psychology*].

are slightly oblique. Consequently the structure is given rigidity in both transverse and longitudinal directions.

As Fig. 5 shows, the hair cells are suspended in this structure with their upper ends at openings in the reticular plate and their hair tufts protruding through. It is believed that normally these tufts are in intimate contact with the tectorial membrane. For the outer hair cells the arrangement seems particularly favorable; their ends rest firmly in the Deiters cups, and their long, slender body portions stand free of any cellular impediment, surrounded only by fluid. The inner hair cells, on the other hand, are closely surrounded by other cells.

The earliest hypothesis regarding the mode of excitation of the hair cells is the one suggested by Hensen and adopted by Helmholtz, that the hair tufts of these cells are thrust against the tectorial membrane as the basilar membrane moves upward. Most subsequent writers have adopted this view. Ter Kuile, however, developed a different conception which he considered more in keeping with the structural peculiarities of the organ. His view was that the foot of the inner pillar cell, since it rests upon the fibrous lip of the spiral lamina, cannot move up and down, but can only rotate. It forms a pivot about which the remainder of the sensory structure turns when the middle portion of the basilar membrane is displaced. At the same time the tectorial membrane swings about its own point of anchorage at the vestibular lip of the limbus, and the result is a relative, sliding motion between it and the reticular surface, a motion in which the hair cells are bent back and forth.

There is much that is reasonable in ter Kuile's formulation of the cochlear mechanics. If the movements of the basilar membrane cause the sensory structure to rotate about the foot of the inner pillar, the peculiar angle of the outer hair cells is accounted for: they stand at right angles to the radius of the rotation, and so in line with the arc of movement. The inner hair cells, on the other hand, stand at a contrary angle and closer to the axis of rotation. Accordingly, the outer hair cells ought to be much more readily stimulated than the inner hair cells. It is well known that on exposure to very intense sounds the outer hair cells are the first to be impaired (Yoshii, Hoessli).

We need not follow ter Kuile in his emphasis upon the sliding movement between tectorial and reticular surfaces. Such movement may indeed occur, but at the same time there will be an up-and-down component, and Hensen's original suggestion of a vertical pressure on the hair tufts as the effective stimulus can be retained.

At this point, however, we leave the Hensen-Helmholtz view —or at least the common interpretation of their very brief statements—which conceives of a single, momentary excitation of the hair cells in the course of a cycle of basilar membrane movement. In this view the tectorial membrane is pictured as normally lying a little distance above the hairs of the hair cells, so that only at the end of an upward excursion is a contact made. For a train of simple oscillations, corresponding to a sinusoidal stimulus, the result would be a series of momentary pulses. Some, as we have seen, have elaborated even further this notion of critical points in the hair-cell excitation: thus Wrightson postulated four excitations per cycle. No such degradation of the vibratory motion into discrete impulses is to be accepted at this stage. Rather, we must conceive that the fluid pressures, which themselves faithfully represent the sound waves, are communicated continuously to the hair cell. We must so conceive the matter on the evidence that the cochlear potentials, which we have traced to the hair cells, are representative of the form of the stimulus. Hence we must picture the tectorial membrane as always maintaining contact with the hair tufts; and the opinion now frequently held that the hairs actually penetrate the lower surface of the tectorial membrane and are firmly embedded therein is consistent with this view. (Almost conclusive evidence of this connection of the hair cells with the tectorial membrane can be found in serial sections of both human and guinea pig ears. With the ordinary histological treatments the tectorial membrane is commonly curled back over the edge of the limbus owing to its shrinkage during fixation, and frequently a hair cell is seen adherent to its tip, obviously having been pulled out of its normal position.)

It has already been mentioned that the cochlear potentials are observed over a wide range of magnitudes, from the smallest that experimental conditions permit—about a tenth of a microvolt—to as much as a millivolt, which is a range of 10,000-fold. Over most of this range the relation to the stimulus is the simplest possible: the potential is directly proportional to the sound pressure. Figure 29 exhibits this relationship. For all sounds within moderate limits of intensity the cochlear response curve is linear: increasing the stimulus by some factor raises the response by the same factor. Ultimately, as high intensities are reached, the curve departs from this linear form. It bends, at first slowly and then more rapidly, and finally attains a maximum from which there is a notable decline.

As non-linearity of the intensity function begins the potential wave itself ceases to be a true copy of the sound wave. It shows a distortion of wave shape, first of mild and then of serious degree as the intensity rises. (For an illustration of this effect, see Fig. 102, page 330.) There is reason to believe that this first stage of distortion, up to the point of the maximum, arises early in the series of actions in the inner ear. It is a reasonable assumption that it is a simple mechanical process.

Since at these high levels the cochlear potential ceases to rise in proportion to the stimulus, we need to look for some process in which a loss of motion appears. Two possibilities easily present themselves. One is that the basilar membrane when displaced too far offers increasing resistance to the pressure. Another is that the cuticular structure that supports the hair cells, though essentially rigid for small displacements, ceases to be so for large ones. More specifically, the Deiters processes probably undergo a small amount of bending when displaced too far, and therefore they do not raise the hair cells as far as they should.

A closer scrutiny of these two possibilities leads us to prefer the second. The first would give a symmetrical kind of distortion, since the resistance would be presented about equally for upward and downward displacement. The second, however, would give asymmetrical distortion, for the yielding of the Deiters processes would occur most noticeably for an upward displacement, whereas in a downward displacement they ought to be pulled along with the basilar membrane more accurately. Now, a symmetrical kind of distortion gives only odd harmonics, whereas an asymmetrical distortion gives both odd and even harmonics. The cochlear potentials for strong stimuli contain odd and even harmonics; the distortion is asymmetrical.

We now have a picture of the hair cell as exposed to varying pressures exerted upon it endwise in close correspondence with the waves of the external stimulus. Next in order is the process

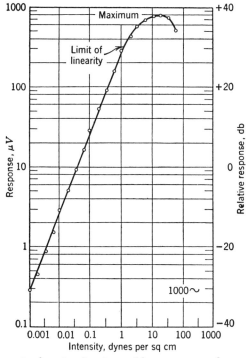

FIG. 29. Intensity function for the cochlear response, observed in the cat.

by which this cell when so acted upon generates the cochlear potentials.

The Electrodynamic Actions of the Hair Cells. The physiological process by which the hair cell generates electrical potentials when subjected to mechanical deformation is not a matter of observation and can only be inferred. There comes at once to mind the action of the piezoelectric crystal, used commonly, as in a familiar type of microphone, to convert sound waves into electric currents; but this on examination seems a poor analogy.

The energy transformation in a crystal depends upon a peculiar structure, which consists of molecules in a rigidly systematic orientation. In the nerve cell no corresponding structure is known.

A better analogy is the giant plant cell, of late the object of extensive study (Osterhout and Hill, Osterhout). Such a cell, as for example one from the common water plant *Nitella*, when bent or pinched produces a large electrical response. This cell is normally polarized, just as a nerve fiber is, because the interior contains positive and negative ions that have different degrees of mobility with respect to the outside membranous wall. Usually (depending upon the fluid environment) the surface is positively polarized, but when a local area is compressed it loses a portion of its charge. This 'negative variation' is relatively enormous and may attain a value of 30 millivolts or more.

How closely the hair cell resembles these plant cells is impossible to say, but it seems safe to assume that its actions similarly depend upon the presence of ions that polarize the surface membrane. Other assumptions regarding the physiological details are less secure; yet it is possible to go farther and on the basis of the phenomena observed in the cochlear activity to indicate many of the characteristics of the process. To aid the understanding, the treatment to follow suggests a specific mode of operation, but the real interest here lies in the more formal characteristics of the behavior, and other specific actions may turn out to be the true ones. (Consider, as other possibilities, Wegel's conception of the action as a strain on the ciliated surface of the cell, and Guild's suggestion that it is a simple bending of the body of the cell; Wegel, 2; Guild, 6.)

Let us picture the hair cell as indicated in Fig. 30, at *A* in the resting condition, and at *B* and *C* when compressed or expanded. It is assumed that positive pressure on the hair tuft pushes the top of the cell inward, compressing the cytoplasm and bulging the cell walls. The reverse pressure raises the top and sucks the walls inward. The changes in the wall alter the surface charge: let us say that they reduce the positivity for expansion and increase it for contraction. The result, for an alternating pressure of not too great amplitude, is a form of electrical response as graphed in Fig. 31a. Note that this is a pulsating direct potential, equivalent to a constant potential E_0 plus an alternating potential E_1. E_0 here is (essentially) the resting potential, that which obtains when no stimulus is present.

The changes in the surface charge might be explained as the result of actual ionic movements through the membrane as the expansions or compressions alter its permeability. This kind of

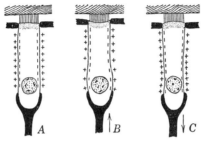

FIG. 30. Theory of the electrodynamic actions of the hair cells. The hair cells are pictured, resting on their Deiters cups below and clasped by the reticular membrane at their upper ends. Their hair tufts are embedded in the tectorial membrane above. A shows the inactive condition, B and C the effects of an upward or downward thrust of the Deiters process as impelled by movements of the basilar membrane below (not shown, but suggested by the arrows). The cell changes in form, and the polarization of its exterior surface alters as indicated.

change would correspond to what we suppose to happen in a nerve fiber in the propagation of an impulse. However, such ionic migrations would have to take place at very high velocities to account for the cochlear potentials recorded for strong high-frequency sounds, and also the cell would have to possess a large reserve of ions to restore those lost in the action. It is more likely that the ions themselves do not move appreciably but are essentially bound to the membrane itself. As the membrane changes it causes variations in the electrical field established outside the cell, by varying the surface concentration of positive ions and perhaps at the same time the degree of isolation of the negative ions in the interior. When the wall is expanded the surface concentration is reduced and its isolating properties are diminished; then the negative ions increase their exterior effects and further reduce the positive field. When the wall is contracted and thickened these isolating properties are increased, and the negative ions have a smaller effect on the outside field.

It is assumed that with moderate stimuli the value of the electrical variation E_1 will increase in amplitude in proportion

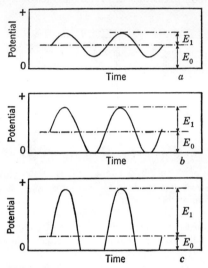

Fig. 31. Further theory of the hair-cell potentials. The three graphs represent potentials generated at three different levels of intensity: a, weak to moderate; b, intense; and c, excessive. E_1 is the alternating component produced by the vibratory movements. E_0 is a positive base potential, normally stable but reduced by overstimulation.

to the stimulus intensity. The base potential E_0 will not be expected to change appreciably. At some level, however, these simple relations cease to hold. A powerful stimulus ought to produce an effect like that represented in Fig. 31b, where E_1 exceeds E_0 in amplitude and the lower peaks of the alternating component of the wave are clipped off. This picture assumes two things: (1) that a stimulus however strong can never do more in its compressional phase than to open the membrane fully and cause a neutralization of the external field—it can never cause the field to grow negative; and (2) that such violent stimulation will reduce the base potential E_0 temporarily either by changing the membrane in some general way or by dispersing the ions, or both. A further stage of overstimulation therefore will be that indicated in Fig. 31c.

Here we conceive what amounts to a rectifier action in the electrodynamic process. The result will be a further stage of distortion, beyond the mechanical distortion already postulated, and this distortion involves not only the enhancement of odd and even harmonics but also an actual reduction in the electrical output.

That there are indeed two stages of distortion in the inner ear has already been inferred from studies of the cochlear potentials. In an investigation of the interaction of two tones simultaneously presented to the ear, Wever, Bray, and Lawrence (4) distinguished two processes that appear in order and show distinctive characteristics. The earlier process accounts for two closely related phenomena, called transformation and interference. Transformation consists in the diversion of a portion of the energy contained in a sinusoidal stimulus into overtones, and when two such stimuli are present into combination tones as well. Interference refers to the fact that the response obtained to a given tone is reduced when a second tone is simultaneously applied. These two are probably different aspects of a common process; at least, when the stimuli are of moderate intensity, the reduction in the response observed to either of them can be accounted for as a diversion of energy to new components, overtones and combination tones, rather than a net loss.

A later process must be called upon to account for the further phenomenon of overloading, which represents an actual loss of response. As we have seen, when the stimulus intensity reaches very high levels the cochlear potential passes through a maximum and then falls rapidly. At this stage the decline of the response cannot be regarded as simply a diversion of energy to overtones and combination tones; the total potential, summated over all these components, is greatly reduced.

It is further observed that stimuli beyond this maximum point are dangerous to the ear; they produce a general impairment of response that is only slowly recovered from, and when a little stronger they are permanently injurious. By an experimental analysis of the relations of the phenomena of transformation and interference to the injury resulting from overstimulation, Wever and Lawrence obtained evidence that the inner ear is the seat of these processes, and that transformation and interference are dependent upon an early, and overloading upon a late, sensory process.

The evidence shows that the first process, identified here as the final phase of the mechanical action through which the hair cells are deformed, follows closely the sensitivity curve of the cochlea (as shown in the cochlear potentials). The second process, on the other hand, adds its own sensitivity effects and somewhat modifies the response curve. Its effect is to discriminate against the very high and the very low tones.

In summary, we see that the two types of distortion contemplated here can account for the form of the cochlear response function in the region of the high intensities. As already noted, the cochlear function is linear at low and moderate intensities, but at high intensities it first bends slowly and then more rapidly until it passes through a maximum and falls. During the early course of distortion, when the departure from linearity is only slight, the overtone functions rise regularly (following various orders of power functions as the transformation theory requires), and when they are added to the fundamental the combined curve is linear, or practically so, indicating a relatively simple process such as the mechanical distortion suggested above. Later, as the maximum of the response function is approached, and beyond, the overtone functions themselves pass through maxima, and the total curve exhibits an energy loss. Here enters the second, electrodynamic form of distortion. The intensity curve for the cochlear responses thus appears to be complex, combining two functions in which the two stages of distortion play their parts, as Fig. 32 suggests.

The two distortion processes described are of the asymmetric type and yield both odd and even harmonics. Moreover, as the theory is developed, the asymmetry is in the same sense in each process, in that the curtailment of wave amplitude in both appears as the basilar membrane is moving upward. A contrary relation would tend to restore symmetry as the second process enters and would then enhance the odd harmonics at the ex-

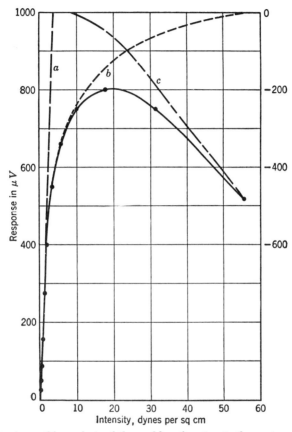

FIG. 32. A possible analysis of the cochlear function in the region of distortion. The solid curve is the observed function, plotted on linear scales; *a* represents the path it would take if linearity were preserved at high levels; *b* suggests a process that is approaching a maximum; and *c* a second process in which the responses are diminished with intensity. For curve *c* use the right-hand ordinate. The sum of *b* and *c* equals the observed function.

pense of the even ones, a circumstance which the observations fail to show. The results do show sometimes (see Wever, Bray, and Lawrence, 1) an instability of the functions for both odd and even harmonics, which perhaps may be traced to slight, varying phase relations between the products of these two distortion processes.

EXCITATION OF THE AUDITORY NERVE TERMINATIONS

Three hypotheses have been advanced to explain the excitation of the auditory nerve fibers. These regard the process respectively as mechanical, chemical, or electrical. According to the mechanical hypothesis the pressures communicated to the cochlea are brought to bear upon the nerve terminations and excite them directly. According to the chemical hypothesis, the hair cell on deformation liberates a chemical substance, and this in turn acts upon the nerve fiber. According to the electrical hypothesis it is the cochlear potential itself that excites the nerve fiber.

This last hypothesis is the one adopted here, for it has certain obvious advantages. We know that the cochlear potential is present and have reason to believe, from its magnitude at a distance where it is picked up by electrodes, that at its site of origin in the hair cells it is of very considerable size. We know further that nerve fibers are easily excitable by electric currents. It seems inevitable that the nerve terminations, entwined about the lower end of the hair cell where the electric field is near its maximum, must be stimulated by these changes. We may even grant the presence of the mechanical and chemical changes as assumed in the other hypotheses. The electrical changes, because they spread with great rapidity, will be effective farther along the dendritic endings than these others in all instances where the excitation is above the threshold. Hence these other changes if they are present will encounter nerve tissue that is already in process of responding, and at best they can have only a facilitative effect.

HIGHER LEVELS OF NERVE POTENTIALS

The fibers of the auditory nerve enter the medulla and promptly end in the cochlear nucleus. Here lie the ganglion cells from which new (secondary) fibers arise that go for the most part to other nuclei of the brain stem, notably the trapezoid nuclei and the superior olivary nuclei. Some fibers run directly upward through the brain stem in tracts known as the lateral lemnisci. These tracts consist mainly, however, of tertiary and perhaps even fourth-order fibers that arise in the trapezoid and the superior olivary nuclei.

The lateral lemniscus runs upward through the brain stem to the midbrain region. A few of its fibers are interrupted in midcourse in the nucleus of the lateral lemniscus; but most proceed to their endings either in the inferior colliculus or the lateral geniculate body. From these two nuclei arise the final fibers that are projected on the temporal cortex of the cerebrum.

Electrical responses may be observed in any of these nuclei and in the tracts that connect them. An electrode in one of the nuclei gives particularly large deflections, because there the electrode can be brought into close relation to the large cell bodies and can more nearly represent the full discharge potential.

In the various tracts the effects are highly localized: the electrode must be placed with great care, and often only a slight displacement away from the proper location causes a marked reduction of amplitude or a complete loss of the responses. At the lower brain-stem levels the contralateral effects are stronger than the ipselateral, on account of the high degree of decussation; but at the lateral lemniscus and beyond the responses appear equal on the two sides.

The central effects are highly susceptible to adverse physiological conditions such as fatigue, anesthesia, circulatory failure, and death. They follow their stimuli with relatively long latencies; and these latencies increase progressively at the higher levels of the nervous system both because the paths of conduction are longer and because synaptic junctions are interposed. Kemp, Coppée, and Robinson determined the synaptic delay as about 0.8 milliseconds.

The limits of frequencies observable in the central tracts vary with the neural level. In general, these limits are well below those obtained at the auditory nerve trunk, and they fall off rapidly the farther we go up the acoustic system. Kemp, Coppée, and Robinson observed synchronous responses up to 2500 ~ at the trapezoid body, but only up to 1000 or 1500 ~ at the inferior colliculus. For frequencies higher than these the impulses were partially synchronous for a time, then wholly asynchronous, and finally vanished altogether.

At the trapezoid body the upper limit for which asynchronous responses were observed was 4000 ~, and at the inferior colliculus this limit was 1500 ~; the higher tones gave no effect as they were introduced and maintained, and they were discerned only as a transient discharge when they were turned off. These results were obtained in the cat. In the opossum, McCrady, Wever, and Bray obtained responses from the trapezoid body up to 9000 ~; the difference is partly due to the greater high-tone sensitivity of this animal and partly to improved recording apparatus.

Gerard, Marshall, and Saul reported synchronous responses in the region of the cortical radiations to a tone of 660 ~. At the cortex itself, Davis found no synchronism to tones, but a series of clicks was reproduced up to 100 per second. Brief tones of various frequencies produce transient cortical effects of a wholly unsynchronized character.

Let us consider the question why the upper limits of synchronism grow less at the higher levels of the nervous system. We might suppose these limits simply to represent properties of the different parts of the nervous system, and in particular the sluggish nature of the synapses, and such conditions cannot be ruled out of account. However, there are two other conditions of a technical nature that we must weigh in this connection. The experiments were carried out on anesthetized animals, and it is the nature of an anesthetic to depress the excitability and conductivity of higher portions of the nervous system. The depressive effect is greater the higher the neural level; and there can be no doubt that the observed restriction of frequency range is in part due to this condition. Then, in the second place, as we progress farther up the nervous system it becomes increasingly difficult to put an electrode in a position that is favorable for recording. The chances are that fibers operating as a group in the transmission of certain impulses become more and more dispersed and intermingled with other fibers, so that an electrode at any given place is unable to record from them suitably. The seriousness of this condition will become increasingly evident as we study the process through which nerve fibers in cooperative action are able to represent the high frequencies.

CHAPTER 7

FREQUENCY REPRESENTATION IN THE AUDITORY NERVE

The study of auditory nerve responses reveals, over the major portion of the auditory range, a faithful representation of stimulus frequency in the nerve discharge. Of particular importance for the theory of hearing is the upper limit of this relationship. This limit has been studied extensively only in the cat. Wever and Bray in their earlier experiments in 1930 obtained synchronous responses up to 4100 ~ and later with improved recording apparatus up to 5200 ~ (2, 4). In repeating these experiments Saul and Davis in 1932 obtained synchronous responses up to 4000 ~ but were of the opinion that the responses were contaminated with cochlear potentials; they attributed to the nerve itself a synchronism to only about 1000 ~. In subsequent reports by Davis and his collaborators (Davis, Derbyshire, Lurie, and Saul; Davis, 1) higher frequencies were ascribed to the nerve, and in 1935 Derbyshire and Davis indicated the limit of synchronism as lying between 3000 and 4000 ~.

The last-mentioned results and those of Wever and Bray seem in good agreement when we consider that synchronism does not fail at any definite point but gives way only gradually to asynchronism. There is a wide area of transition, and observers may differ in what they regard as a reasonable representation of the stimulus frequency. In my opinion, here is an occasion when it is proper to assume a generous attitude and to accept as the limit of synchronism the highest point where the observer, either by eye or by ear, can make out a definite frequency. If the observer can perceive a frequency pattern, then it is likely that the animal on which the observation is made, through his nervous analyzers, can make equally good use of the information.

Asynchronous impulses continue to still higher levels. Unquestionably they extend to the upper limit of hearing in the animal, but here direct evidence is lacking. A difficulty is that as the stimulus frequency is raised the responses fall off rapidly in strength and finally become submerged in the irregular discharge that constitutes the physiological background. In the opossum, which is a particularly favorable animal for this observation on account of its great sensitivity to high tones, asynchronous responses have been obtained to tones as high as 15,000 ~ (McCrady, Wever, and Bray, 1).

The synchronous discharges of 4000 or 5000 per second, observed in the nerve responses of the cat, though they fall short by two octaves or more of reaching the upper limit of hearing of the animal, are nonetheless very high rates for nerves to represent, and their observation forces us to consider, in the light of the most recent evidence on nerve action, the question how such rates can be established and maintained.

THE SINGLE-FIBER HYPOTHESIS

The direct and simple explanation of these results is of course the one that has been the traditional assumption of the frequency theories: that the fibers of the auditory nerve possess a special capacity for rapid recovery and that a single one of them can carry impulses at the rates recorded. Again, the traditional point of attack upon this explanation has been that it incurs the restriction of refractory phase. Wever and Bray in 1930, on making their first observations of the frequency relationship, were disposed to reject this explanation and to seek another—subsumed in the volley principle—that would avoid such a restriction.

Now, in the light of further knowledge of sensory nerve action in general, and some particular study of the auditory nerve processes themselves, the single-fiber hypothesis appears even less probable than before. Many more nerves have been investigated, yet without any appreciable extension downward of the range of refractory periods. The measurements show usually, for the fastest type of mammalian fibers, a range of absolute refractory periods of 0.6 to 0.9 milliseconds, and the shortest periods so far found, measured by Gasser and Grundfest for 'type A' fibers in spinal and peripheral nerves in the cat, are 0.41 to 0.44 milliseconds. If we calculate a maximum frequency on the basis of the smallest period cited, 0.41 milliseconds, we obtain a figure of 2439 per second, which is about half the limit observed in the auditory nerve. More serious still, the calculation of a maximum in this way, as the reciprocal of the absolute refractory period, fails to take cognizance of the fact that a nerve fiber is adversely affected by continuing stimulation and does not maintain an optimum performance.

In hearing we have to deal with sounds that go on for long periods of time—for seconds, minutes, and more. The auditory nerve discharges are correspondingly prolonged, and yet throughout their course these discharges continue to give a faithful representation of the stimulus frequency.

Let us look further into this matter of the limitations on nerve action that come from changes in the condition of the fibers due to continuing stimulation. There are two changes that are of significance here. One is a prolongation of the absolute refractory period and the other is an impairment of excitability; and of these two the second is by far the more important.

Formerly it was believed that severe and continuous stimulation of a nerve fiber would produce a marked extension of its absolute refractory period. Field and Brücke in 1926 reported that the excitation of a nerve for 1 or 2 min by 'tetanizing' shocks caused an increase in this period up to 9- or 10-fold. Further investigations have led to a reinterpretation of these results as indicating not so much an alteration of refractory phase as an impairment of excitability.

The confusion here arose from a failure of Field and Brücke in their experimental arrangements to meet the strict definition of the absolute refractory period as the period after excitation during which *no stimulus whatever* will elicit a response. Their determinations of refractory phase were made with two stimuli each only a little above threshold, and for this condition the second must indeed be delayed for a long interval if the nerve has recently been tetanized. But if the second stimulus is raised in intensity it will be effective earlier; and if it is raised to a very high level it will require only a little more than the normal interval. Woronzow, using a second stimulus of 'supramaximal' intensity, obtained only a 1½- to 3-fold extension of the absolute refractory period after 4 hr of continuous tetanization. Under his conditions of testing, a more moderate stimulation, such as that employed by Field and Brücke, caused no detectable change.

These results show that after a period of tetanization the first of a pair of stimuli has a profound effect upon the excitability of a nerve fiber. It has been found further that such an effect is present also, though in mild degree, when the nerve is unfatigued. Therefore it has become customary to measure the absolute refractory period by applying the first stimulus at an intensity barely above threshold, thereby minimizing its depressive effects, and then to overcome as far as possible the depression that does appear by presenting the second stimulus at a high level—at least 5 times the threshold intensity. This is the procedure used by Gasser and Grundfest in obtaining the brief periods cited above.

Though the results of Field and Brücke cannot be accepted for the behavior of the absolute refractory period in the strict sense, they do indicate validly the limitations of nerve action in the face of sustained stimulation at a constant level. The excitability of a fiber falls off markedly and restricts its capacity of continuous response at high rates.

It is apparent that under practical conditions of hearing, when the stimulus usually is continued for an appreciable time at one intensity, the frequency of nerve response will depend upon the course of recovery of excitability in the relative refractory period.

A further consideration is the magnitude of the impulses aroused in the early portion of the relative refractory period. When the excitability has barely returned to the point where the stimulus can be effective the spike that is produced is of small magnitude, and it proceeds along the fiber only a short distance and then disappears. For the effective propagation of impulses a minimum of excitability is not enough: the recovery must proceed well into the relative refractory phase. This condition, together with the persisting effects of earlier impulses, makes it hazardous on the basis of the refractory phase data to attempt to predict the maximum frequency of a nerve fiber except in the most general terms. For precise indications we must turn instead to the direct observation of serial impulses.

It would seem a simple matter to apply continuous or rapidly recurrent stimuli to a nerve and to ascertain the frequency of the impulses excited. Yet an observation of this nature is a difficult task, far more complicated technically than the determination of refractory phase. The refractory phase experiments are carried out in whole nerves containing many fibers of various kinds, yet the measurements concern only one fiber or at most a small group of fibers with the shortest refractory properties and the highest recovery powers. The limitation of the intensity of the first stimulus and the reduction of the time interval before presentation of the second result, fortunately, in the exclusion of the remaining elements. In the direct observation of frequencies in nerves no such easy simplification is possible, and a stimulation of the entire nerve sets many of its fibers in operation, resulting in a complex discharge in which no determinate frequency can be found. The most that can be done with a whole nerve is to count impulses over a brief period and ascertain a crude composite frequency. The precise study of serial discharge frequencies depends upon the isolation of single fibers.

The isolation of single nerve fibers was first achieved by Pratt in 1925 by the use of an electrode so small that when it was inserted into a nerve it made contact with only a few fibers, or at times when the placement was especially fortunate with only one. When the nerve was stimulated many of its fibers were set in action, but the recording—in the more successful trials—included only the impulses of a single one of them.

In the year following Pratt's experiment a like result was obtained by Adrian and Zotterman (1) by different means, by limiting the number of fibers excited to activity. They worked with the sterno-cutaneous muscle of the frog, which contains but three or four end organs stimulable by stretching the muscle, and then they reduced this number of organs to one by trimming away strips of the muscle. A load applied to the muscle thereupon produced impulses in only the one nerve fiber attached to the ending that remained.

These experiments represent the two general approaches that may be made to the problem of obtaining single nerve fiber preparations—one by a restriction of the fibers set in action and the other by a limitation of those tapped for recording. Additional techniques have been developed under these two general headings and are employed in different situations according to the anatomical conditions. For senses like the eye and the skin senses where the endings are areally distributed and readily accessible the sensory limitation can be achieved at least in part by a careful focusing of the stimulus. Another method makes use of a fortunate anatomical situation. Matthews (1) after a deliberate search discovered a small muscle in the frog's toe that contains only a single stretch receptor. Stimulating the muscle gives a simple train of impulses in its nerve with no need of special dissection.

Another situation that Adrian (4, see also Adrian, Cattell, and Hoagland) discovered by chance provides the neural kind of limitation. He found that once in a while a sensory fiber in its upward course sends off a branch that runs down a motor nerve and thereby becomes anatomically separated from its fellows. This is called an antidromic fiber. Sensory stimulation then produces a direct effect in the motor nerve, which can be observed uncomplicated by reflex reactions after severing the motor root. The response obtained is usually a single-fiber response simply because this kind of branching is rare.

When all else is unavailing there is the direct form of limitation, first carried out by Adrian and Bronk, which consists of meticulously cutting down the nerve until there remains only a minute strand containing a single active fiber.

Several kinds of sensory nerves have been investigated by one or another of these methods; the results are given in Table I. This table shows in the first three columns the investigators, the types of nerves studied, and the stimuli employed, in the fourth column the frequencies obtained when many fibers were operating, and in the last two columns the frequencies obtained when only a single fiber was operating.

TABLE I

Investigators	Nerve	Stimulus	Many Fibers	Single, Momentary	Single, Adapted
Adrian and Zotterman 1926 (1)	brachial (frog)	stretching muscle	400	190	120
Adrian and Zotterman 1926 (2)	internal plantar (cat)	pressure on skin		150	
Adrian and Bronk 1928 (1)	phrenic (rabbit)	breathing	90	80	
Adrian and Bronk 1929 (2)	peroneal (cat) tibialis (cat)	pressure pressure		25 44	
Adrian 1930 (5)	various	nerve injury	800	150	
Matthews 1931 (1)	peroneal (frog)	stretching muscle		260	
Adrian, Cattell and Hoagland 1931	dorsal cutaneous (frog)	air blast on skin		300	150
Cattell and Hoagland 1931	cutaneous (frog)	air blast on skin		400	
Hartline and Graham 1932	optic (limulus)	light		130	
Hoagland 1933	lateral line (trout)	spontaneous	600	120	
Matthews 1933	motor (cat)	stretching muscle		500	
Pumphrey and Rawdon-Smith 1936 (1, 2)	cercal (cockroach, cricket)	sounds	800		
Echlin and Fessard 1938 (2)	sciatic (frog) (cat)	stretching muscle (vibratory)	440 530	330 240	
Brown 1939	saphenous (cat)	vibration on skin	450		
Pfaffmann 1939	trigeminal (cat)	vibration on tooth	1500	1000	
Galambos and Davis 1943 (1)	auditory (cat)	sounds		450	200

As the table shows, Adrian and Zotterman were the first to report on the frequency of discharge of single fibers. From a fiber of the brachial nerve supplying an isolated stretch receptor of the sterno-cutaneous muscle of the frog a maximum discharge of 190 impulses per second was obtained. This rate was not steadily maintained, however, but fell away almost at once, and after 10 sec it had been reduced to about 120 per second.

This decline in response frequency during activity is typical of single-fiber preparations, and therefore it is necessary to distinguish clearly between a maximum discharge rate, which is momentary only, and a rate that can be maintained over a period of time. In the table one column gives the maximum, instantaneous frequency, and another a sustained or 'adaptation frequency'—one to which the fiber settles down after a few seconds of activity. The designation of an adaptation frequency is sometimes rather uncertain, because in many of the experiments the action of the fiber under continued stimulation was not given particular attention. The figures show in a general way the operation of the fiber after it has reached a steady state.

An examination of the results reveals that most of the fibers so far studied have maximum rates that are below 300 per second. On continued stimulation we may expect a decline to about half this rate. Among the more rapid rates are those obtained by Adrian, Cattell, and Hoagland and by Cattell and Hoagland for cutaneous fibers, and by Matthews for fibers supplying stretch receptors; for these the initial frequency is 300 per second or over. The highest frequency of all is that observed by Pfaffmann in a fiber of the trigeminal nerve, excited by applying a vibratory stimulus to a tooth, which at times gave a momentary discharge as rapid as 900 to 1000 per second.

The last entry of the table comes from an experiment by Galambos and Davis on the auditory nerve. They approached this nerve intracranially where it passes out of the internal auditory meatus to the medulla oblongata and inserted a microelectrode in the attempt to record from single fibers. On stimulating the ear with sound they obtained simple series of spikes that at first they took to represent single-fiber activity. A number of persons, however, have questioned whether their electrodes were in contact with nerve fibers or were displaced so far medially as to be in the cochlear nucleus and to be recording from the second-order nerve cells there. Galambos and Davis (3) now accept this latter explanation. Still, the results may be taken as establishing a minimum performance for the cochlear fibers: these fibers must do at least as well as the second-order elements that they are themselves exciting.

The auditory elements studied by Galambos and Davis developed a maximum instantaneous frequency of 400 to 450 per second. They then quickly adapted to a sustained frequency around 150 to 200 per second. If we take these results as characteristic of the cochlear fibers themselves, then they fall among those for the more rapid-acting of the various sensory fibers studied, but bear no special distinction in this respect.

All this evidence is in agreement in indicating that the single-fiber hypothesis cannot be accepted in the explanation of the high rates of discharge observed in the auditory nerve as a whole. A single fiber is limited to a few hundred impulses a second and cannot by itself attain rates in the thousands as observed. We are forced to the conclusion that the high rates are a result of a combined action of many fibers working in concert. This conception of auditory nerve action constitutes what has been called the volley principle. This is a principle of action that was predicated for the auditory nerve by Fletcher, and independently by Troland, in the interests of a theory of phase localization, and then developed by Wever and Bray to explain their observations of auditory nerve impulses.

CHAPTER 8

THE VOLLEY PRINCIPLE

Consider a group of auditory nerve fibers that are exposed to rapidly recurring excitations of a constant magnitude such as we may assume to be afforded by a pure tone acting on the ear. A particular fiber after being stimulated responds and then goes into refractory phase. For a time represented by the absolute refractory period, and in addition part of the relative refractory period, the fiber cannot again be set in action. Excitations occurring during this interval are ignored. After the time is past, and the depression left by the first excitation is sufficiently recovered from, another of the serial excitatory pulses will be effective, and the fiber will fire again. Another resting period will ensue, and another impulse, and so on as long as the stimulus is brought to bear. The result will be a series of impulses in the fiber, not at the rate of the excitations but at some slower rate.

A second nerve fiber, meanwhile, if it is exposed to the same series of excitations, will be doing much the same thing. Let us suppose, without concern just now with how it is brought about, that the second fiber comes into action a moment later than the first fiber and responds to an excitation that occurs during the time when the first fiber is inoperative. The silent intervals in the discharge of the first fiber will then be filled in, at least in part, by firings of the second. Additional fibers may fill in this interval completely, if they enter the action at the proper times. So a group of fibers, if they work in rotation, can respond to every single excitation of a rapid series, without an excessive requirement being placed upon any one of them. This production of a rapid rate by the combination of slower rates has a simple analogy in the beating of a drum. A roll is produced with two drumsticks by rattling them in alternate rhythm, so that the resulting frequency is double that of either stick alone. If the drummer had more hands and the muscular coordination to go with them he could attain rates as rapid as he pleased.

The action is illustrated in Fig. 33. The curve at the top represents a sound whose waves appear at a rate too rapid for a single fiber to follow—let us say five times the maximum rate.

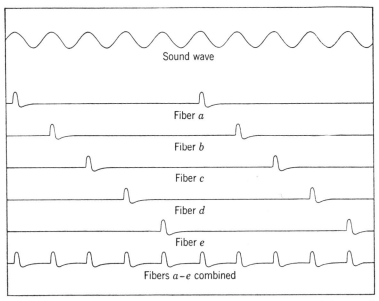

FIG. 33. The volley principle. Each fiber responds to certain of the sound waves, and their total responses represent the full frequency of the wave.

Below is represented in turn the action of five different fibers, with 'spikes' appearing at every fifth wave. Fiber *a* is shown as responding to the first, then the sixth, then the eleventh wave, and so on; while fiber *b* responds to the second, seventh, twelfth, etc., and similarly for the others. Finally, at the bottom of the figure is pictured the effect of combining the discharges of all five fibers: the total response reproduces precisely the frequency of the stimulating sound. A still larger number of fibers, several hundreds, say, would give a similar picture, except that the magnitude of the discharge wave would be increased.

THE BASIC CONDITIONS

This conception of auditory nerve action rests upon three fairly simple conditions, already implied in the foregoing statements.

Phasic Character of Excitation. The first condition is that the excitatory process is phasic: that a sound wave produces a series of regularly recurrent pulses of excitation in which the periodic character of the sound wave is preserved. More explicitly, this means that there is one excitation during every cycle, and only one, and that it appears at some reasonably regular phase position in the cycle. In the process of transformation of the pressure changes of the conducted sound into an excitatory process there can be no long latencies and no accumulation or storing of energy over times that are appreciable with respect to the periods of the stimulus: the energy must be consumed or dissipated practically as fast as it is received. This condition obviously depends upon the process of excitation already considered in the treatment of the functions of the hair cell.

Multiplicity of Nerve Fibers. The second condition is that many nerve fibers are exposed to the excitatory influences of even the simplest acoustic stimulus. This condition is assured by the inevitable spread of action of the stimulus within the cochlea, which will expose a multiplicity of receptor cells to its influence, and further by the diffuseness of innervation, in which each segment of the basilar membrane is served by a considerable bundle of nerve fibers.

Differences among the Nerve Fibers. The third condition is that there are differences in the properties of the nerve fibers, and differences in the excitatory influences brought to bear upon them, sufficient to get the fibers out of step with one another. There are several variables in the situation that almost inevitably must operate to produce this result.

1. Refractory Phase. Unquestionably the fundamental variable here is refractory phase. Though the auditory fibers are of fairly uniform size and presumably therefore have refractory properties of the same order of magnitude, they are certain to vary in some degree. A group of fibers exposed to the same excitatory influences may at first respond together, but eventually, if the

excitations recur at a rapid rate, a time will come when even slight variations of excitability will be critical, and at a given excitatory pulse some fibers of the group will be just sufficiently recovered to respond and the others will not. These others will miss that pulse and wait for the next, thereby beginning a new rhythmic group. These two rhythms then will go on together until by the same process still others appear. Eventually there will be some fraction of the fibers responding at every pulse of excitation, and therefore in the aggregate they will represent the frequency of the stimulus as indicated in Fig. 33.

2. Availability. A rotational action will be established more quickly if different fibers in the group under consideration are not at the same level of excitability at the outset. We know that fibers are subject to considerable independent variability in excitability (cf. Blair and Erlanger). If on account of some previous activity, acoustically or otherwise aroused, some of the fibers are refractory when the excitatory series begins, then the remaining, fresh fibers will set out on their rhythm at once, and the previously active fibers will join in a bit later when ready. Under such conditions the chances are that these two groups will be out of step with one another.

Temporary differences in availability such as are in consideration here might be produced by various kinds of activity. As will be brought out later, it is probable that some (but not usually all) of the fibers excited by one tonal stimulus will be excited by other stimuli also, so that when one sound follows quickly upon another only a portion of the normal complement of nerve fibers may be available to the second stimulus at the first instant. Other fibers will straggle in as they recover sufficiently from their preceding activity.

Spontaneous activity of nerve fibers is common and possibly is present in the auditory nerve itself; the cause is unknown, but it may be related to metabolic conditions, circulatory changes, and the like. A fiber that from some such cause is already discharging, or has just ceased to discharge, would be slow to take up a new rhythm and hence would get out of step with fibers not involved in such activity.

3. Level of Excitation. So far in this discussion, excitation has been spoken of as though it were equal for the various fibers

responding to a given tone, but this is hardly a likely state of affairs; indeed, it is more reasonable to suppose excitation to be different for every fiber.

We think of the effects of a stimulus as distributed somewhat within the cochlea, but not distributed in a uniform manner. Most generally, the action of a simple stimulus is pictured as maximal in a given region of the basilar membrane, and grading out continuously on either side.

Besides this general, areal variation, there is likely to be some variation of excitation even within a narrow band of the membrane. The various hair cells are differently situated on the membrane so that some appear more easily affected by a stimulus than others. Many have emphasized the difference between outer and inner hair cells: the outer hair cells lie on the middle and more mobile part of the membrane and are suspended lightly at their two ends, but the inner hair cells are at the edge of the membrane and are closely surrounded by other cells. Therefore the nerve fibers that supply the outer hair cells ought to be more rudely exposed to the effects of a stimulus than fibers running to the inner hair cells of the same level. Certainly we know that the outer hair cells are more susceptible to damage by overstimulation. Small differences may be expected also among the outer hair cells themselves because they occupy different transverse positions on the membrane and therefore are subjected to different amplitudes of displacement.

Further differences that ought to be reflected in variations of excitability are differences in the individual constitution of hair cells, such as differences in size or elasticity.

A group of nerve fibers, even if their refractory properties were identical, would ultimately fall out of step if exposed to different degrees of excitation, because those excited the more strongly could respond earlier in the relative refractory period, and under critical conditions would respond to an excitation to which fibers less advantageously placed must fail.

4. Phase of Excitation. A final source of variation concerns the time or phase of excitation of different nerve fibers. If a given stimulus involves an extended area of the cochlea, then the stimulus wave will reach different sensory elements at different times owing to differences in the lengths of the paths of con-

duction. Differences of this sort may be small but nevertheless under critical conditions will have an effect. Moreover, if there is resonance in the cochlea, even highly damped resonance, there will be differences of phase in elements that are differently tuned; and on the assumption that nerve excitation occurs at some given phase position these differences will be translated into time differences.

All these types of variation—of rates of recovery, of availability, of excitatory intensity, and of time or phase of excitation—will operate concurrently to disperse the operating fibers into separate rhythmic groups.

Regularity of the Rhythm. In the foregoing discussion, and in Fig. 33, each nerve fiber has been represented as responding at a regular rate, which is some simple fraction of the stimulus frequency. Such regularity of discharge in the individual fiber may sometimes be present, yet is not essential. Indeed, some fluctuations of rhythm are to be expected, from variations occurring from time to time in any or all the conditions mentioned above that bring about rotational activity of the fibers; and these fluctuations ought to become marked under certain conditions, as when the fiber is being stimulated at an intensity close to its threshold, or is being driven at a rate approaching its maximum capabilities.

A fiber might respond for a time, say, at every fifth wave, then drop to every sixth, and possibly after a while return to the faster rhythm. Such variations will matter little so long as the synchronous relation to the stimulus is maintained. In the response of a large group of fibers the ups and downs in the rhythms of individual fibers will be averaged out, and the total discharge will be held at a reasonably uniform level.

A more significant alteration in response is expected from the effects of continued stimulation, especially when the stimulus intensity is great. As already brought out, such stimulation of a fiber produces a small extension of refractory period and particularly an impairment of excitability; and these changes are progressive as the stimulation is continued. Therefore, it is to be expected that under conditions of forcing the fiber will respond at a rapid rate when the stimulus is first applied, and then at a lower and lower rate as time goes on. This kind of action will not interfere with the representation of the stimulus rhythm any more than will the minor fluctuations just mentioned, though if it takes place in many of the fibers it will cause a decline in the over-all magnitude of the discharge.

THE EFFECT OF INTENSITY

When stimulation is at threshold intensity a given nerve fiber can be excited only at a slow rate, for each of its responses must be followed by full recovery, which requires the entire period of its absolute and relative refractory phases. Under this condition the fiber can make only a minimum contribution to the total discharge. At a slightly higher intensity, however, the fiber will no longer require complete recovery but can respond sometime during the relative refractory period, and as the intensity is raised further its excitation can come earlier and earlier. Therefore the rate of firing of a fiber will increase with the stimulus intensity, up to a limit imposed by the length of the absolute refractory period. This is the intensity-frequency principle already referred to, and demonstrated for a great variety of sensory nerves (Adrian, 3).

Let us suppose, for example, that at threshold intensity a given fiber responds at every sixth wave of a stimulus. At a higher intensity it may fire at every fifth wave, and at one still higher at every fourth, and so on until the absolute limit is reached. This effect of stimulus intensity on the pattern of response of a group of nerve fibers is illustrated in Fig. 34. The upper part of the figure shows the discharge of a few fibers at a relatively slow rate, as stimulated by a faint tone: each fiber fires at every sixth wave. The lower part shows the pattern of action for a considerably stronger tone: now each fiber fires at every third wave. At the fainter intensity the total discharge of these few fibers gives only one impulse per wave, which is barely sufficient to represent the stimulus frequency. At the greater intensity there are two impulses per wave, yet the composite frequency is unaltered.

In this diagram, for sake of simplicity, the fibers have been pictured as firing at a uniform rate. The principle of intensity representation holds just as well, however, if as suggested above there is variability in the firings of individual fibers. It is only

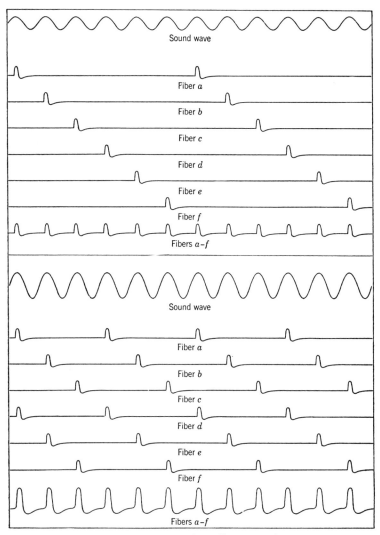

FIG. 34. Intensity representation in the volley principle. Above, the pattern of discharge in a group of nerve fibers at one intensity; and below, this pattern at a higher intensity. The frequency is represented in both patterns, but the discharge is larger in magnitude in the second.

necessary that a good many fibers be included so that their irregularities become ironed out in the total discharge.

A BROADER CONSIDERATION OF THE PRINCIPLE

Although the volley principle was conceived and elaborated in the service of audition, it immediately is evident that it merits a wider application as a principle of nerve action in response to any kind of rapidly recurring stimulation. There are many vibratory receptor organs besides the ear. Indeed, any mechanical receptor accepts that role in the presence of the proper stimulation. The touch spots of the skin, the pressure endings in the subcutaneous tissues, the stretch receptors of muscle and tendon, and certain specialized receptor elements of insects all respond to mechanical vibrations that fall within suitable limits of frequency and intensity. Let us consider the phenomena that appear on stimulation of these organs and the applications of the volley principle in their interpretation.

Vibratory Sensibility. When a vibrating object like the stem of a tuning fork is brought into contact with the skin, a sensation of a peculiar intermittent quality is aroused. There is a dispute of long standing whether this sense of vibration is dependent upon the purely superficial endings of cutaneous touch or upon more deep-lying organs as perhaps the endings of subcutaneous pressure or endings in the muscles and tendons. A decision is made difficult by the fact that stimuli applied to the skin are readily conducted through it to the tissues below and at the same time are radiated in all directions to surrounding areas. The evidence now indicates that both the superficial and deep endings mediate vibratory sensibility, and that whatever the endings the phenomena follow the same general pattern, though they differ somewhat quantitatively. For present purposes there is no great drawback in dealing with what may at times be a composite result of the action of different types of endings stimulated simultaneously.

In the repetitive stimulation of cutaneous areas there are many points of similarity with hearing. Vibratory sensations appear between lower and upper frequency limits and vary in quality as a function of frequency. The upper limit varies for different subjects and for different bodily areas, and particularly, just as in the case of hearing, it is dependent upon the stimulus intensity. On account of the intensity relationship and the technical difficulty in obtaining large amplitudes of vibration at high rates, a determination of the upper frequency limit is not easy. The reports of various investigators show little consistency. Knudsen in 1928, working on the finger tip, observed results for frequencies up to 1600 ~ but was convinced that larger amplitudes would show a higher limit. Gilmer in 1935 obtained a limit of 2600 ~ for his most sensitive subjects, and Setzepfand in the same year mentioned effects up to 3000 ~. Others by the use of a high degree of amplification to obtain powerful stimuli have observed limits even beyond. Gault and his associates found vibrations to be present at 8192 ~ (see Goodfellow's summary); and Geldard and Weitz with further improved equipment observed them up to 12,000 ~.

Because more is known of peripheral nerve activity in the lower animals than in man, it is especially helpful for theoretical purposes to consider the vibratory sensitivity of these animals. Skolnick investigated the upper limits of response in the rat by training the animals to discriminate between two platforms, one of which was vibrating and the other stationary. The rats learned to test the two platforms by reaching out and touching first one and then the other with a forepaw, and they were able to make a choice with nearly perfect accuracy for vibratory frequencies up to 1600 ~. Beyond that frequency the performance deteriorated until it became only a matter of chance around 2400 ~. The threshold, taken as the frequency giving 75 per cent accuracy, was in the region of 1800 to 2000 ~.

These observations, like those on man already mentioned, were limited by the intensities with which the platforms could be set in vibration. At high frequencies a great deal of power is required to move even a light body, and there is little doubt that in Skolnick's experiment greater intensities would have extended the frequency limit. At any rate, the performance of the rats compared favorably with that of human subjects under similar conditions. Persons tested by placing their finger tips on the same platforms used for the rats were able to perceive the vibrations only up to 1600 to 1700 ~. It seems, then, that vibratory sensitivity in the rat is at least as keen as it is in man, and perhaps a little keener.

As already mentioned, the vibratory experience varies in quality according to the vibration rate. At the lower frequencies it is a slow trembling in which the individual pulses can be made out, and then as the frequency rises it becomes a rapid vibration characterized by roughness, until finally it fades out to imperceptibility. An index of the alteration of quality within this range is the change of vibration frequency that is just perceptible. All the work on this problem has been done on man. Knudsen in a short series of tests found that his two subjects in the region of 256 ~ could appreciate a frequency change of 8 to 10 per cent, and an octave higher, around 512 ~, a change of 20 to 35 per cent. Roberts carried on a more intensive investigation of this capacity, though only for frequencies in the region of 400 ~, and obtained considerably finer discrimination. His subjects achieved a discrimination of 2.5 per cent, and that despite a systematic variation of intensity designed to prevent its operating as a cue.

Vibratory sensitivity is dulled by fatigue. An exposure to a vibratory stimulus for a brief period elevates the intensity threshold for several minutes thereafter. Wedell and Cummings observed impairments of sensitivity that amounted to 10 to 15 db immediately after stimulation for 3 min with a vibration of medium intensity, and the effects were still detectable at the end of 9 min. The fatigue effect varies as a function of frequency and intensity: the impairment of sensitivity is greater the higher the frequency and the more intense the fatiguing stimulus.

These phenomena of vibratory sensibility present a problem akin to that in audition, the problem of the mode of representation of the stimulus in the nerve response. We have seen how the auditory problem has been dealt with, in the development of place and frequency theories, with the place theories traditionally in the more favored position. Curiously, for there is much the same occasion for it, there has been far less theorizing regarding the vibratory sense.

There does not seem to be much ground for a place theory of vibratory discrimination. Whatever may be the endings in the skin or adjacent tissues that are responsible for vibratory perception, they doubtless fall short of the degree of elaboration, and possibly even of the numbers, that a place theory would require. A frequency theory, in which the vibratory frequency is assumed to be immediately represented in the nerve discharge, seems both the simplest and the most adequate basis for an explanation of vibratory phenomena.

We can evaluate such a frequency theory of vibratory sensibility by reference to the results on cutaneous and kinesthetic fibers already indicated in Table I. Adrian, Cattell, and Hoagland stimulated an area of skin in the frog with an intermittent air blast and recorded the impulses set up in a single (antidromic) fiber of the cutaneous nerve supplying the area. A synchronized response up to 250 to 300 per second could be obtained for short times, and a response around 150 per second over several seconds. These observations were extended by Cattell and Hoagland, who obtained a maximum regular rate of 354 per second for a train of 10 impulses. They found that as the stimulating frequency was raised above this maximum the response was interrupted by the frequent dropping out of impulses, until ultimately all response disappeared. The same kind of deterioration of the response occurred on the maintenance of a stimulus well below the maximum, evidently as a result of adaptation of the sensory endings.

In an experiment performed by G. L. Brown (as reported by Newman, Doupe, and Wilkins), synchronous potentials up to 450 per second were obtained from a cutaneous branch of the saphenous nerve of the cat on the application of vibratory stimuli to the skin. The experiment is reported only briefly, and there is no indication whether higher frequencies were tried. It is important to note, however, that in this case the recording was from the whole nerve, and hence the synchronism was maintained in a multiplicity of fibers. It would be helpful to know whether a single fiber could maintain an equally high rate under the same conditions, but from the general evidence it seems unlikely.

These experiments are in good agreement in showing that the maximum frequency for cutaneous nerve fibers is of the order of 300 or 400 per second. These rates are so far below the upper limit of vibratory sensibility of some thousands per second as to rule out a simple frequency theory of their representation. If we are to have a frequency theory of vibratory sensibility—and as already brought out there seems no reasonable alternative— it is necessary to invoke the volley principle.

A theory of vibratory sensibility in terms of the volley principle is fully adequate to account for the phenomena. The degree of discrimination of vibratory frequency, and also the phenomena associated with fatigue, are consistent with expectations on the basis of this principle. If the stimulus frequency is represented in the nerve discharge, then its variations in frequency ought to be appreciable. A fatigue effect is to be expected, for, if threshold sensitivity is determined by the transmission of some minimum number of impulses, then previous exposure to strong stimulation ought to impair the excitability of the elements and thereby alter the threshold.

Impulses in the Stretch Receptors. In experiments carried out on frogs, rabbits, and cats, Echlin and Fessard observed that the stem of a tuning fork when held firmly against almost any bony part of the leg produced impulses in the nerve supplying the region at a frequency corresponding to that of the fork. The effects were especially strong when the leg was manipulated in such a way as to stretch the tendons. Removing the skin had no effect upon the phenomena. It appeared, therefore, that the stretch receptors—the endings in muscles or tendons—were responsible for the phenomena.

When in a refinement of these experiments a string was tied to a tendon and a weight attached so as to produce a steady tension, the nerve discharge was complex and irregular, but when a tuning fork was held against the string so as to add an alternating tension the discharge became simple and reproduced the frequency of the fork. In frogs, such synchronous responses were obtained up to 440 per second, and in cats up to 530 per second.

For a study of the behavior of single nerve fibers, mostly carried out in the frog, they employed the toe-muscle preparation discovered by Matthews, a preparation that often contains but a single muscle spindle stimulable by stretching the muscle. When the muscle was first given a steady stretch and then vibratory stimuli were superimposed, synchronous responses were obtained for all frequencies up to 330 per second. Under particular conditions, as the stimulation was continued and adaptation supervened, the discharge did not always continue to represent the stimulus in this exact manner. Often it fell suddenly to a half or a third of the stimulation rate. For example, if a fork of 232 ~ was used, the discharge often had this frequency in the beginning, and then fell to 116 or even to 77⅓ per second. The continuing stimulation reduced the excitability of the fiber so that it required more time after each impulse before it could fire again, and when this change became critical the response fell to a submultiple rate.

Especially illuminating was an experiment that made use of a preparation containing two endings. In one trial, when a fork of 232 ~ was applied, a response of that rate was observed, but its amplitude, because it was double that typical of one fiber, showed that both endings and hence two nerve fibers were adding their responses in precise synchronism. Later, after some adaptation had occurred, a second application of the stimulus gave a response of 116 per second, where again both fibers were acting concertedly but were coming in only at each alternate cycle of the stimulus. Finally, it was found that on some occasions the two fibers produced a frequency of 232 per second, in which each fiber again was responding at every alternate wave, but the two were out of step with one another so that both rates summated to represent the full frequency of the stimulus. Here was a direct demonstration of the volley principle.

Of special interest in this experiment is the observation of a fiber when being driven near its maximum frequency, and just at the point of passing over to a submultiple rate. The first sign of deficiency is a lag in phase of the spikes, and then an occasional dropping out of one. After a spike is dropped the fiber recovers, and the phase lag disappears momentarily. This behavior continues and grows more prominent as the stimulus is maintained, until at last every second impulse is omitted, and the fiber fires in simple alternation.

Figure 35 shows this phenomenon in one of two fibers in a two-unit preparation. Fiber *a* is not yet near its limit of response and fires regularly, but fiber *b* shows the signs of difficulty already described.

Impulses in the Dental Nerves. Further results of similar nature were obtained by Pfaffmann in a study of impulses in a branch of the trigeminal nerve of the cat during stimulation by mechanical vibrations applied to a tooth. When the nerve was intact, very slow vibration frequencies usually gave responses in which two or more deflections could be observed in a single

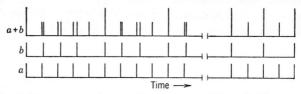

FIG. 35. Volley action in the stretch receptors. The vertical lines represent nerve impulses. Fiber *a* responds regularly to every stimulus wave; but fiber *b* shows signs of difficulty, in the form of phase retardation and skipping of impulses. On the right, the action is shown after a lapse of time, when fiber *b* had stepped down to the half frequency. The upper line of the diagram shows the pattern produced by combining the responses of the two fibers. After Echlin and Fessard [*Journal of Physiology*].

cycle, but high frequencies gave only single deflections. The responses followed the stimulus frequency faithfully up to a maximum of about 1500 per second.

Single-fiber preparations were obtained by cutting down the nerve trunk until only a simple series of impulses was obtained on stimulating some one tooth. These preparations gave synchronous impulses, at least for a time, at all vibration rates until the maximum frequency was approached. This maximum frequency of synchronism varied considerably for different preparations; some gave responses only up to 350 ~, and others went as high as 1000 ~.

The maintenance of synchronism was found to depend upon individual peculiarities of the preparation on the one hand, and on the intensity, frequency, and duration of the stimulus on the other hand. When, with rather strong stimuli, the frequency was progressively raised, the response continued for a time to follow the frequency, but a diminution of the spike height indicated that the impulses were falling in the relative refractory period. With still higher frequencies there was a transition to a frequency of one-half that of the stimulus, a transition marked by several swings back and forth between complete and half-frequency stages. With further increase of frequency, still lower submultiple rates appeared.

A similar behavior was exhibited if a medium-frequency stimulus was first presented at a high intensity and then was gradually weakened. The response at first showed full synchronism, then fell to a 1:2 relation, and later to a 1:3 relation.

If a strong stimulus of a frequency just below the maximum synchronous frequency was applied and maintained, the response for a brief time reproduced the stimulus frequency fully and then as adaptation set in it fell to one of the submultiple rates.

It is to be noted that the frequency observed in the intact nerve was higher than that of which any single fiber was capable. The results thus show that the dental nerve fibers operate according to the volley principle in representing a high-frequency stimulus. It is probable that a tooth provides a particularly favorable condition for the simultaneous stimulation of several receptors, for it vibrates bodily and forms a high gradient of pressure on the endings in its socket.

Impulses in the Cercal Organs. Many insects bear at the end of the abdomen a pair of antenna-like organs called cerci, which have long been considered to have a sensory function. In the cockroach and cricket the cerci are provided with several hundred sensillae, each of which consists of a slender chitinous hair connected at its base with a ganglion cell and nerve fiber. Pumphrey and Rawdon-Smith observed the impulses excited in the cercal nerve on mechanical stimulation. They found the cercal organ to be stimulated by gentle air currents, and also by sounds over a considerable range of frequencies.

Low sound frequencies, up to about 400 ~, usually produced a synchronous discharge in the nerve. Occasionally, for a brief time at the beginning of stimulation, the lower frequencies gave a response of double the frequency of the exciting sound, and then thereafter the discharge reproduced the frequency exactly. Also, if the stimulus frequency was in the region of 400 ~, a reduction in the intensity caused the discharge to drop to one-half the stimulating frequency, and sometimes to a smaller fraction.

Stimuli between 400 and 800 ∽, even when intense, produced discharges at full synchronism only momentarily and then gave a discharge that was increasingly asynchronous, but in which a submultiple rate could be discerned. Beyond 800 ∽ the discharge was altogether asynchronous, though some response continued to at least 4000 ∽.

A drop in the magnitude of the discharge in the region of 200 ∽ suggested that above this frequency the individual nerve fibers were no longer able to represent the stimulus frequency but were forced to go into alternate or slower rhythms. Synchronous discharges above this critical rate therefore are to be interpreted as the result of the combined action of many fibers, acting according to the volley principle.

These results demonstrate the validity of the volley principle in the action of several types of mechanical receptors under rapid repetitive stimulation. In these forms of sensitivity the frequency range is so high, and the discrimination so acute, as to make it more than improbable for the response to be represented by a single fiber, or even by many fibers operating in a random and disorderly fashion. Only the systematic action predicated in the volley principle can achieve the results.

All three of the basic conditions set forth as required for volley action are in evidence. Excitation, even under the simple conditions provided by these receptors, is phasic in character, at least within a particular range of frequencies and intensities. Many elements are brought together in such a way as to be affected as a group by a single stimulus. And finally, variations appear, even in these simple groups, and these variations give some degree of differential action of the several elements. The observations show clearly that over a considerable range of frequencies the receptors and their nerve fibers respond synchronously to the stimulus, and under some of the conditions—when the frequency exceeds that for which a single unit is capable—they respond in this way by the rotational kind of action subsumed in the volley principle.

The behavior of these organs is often imperfect. At times a good many of the elements remain outside the synchronous volleys, or the elements soon reach their frequency limits, or they fail to get out of step sufficiently to give the full frequency. These limitations do not impair the validity of the volley principle, but only emphasize the difference between these more primitive forms of vibratory sensitivity and the refined form mediated by the ear.

THE STUDY OF SINGLE AUDITORY ELEMENTS

Further evidence on the principle comes from the ear itself, in a study of the responses of single neural elements made by Galambos and Davis.

As already reported briefly, these investigators used an electrode of microscopic dimensions inserted into the root of the

FIG. 36. Impulses in single elements of the auditory nervous system. The vertical deflections represent successive firings of an element, on stimulation with a tone of 9800 ∼. The time increases from left to right. From Galambos and Davis (2). [This figure and the two following are from the *Journal of Neurophysiology*, courtesy of Charles C Thomas, publisher.]

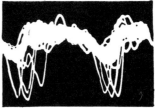

FIG. 37. Synchronization of neural activity. Cochlear and nerve potentials were recorded simultaneously during stimulation with 550 ∼. The cochlear potential is shown by the thick wavy line, and the nerve spikes by the sharper downward deflections. This is a cathode-ray pattern in which many successive wave sections were superimposed; that is why 4 or 5 spikes appear at each cochlear wave. Note the slight variations in synchronism. From Galambos and Davis (1).

auditory nerve of the cat as exposed in the cranial cavity. They intended to make contact with the auditory fibers themselves, but there is now some doubt whether they were actually doing so. Rather, it seems that they were encountering cell bodies of the cochlear nucleus. The large magnitude of the recorded potentials favors this latter explanation. However, this consideration is no impairment of the results and does not prevent our use of them as indicating the behavior of the cochlear fibers proper; it only requires that we take the results as conservative. The cochlear fibers must perform at least as well as these second-order neurons; they may do better in their representations of the stimulus, but they cannot do worse.

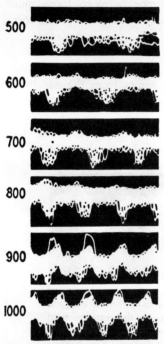

FIG. 38. Synchronization of responses in a single neural element in response to various tones. This element maintained its synchronism for all the tones shown. From Galambos and Davis (1).

The observations made on these single elements correspond in every essential feature with the picture of auditory nerve action that has been presented under the volley principle. A regular series of impulses, as shown in Fig. 36, appears in an auditory element when the ear is stimulated with a pure tone. The rate of these impulses varies as a function of intensity up to about 450 per second.

By recording the cochlear response and the nerve spikes at the same time it was proved that the nerve response is well synchronized with the cochlear potentials and hence with the stimulating waves. Figure 37 shows a record of the responses to a tone of 550 ⁓; here the cochlear potential is represented by the heavy wave and the nerve spikes by the deflections that group themselves mainly about the lower half of each cycle. Similar results on a particular element, stimulated by six different tones, are shown in Fig. 38; in every case the nerve response is in synchronism with the sound. The highest frequency for which the synchronism was demonstrated in this experiment was 1050 ∼, but the authors concluded from indirect indications that a satisfactory degree of synchronism will be maintained up to about 4000 ∼.

From the evidence presented the volley principle may now be accepted as firmly established in the physiological action of the ear. There remains the question of the role it plays in hearing. There is no absolute necessity that it have any role at all, as some have contended; but the thesis of the following pages is that it occupies a position of fundamental importance.

Part III
The Volley Theory

CHAPTER 9

THE VOLLEY THEORY: THE BASIC EVIDENCE

In the historical treatment of the first four chapters the place and frequency theories of hearing were developed as they came into being, as exclusive and vigorously opposed conceptions of the action of the ear. In the chapter following, where these types of theory were examined critically in their more modern forms, it became evident that each conception possesses certain advantages yet at the same time suffers serious faults; and though each has distinctive explanatory powers as regards some of the manifestations of hearing, neither provides a full account. And so the two views have persisted as alternatives, with neither able to demonstrate an overwhelming superiority.

The volley theory represents a new departure in this field, in which the two traditional conceptions are combined and compromised so as to retain the positive features of each and fill out their deficiencies. It is a curious fact, in view of their history of bitter adversity, that these conceptions and the principles that they embrace are not mutually exclusive or contradictory but readily lend themselves to fusion into a single harmonious theory. Rutherford asserted as much as long ago as 1898 in presenting his own theory, pointing out that it was quite compatible with the one that Helmholtz had championed; but he did not develop this amiable suggestion, and evidently no one else in his time became interested in doing so.

This new theory, which on occasion has been called the resonance-volley theory to accent its dual character, accepts the idea of resonance in a particular sense as a means of distribution of response over the basilar membrane according to the stimulus frequency, and at the same time it embodies the volley principle for the representation of the stimulus in the pattern of nerve impulses. Pitch therefore has a twofold representation, in terms of place on the basilar membrane and hence of particularity of nerve fibers, and in terms of composite impulse frequency.

189

Many further aspects of hearing—loudness and tonal interaction among them—likewise are best explained by the concurrent operation of place and frequency principles, while some are based more simply upon the one or the other of these principles. It will be the object of this and the chapters following to develop this theory in its full details, and to attempt within its framework a comprehensive account of the phenomena of hearing. It will not be found a simple theory, and objections may be voiced on that account, but hearing is not a simple matter either, and no theory that is truly simple can be even halfway adequate in dealing with its phenomena. The older theories, elementary though they appear as they confront the problems of pitch, are distractingly complex when they face remaining issues, and even with pitch they are not ever in fact as simple as they seem.

THE FRAMEWORK OF THE THEORY

In the volley theory, the place and frequency principles are accepted, not in their most inclusive forms of operation as conceived in the classical hypotheses where they arose, but subject to certain restrictions. In the first instance, the roles to which they are assigned in pitch perception vary according to the tonal region. Frequency serves for the low tones, place for the high tones, and both perform in the broader ground between. This allocation follows the evidence that volley action is faithfully representative for low and intermediate frequencies but becomes inaccurate and fails for the high frequencies; and on the other hand that place representation is discriminatory in the upper and middle portions of the auditory scale but on account of spread of response is decidedly less so at the lower end. The two variables thus are in part auxiliary and in part complementary in their determination of pitch.

We here distinguish three regions of the auditory scale, the low, middle, and high-tone regions, as the two modes of tonal representation are brought into play singly and in combination. As just suggested, the low-tone region is that in which frequency holds sway, the high-tone region that for place representation, and the middle-tone region one where both frequency and place work side by side. The boundaries of these regions can hardly be precise, for a given mode of representation will not begin or cease abruptly, but will fade in and out gradually. Therefore they can be located only in a rough and tentative fashion. The primary evidence for this location comes from two experimental observations on the auditory nerve already described. The first is that frequency representation is accurately maintained from the lowermost end of the scale up to somewhere approaching 5000 ~ but ceases thereafter. The second is that a specificity of nerve fibers, and thus of place representation, is found over a range from about 400 ~ upward, but not below.

Consequently it is suggested that the first transition, where place joins frequency, lies probably in the region of 400 ~; and the second, where frequency fails, leaving place to hold the field alone, is in the region of 5000 ~. If 15 ~ and 24,000 ~ are taken as the extremes of the pitch scale, then we have 15 to 400 ~ as the low-tone range, 400 to 5000 ~ as the middle range, and 5000 to 24,000 ~ as the high-tone range. These ranges are represented in Fig. 39 along with other pertinent data.

Loudness depends upon a duality of processes just as pitch does, though here, as will be seen, the two can be resolved into one in the end. Even more important—and this may seem confusing at first—loudness involves the same physical dimensions of time and space that pitch does, though in distinctive modes of variation.

One process of intensity representation has already been brought out in the discussion of the volley principle. It was shown that an increase of intensity will lead to an increase in the rate at which a given nerve fiber contributes to the total nerve discharge. Also it was pointed out that such a change can occur without altering the composite rhythm established by the group of fibers of which this one is a member. Therefore it is possible for one kind of temporal variation to operate for pitch and another for loudness without essential contradiction. To avoid confusion, the terms 'frequency' or 'volley frequency' will be used to refer to the synchronized discharge, and 'rate of impulses,' 'discharge rate,' or 'magnitude of discharge' will be used for the amount of the contribution of the several fibers to the discharge irrespective of the volley frequency.

The second intensity variable depends upon the spatial extent and distribution of the action in the cochlea, and consequently in the auditory nerve. It has already been suggested that any tone involves an extensive area of the basilar membrane, yet varies in its degree of involvement of different portions of this area. We picture a certain central region as most strongly stimulated, and other regions as stimulated less and less as we

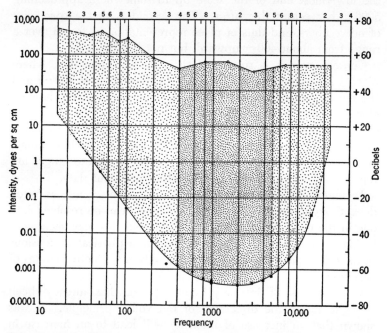

Fig. 39. The auditory area. The lower boundary is the curve of threshold sensitivity, and the upper boundary is the limit at which pain, pressure, and other sensations supervene. Data from Wegel (2).

proceed up and down the cochlea. If the stimulus intensity is low, it may be that only in the central region is the sensory action strong enough to excite any nerve fibers; for the fibers elsewhere the excitation is below threshold. A rise in the intensity will increase the sensory action everywhere, and some of the nerve fibers previously inactive will now be brought into play.

Another condition probably contributes to this relation between intensity and the number of active fibers. In a given region, as already suggested, there may be differences in the stimulation of sensory cells, because some are more favorably situated than others with respect to the vibratory motion. These differences will naturally be reflected in the excitatory effects that these cells present to their nerve fibers. So it may happen that within certain regions, particularly where the stimulation is only moderate, there will be some fibers that are excited and others that are not. A rise of intensity will bring in these less favored elements.

Both these forms of spatial variation, the effective breadth of the stimulation pattern and what may be called the excitatory density within it, will determine the number of nerve fibers set in operation by a stimulus of a given intensity.

According to this theory, then, the stimulus intensity is represented by the number of nerve fibers acting and also by the rates at which they act. These two modes of variation can be subsumed in a single variable as the number of impulses per unit of time in the total discharge, or, what amounts to the same thing, the average number of impulses per volley.

Further Consideration of the Resonance Principle

It has just been pointed out that resonance as conceived in the volley theory is subject to certain restrictive conditions, and it is well at this stage to examine in detail the nature of these conditions and their consequences for the behavior of the response mechanism. As will be seen, the type of resonator action contemplated is different from that familiarly portrayed in the classical resonance theory. The difference is so great, indeed, that though it is technically correct still to speak of resonance in this connection there is perhaps some risk of misunderstanding in doing so.

The two restrictions that have the most far-reaching consequences are (1) the admission of heavy damping in the cochlea and (2) the limitation in the scope of specific resonance already referred to.

THE EFFECTS OF DAMPING

Already, in earlier discussions of the resonance theory and its principles, repeated reference has been made to damping and its significance in determining the behavior of acoustic systems. Here once more we need to consider this condition of resonance, and with special regard to the case in which the damping is great. Let us first review the general principles in the action of simple vibratory elements under heavy damping.

1. A vibratory element shows the effect of damping most obviously in a limitation of its amplitude of response. Damping thus imposes a check upon what tuning can gain in the direction of sensitivity.

2. Damping at the same time makes the element responsive to frequencies other than that to which it is tuned. This spread of resonance first extends to the near-by frequencies and then becomes more marked as damping mounts until frequencies well removed from the natural frequency are nearly as effective as it is itself. Thus the selectivity of a resonator is reduced to a low degree.

3. The spread of resonance is a function of frequency also. For constant damping, the lower the tuning of an element the greater the effectiveness of adjacent frequencies.

4. A further effect of damping refers to the character of the response of a resonator at the beginning and end of an excitation. When the imposed vibration is different from the natural frequency its first impact sets up a response not of its own frequency but of the natural frequency. This in-tune vibration dies away, at a rate determined by the damping, and is gradually replaced by the forced frequency, but during the transition period both frequencies are present and the response is correspondingly complex. When after a time the external forcing is stopped the imposed vibration ceases at once, but the resonator now vibrates at its own frequency, and continues to do so until finally the damping brings it to an end. When the damping is high both the transients of onset and the terminal persistence of the vibrations become small, perhaps so small as to be negligible.

Now let us contemplate an array of elements tuned progressively so as to cover a range of frequencies, and all under heavy damping. It is obvious that they will not respond discretely to an imposed frequency. If this frequency falls somewhere well within the range covered by the array it will arouse a maximum of response in those elements in best agreement with it, and a decreasing response in the ones more distant. As the imposed frequency is shifted upward or downward the curve of response shifts accordingly. A frequency even outside the range of tuning will have an effect, most marked of course in the elements on the end nearest it and diminishing from there across the series.

If for this array the damping is constant the curve of response will change somewhat in form according to the imposed frequency: the lower the frequency the broader the response pattern. In the cochlea, this effect will be complicated by local variations in the amount of damping, resulting either from variations in the size and form of the moving parts or from a possible dependence on the velocity of the motion.

From these considerations it is clear that if the ear contained isolated elements they would not behave as such under heavy damping but would operate together in a broad pattern. Therefore the picture that has been drawn does not require any essential alteration as we turn to the actualities of the anatomical situation in the ear.

As we know, the ear contains no isolated elements. The basilar membrane is not segmented, and it is neither realistic nor reasonable to suppose that it can act as if it were. We must treat it for what it is: a long, continuous ribbon, well loaded with cellular masses, exposed to damping, and only somewhat differentiated in mechanical properties. The physical principles that truly apply to simple resonant elements apply to this kind of structure also, only we must not seek to simplify the mechanics by neglecting some of the conditions as so often is done in treating the isolated, undamped resonator. If all conditions are observed—internal and external damping, the intercoupling of parts of the structure, the frictional resistances of the confining bony walls, and the rest—then it should be immaterial as far as theoretical adequacy goes whether we develop the problem as the vibration of a stretched string or membrane, or of a tube with yielding walls. Which development may turn out finally to be the most convenient or the most practical to handle is another matter. Just now the stretched-string formulation is emphasized because it is the traditional one and the one for which the physical laws are most thoroughly worked out. The point at present is that whatever our approach we must conceive of a broad pattern of action, far removed from the old 'pitch to a fiber' idea.

This conception of cochlear mechanics receives theoretical support and clarification in a further contemplation of the form of the cochlear response function and the electrodynamic actions of the hair cell. In Chapter 6 it was suggested that the electrical response of the cochlea represents a summation of potentials generated in all the hair cells exposed to the stimulus. The magnitude of this response for any given stimulus intensity evidently depends upon two things, the size of the response in each hair cell and the number of hair cells in operation.

It is usual, in dealing with the electrical behavior of nerves and sense organs of all kinds, to take it for granted that the potentials produced by the different active elements are simply additive. Yet it is necessary to explain why this may be so; such a form of combination of the output of potential generators in parallel is not a necessary one, and indeed it is not even usual in our general experience with electric circuits. It occurs when the generators have an internal impedance that is very large with respect to the other impedance in the circuit. We must suppose that the impedance of the hair cells greatly exceeds that of the path of conduction to our electrodes and measuring equipment.

Now it was suggested in the theory of hair-cell action that the production of the electrical potential in the individual cell is a simple process and (below the level of distortion) follows a linear form. If this suggestion is accepted, and is added to the fact that the cochlear response function itself is linear (over the same range), a remarkable conclusion emerges, namely, that the number of hair cells stimulated by a given tone does not vary with intensity. This conclusion is necessary because if each of a group of hair cells is responding linearly any progressive addition to the number in the group must give a total response that is not linear but is accelerated in form.

Let us consider the alternative to this conclusion. It is that the electrodynamic process in the individual hair cell has a decelerated rise with intensity, and that the spread of response with intensity has such a form as exactly to compensate for this deceleration so that the total potential shows a linear form. Such a coincidence of processes might be conceived of in a limited region of intensity, but its maintenance over a range so extensive as that for which the cochlear function is linear—a range of over 60 db—is so improbable as hardly to invite further consideration.

The simplest form of the conception of invariable spread is that every stimulus, even at threshold, extends its effects throughout the entire cochlea and reaches every hair cell. This does not mean, however, that every cell is equally involved—far from it. It is still reasonable to suppose that cells more favorably situated make the major contribution to the recorded activity, and other cells on the fringes add only slight amounts. Also it is well to remember that these latter cells, in which the excitation is feeble, may fail to excite their nerve fibers and hence may not be concerned in the ultimate loudness of the sound. It is necessary therefore to distinguish two kinds of spread of stimulus action, the true spread which is now conceived as always maximal in extent, and a relative or effective spread in which the varying magnitude of the response is taken into account. The relative spread will be reflected in the neural excitation.

THE SCOPE OF SPECIFIC RESONANCE

As the discussion of Chapter 5 has brought out, one of the most difficult problems of the traditional resonance theory is the differentiation of cochlear elements over a range so extensive as $10\frac{1}{2}$ octaves. This problem is made easier by even a moderate curtailment in the scope of specific tuning demanded.

Since in the volley theory the low tones are suitably represented by the volley frequency it is not necessary to allocate specific spatial representation to them; no regions need be precisely tuned to their frequencies. Stimuli at the lower end of the auditory range can operate by forcing the vibration of regions tuned to the middle frequencies. The only sacrifice here will be in sensitivity.

It is further possible, and even likely, that some curtailment of tuning is present also at the upper end of the auditory range. Precise tuning need not continue all the way to the upper limit of hearing but may cease somewhat before this limit is reached. The stimuli of highest frequency then would operate by the forcing of regions tuned to frequencies somewhat below. Here the sacrifice will be in sensitivity and also in pitch discrimination.

It is possible along the lines of this argument to dispose of 4½ to 5 octaves of tuning at the lower end of the auditory range, and perhaps ½ to 1 octave at the upper end. We are left with a requirement of tuning over but 5 or 6 octaves, something like half the extent ordinarily reckoned with.

This modest requirement makes cochlear differentiation a relatively simple matter, regardless of the particular factors of differentiation that are accepted. For illustration, consider the Helmholtz type of theory in which differentiation is attributed to variations in the length, tension, and mass of the basilar membrane fibers according to the laws of vibrating strings. The variation in width of the basilar membrane (length of the transverse fibers) of about 6-fold will account for 2½ octaves, leaving only 2½ to 3½ octaves for the remaining factors of tension and mass. According to results already presented, the cells lying on the basilar membrane exhibit about a 4-fold variation in bulk. The mass factor therefore can give a differentiation of $\sqrt{4}$, or 2-fold, and will account for another octave.

Following the traditional treatment, we may call upon the factor of tension to handle the remaining 1½ to 2½ octaves. If the tension varies in proportion to the size of the spiral ligament, or about 15-fold, then it may reasonably be supposed to contribute $\sqrt{15}$ or nearly a 4-fold variation to the tuning, which is two octaves. Compare this amount with Wilkinson's calculation of a variation in tension of several thousand fold!

In view of the fact that no one, from Helmholtz on, has obtained any visible evidence of an active tension in the basilar membrane, it is more reasonable to speak of a factor of stiffness rather than one of tension. In doing so we depart from the usual vibrating-string formula, in which stiffness is neglected for the sake of simplification. If the ligament adds stiffness in relation to its bulk we shall have a differentiation in the desired direction. There is also a variation from base to apex in the thickness of the basilar membrane and its parts, contributing further to the stiffness differentiation. Békésy, we recall, obtained indications of a considerable variation in stiffness, one of about 100-fold.

It is even possible to avoid any assumption of differentiation by either tension or stiffness, for as already suggested it is likely that damping varies throughout the cochlea. If its variation on account of local conditions amounts to as much as 3- to 4-fold we shall have the final differentiation needed.

We now have before us in general form a conception of cochlear action that differs significantly from that commonly represented in resonance theories. The principle of place representation, though still accepted, is profoundly modified by the restrictions in the scope of tuning and particularly of the specificity of response. In consequence, this principle by itself cannot satisfy the requirements of pitch recognition and discrimination. At the low-frequency end of the scale, and probably in the intermediate range also, the supplementary operation of the volley principle becomes indispensable.

From a consideration of cochlear mechanics alone we can not fill in the details of this conception because the physical conditions, and even the principles of the action, are insufficiently understood. For a further development of these ideas therefore we turn to the functional evidence: to clinical and experimental data obtained from the ear in operation.

The Localization of Response in the Cochlea

The evidence first to be considered has been developed very largely about the problem of the localization of response in the cochlea. In our present contemplation of this evidence we ought not to restrict ourselves, as was done so often in the past, to the simple question whether such localization exists. Rather, we need to inquire within what regions of frequency the localization holds, and within these regions how specific it is in its operation.

CLINICAL OBSERVATIONS

Valuable evidence on the question of the localization of response in the cochlea comes from clinical observations of local injuries and degenerations. First deserving of mention, at least for their historical interest, are the observations of Gruber and Stepanow (1), made on patients who had lost the apical portion of the cochlea. In Gruber's patient an operation was performed to remove a growth deep in the ear, and then in the course of further probing there was found in the middle ear cavity a bony fragment that turned out to be the upper two turns of the cochlea. Stepanow's experience was similar, except that in his patient the cochlear fragment represented one and a half turns. In each instance the ear was reported to be only partially deaf, and loud sounds of various sorts, including speech, were perceived. For Stepanow's patient, indeed, hearing was indicated for all tones of the piano. We can not attach much significance to these results, however, because we can not be certain that the hearing tests were properly conducted and that the persons were really doing their hearing with the affected ear and not with the other.

Apart from these unusual instances the correlation between hearing and a cochlear defect can be made only by means of a microscopical examination after the person's death. One of the earliest observations of this kind was made by Moos and Steinbrügge on a patient who before death had suffered a loss of hearing for high tones and whose cochlea later was found to have an atrophy of nerve fibers in the basal turn. There have been a good many observations of this kind, mostly of isolated cases, but variations in methods of testing the hearing and also in preparing the ears for microscopical examination make it difficult to combine the data in any meaningful way.

Only recently has this problem been approached systematically and on such a scale as to yield definitive results. Since 1924 a program has been carried out in the Otological Research Laboratory of the Johns Hopkins Medical School for the collection and preparation of the temporal bones of persons whose hearing had been tested before death; and by the routine testing of large numbers of hospital patients this material has been assembled in such quantity—at this writing some 2100 ears—as to permit a statistical treatment of the problem of pathological condition in relation to auditory defect.

The principal report was made by Crowe, Guild, and Polvogt in 1934 (see also Guild, 4) and was based upon an examination of 79 ears in which the audiometer tests had shown a loss of acuity for high tones. Two forms of such loss were distinguished as abrupt and gradual high-tone loss, as illustrated in Fig. 40. Serial sections of these 79 ears were studied by Guild's graphic reconstruction method, mentioned earlier, in which a scale diagram is made to represent the basilar membrane and the condi-

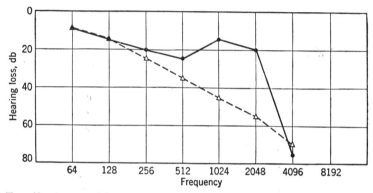

Fig. 40. Types of high-tone loss. The solid line represents the abrupt form of high-tone loss, and the broken line represents the gradual form. Data from Crowe, Guild, and Polvogt.

tion of its various structures. It was found necessary in this study to map in detail only the basal turn, as with rare exceptions this was the only region in which abnormalities appeared. Figure 41 illustrates the procedure. The inner ribbon of the diagram represents the nerve fibers as seen in their bony channel running under the limbus; when this channel contains a normal number of fibers the ribbon is fully filled in with black, and when the number of fibers is below normal the filling is proportionately less. In the example shown there was total atrophy at the extreme basal end and then partial atrophy of a patchy sort for about 5 mm, beyond which the condition was normal. Next is shown the condition of the organ of Corti, with pictorial symbols to indicate the structural framework and the number of hair cells present; here abnormality of the sensory structure was present at the basal end only. The two remaining ribbons of the diagram represent the condition of the external sulcus cells and the stria vascularis.

Among the 79 ears studied by this method were 41 of the type suffering a gradual high-tone loss. Of these, 24 showed a considerable degree of atrophy of nerve fibers, most noticeable at the lower basal end but often extending into the upper basal region as well. In most cases there was also some slight abnormality of the organ of Corti, generally limited to the lower basal end. In the remaining 17 ears of this group the atrophies of nerve and organ of Corti were hardly greater than those observed in normal ears; and other conditions not revealed to view and possibly existing in the central auditory pathways must be supposed to account for the hearing loss.

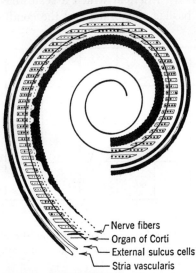

Nerve fibers
Organ of Corti
External sulcus cells
Stria vascularis

FIG. 41. Spiral diagram of the basal turn of the cochlea, showing the condition of the sensory structures. From Crowe, Guild, and Polvogt [*Bulletin of the Johns Hopkins Hospital*].

There were 24 ears of the type suffering an abrupt high-tone loss. These showed even more serious atrophy of nerve, again most prominent in the lower basal region, and in addition there was serious atrophy of the organ of Corti in this same region.

These results clearly indicate a relationship between a loss of acuity for high tones and the atrophy of nerve fibers and of organ of Corti in the basal part of the cochlea. The association of atrophies of the organ of Corti with the abrupt form of high-tone impairment suggests that there is a greater specificity in the sensory action than there is in its neural representation.

A detailed consideration of certain of the cases, and a statistical analysis of the data by Ciocco, lead to more specific inferences regarding cochlear localization. As Fig. 42 shows, the area most important for the reception of 8192 ~ seems to lie about 5 mm from the basal end, and that for 4096 ~ about 8 mm from the basal end. The tone 2048 ~ is less exactly located, but it probably depends upon the region 10 to 12 mm or more from the basal end. These are only general indications, and the data do

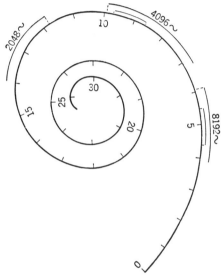

Fig. 42. Cochlear localization for high tones, based on the pathological observations of Crowe, Guild, and Polvogt. From their paper. The scale shows distances in millimeters from the basal end of the basilar membrane.

not make possible any further determination of the degree of the localization.

Now as we turn to the low tones and consider the evidence on their localization afforded by this same collection of clinical material, the picture is strikingly different. In the first place, a loss of hearing for only the low tones is unknown. When acuity is impaired for the low tones it is impaired for the middle and usually the high tones as well. Often, when the curve of hearing is depressed at the low-frequency end, it continues to fall, either gradually or precipitously, as the high frequencies are approached. In many cases the curve is roughly horizontal: all

tones are about equally affected. Only rather infrequently does
the curve ascend from low to high, and then the middle tones
are poorly heard, and usually the high tones are below normal
also, though relatively they are better heard than the low tones.
Consequently a study of low-tone hearing strictly comparable to
that just described for high tones is not possible, and it is apparent here, apart from any special consideration of theory, that
there exists some important, even fundamental, difference in the
ear's behavior toward the high and low frequencies.

Another circumstance is that, whereas basal atrophies are
common, local atrophies elsewhere in the cochlea are extremely
rare. Now it may be conceived that this regional difference in
the cochlear pathology supplies the reason for the observed
difference in the clinical picture for high and low tones, and
some relation here can not be ruled out. Yet that this is not the
whole and possibly not even the major explanation is indicated
in a study of those unusual cases where atrophies in the apical
and middle regions are present. Guild (5) found in the Hopkins
collection of material 5 ears (from 4 individuals) with circum-
scribed atrophy of nerve in the upper middle and lower apical
regions. In three individuals the condition was unilateral, and
the opposite ear was normal in the corresponding region, yet the
acuity of the two ears was practically identical. In the remaining
patient the condition was bilateral, and rather more extensive
than in the others; and in this case the acuity in both ears was
slightly below normal for the low tones, but because poor concentration on the part of the patient was reported at the time
of the examination an evaluation of this result is somewhat uncertain. Taken as a whole these observations show that a
considerable amount of nerve atrophy in the upper regions of
the cochlea does not have any marked effect upon the acuity for
low tones.

In his search for other cochlear anomalies outside the basal
region Guild discovered 7 ears with the structural defect known
as scala communis cochleae, a condition in which the bony
septum between middle and apical turns is lacking and the scala
vestibuli communicates freely with the scala tympani. This condition would allow the sound pressures present in the upper
part of the scala vestibuli to extend immediately to the scala

tympani without passing through the basilar membrane, and on any of the simpler conceptions of cochlear mechanics like the Helmholtz resonance theory this by-passing of the membrane ought to have a profound effect on sensitivity to some or even all of the low tones. Yet every one of these ears had good hearing for low tones—and most of them for the high tones too. Still another condition that Guild occasionally encountered in the middle and apical regions was an aberrant blood vessel that stretched across the scala tympani and made contact with the basilar membrane; yet the constraint on the movement of the membrane so applied had no observable effect upon hearing. It is apparent that these observations lend no support to a theory of restricted response to low tones.

In pursuing further this question of low-tone localization, Oda studied a group of 35 ears of the Hopkins collection in which there was impaired hearing for both low and high tones. This group was selected with the intention of excluding the major middle ear lesions as well as other impairments of conduction. This was done on a basis of the Rinne test: it was required that a tuning fork held opposite the ear be heard for a longer time after it was struck than if the stem of the fork were applied to the mastoid bone, or in other words that air conduction be better than bone conduction for the same fork. It is expected that a blocking of the aerial pathway or interruption of the ossicular chain would seriously impair air conduction but not conduction through the bones of the head.

In practically all of the 35 ears examined there were lesions of nerve and often of the organ of Corti also in the basal turn, as would be expected in view of the poor hearing for high tones. In only 7 ears, however, did these lesions extend into middle and apical regions and thereby provide an explanation of the low-tone losses. In all these 7 there was a spotty or continuous atrophy of nerve fibers all the way to the apex, and amounting to 40 to 80 per cent of the total nerve supply.

Of the remaining 28 ears, it was found that despite the preliminary selection by the Rinne test, 7 had conductive lesions of perhaps enough severity to account for the low-tone losses. In 5 others these lesions were milder and were not deemed sufficient in themselves to cause the losses, but, Oda believed, in combination with the cochlear atrophies that were present in the basal turn they may have done so. This last conclusion of course implies that the basal turn of the cochlea is involved in low-tone reception.

This implication is fortified by a consideration of the results of this study in relation to those of Crowe, Guild, and Polvogt, especially for those ears with abrupt high-tone loss. Oda pointed out that in a significant number of his cases the nerve atrophy extended farther into the upper basal turn than it did in the ears with normal low-tone acuity. This evidence, then, more specifically indicates the upper basal region as involved in the hearing of low tones. Certainly, taken as a whole, the evidence does not favor the view that low tones have any restricted representation in the cochlea, but indicates them instead as spreading over all the area from the apical end at least as far as the upper basal turn, or in other words throughout one-half or more of the length of the cochlea. And this, it must be emphasized, is said of tones that are only of threshold strength.

RESULTS OF EXPERIMENTAL INJURY

Many attempts have been made to supplement the clinical data on localization by the deliberate destruction of parts of the cochlea in experimental animals. Nearly all these experiments have been carried out on guinea pigs, largely because in this animal the cochlea, instead of being embedded in solid bone as in most other mammals, juts into the middle ear cavity with a bony covering so thin that the various turns and even the location of the spiral ligament can be discerned. Also, this animal responds to sounds with a reflex twitching of the pinna, and this response gave promise of usefulness as an indicator of hearing.

In the early experiments the injuries were gross. Baginsky, for example, destroyed the entire apex of the cochlea and then observed that the reflex responses to low tones vanished, while those to high tones remained. On the other hand, Stepanow (2) after a similar destruction obtained responses both to high and low tones. We must prefer Stepanow's result here, because as he pointed out a positive response is evidence of hearing but a failure to respond is inconclusive: the animal may hear the sound but ignore it. This is the drawback to the use of the pinna reflex: the reaction is not a compulsory one. A more positive indication of hearing is afforded by the conditioned response method, in which continued training can develop the desired degree of regularity of reaction. Wittmaack (4) reported results on a dog trained by this method. Before operation the animal responded to all tones from 50 to 30,000 ~. Then one cochlea was totally destroyed, and the other was damaged in all but the basal part. At first the animal responded only to high tones, but as time went on it recovered much of its former range, until after a year it gave evidence of hearing tones from 340 ~ upward and also from 250 ~ downward. Wittmaack suggested that the response to the lowest tones was by means of their overtones and that the deafness really included everything below 340 ~. Histological examination revealed that the whole apical portion of the cochlea had been destroyed and that only a fragment of normal organ of Corti and nerve remained in the basal region.

Some have attempted to produce more limited cochlear lesions. Held and Kleinknecht, working on guinea pigs, drilled minute holes through the bony wall in the region of the spiral ligament, in the intention of injuring this ligament sufficiently to reduce the tension on the basilar membrane at a particular spot and thereby to cause a local impairment of tonal response. They reported that such drillings at the beginning of the middle third of the basal turn (i.e., about 2.5 mm from the basal end or $\frac{1}{7}$ of the way to the apex) caused a loss of hearing, as shown by absence of the pinna reflex, for tones around 5214 to 5424 ~. Only a few animals gave satisfactory results, and the drillings in more apical locations produced general losses because, as they supposed, the more fragile condition of the cochlea there caused it to be more extensively damaged.

In more recent years the experiments to determine the effects of local injury have employed the electrical responses of the cochlea. Hughson, Crowe, and Howe were first to use this method. In cats they drilled part way through the cochlear wall and then used a high-frequency cautery to scorch the tissues beneath. This operation in the basal turn caused a general reduction in responses, with the most serious effect upon the high tones. Others who have repeated these experiments, with minor differences in the manner of producing the damage, have obtained various results, but usually all tones are affected somewhat by the more drastic injuries. Notably lacking in many of the reports is a histological check on the locus and extent of the cochlear insult. Stevens, Davis, and Lurie stated that in their experiment such a check was made, but they gave no details. Their sample results on the changes in the cochlear responses indicate rather general and irregular losses as a result of drilling through the cochlear wall.

A well-controlled study was carried out by Walzl and Bordley on cats. They developed a technique to avoid a general traumatizing of the cochlear structures or a loss of endolymph. After carefully grinding away the bone over the spiral ligament in a selected spot they used a blunt needle to push the ligament inward and thereby crush or dislodge the organ of Corti immediately adjacent. Before and after the damage they measured the electrical responses for various tones over a wide range. Then they made graphic reconstructions based upon serial sections of the ears to determine the locations of the lesions. For small lesions in the basal part of the cochlea there were fairly restricted depressions of sensitivity, and the frequency regions in which they were found varied systematically with the site of the lesion. The more basal lesions caused high-tone losses, and those somewhat higher in the cochlea caused losses of lower frequencies. However, lesions in the apex gave no noticeable impairments when they were small, and then when they were enlarged they caused rather general losses. The most apical lesion yielding restricted losses was 15 mm from the basal end, which is about $\frac{2}{3}$ the length of the cat's basilar membrane, and it had its maximum effect upon a tone of 256 ~. This depression amounted to 20 db, and it is important to note that other tones, all the way to 724 ~, were affected also though in lesser degree. In general, the smaller lesions had effects over 1 or 2 octaves, and somewhat larger ones had far wider effects. Thus damage near the basal end of about $1\frac{1}{2}$ mm in extent affected all tones above 512 ~. Although in these lesions the destruction of the organ of Corti was complete within the affected area, it is significant that the depression of sensitivity was only moderate, of the order usually of 10 to 20 db. Obviously there is a great residuum of function, afforded by other areas that participate in the response to a given tone. The study of larger lesions and also of multiple lesions added further information on the degree of spread over the basilar membrane. After a lesion was produced in the basal region, and caused a loss for high tones, a second lesion near by caused a further reduction in the high-tone response. Areas in the basal turn as much as 3 mm apart thus were found to serve particular high tones in common. If the second lesion was made in the middle turn, some 10 mm away, the high tones were not depressed much further, though the low tones were widely affected. Therefore it appears that the high tones do not spread very far toward the apical end at the stimulus intensities used. On the other hand, if the lesion was first made in the middle region, where it depressed the low tones, a second lesion in the basal turn caused a further loss of low-tone response as well as a depression of high tones. Plainly, the low tones extend into the basal region. Specifically, the evidence indicated that tones of 256 ~ and below extend from the apical region at least as far as 5 mm from the basal end of the cochlea. These results therefore show clearly that localization is not highly specific, but all tones, even at moderate intensities, spread somewhat over the basilar membrane; and the low tones spread much more widely than the high tones.

THE STIMULATION DEAFNESS EXPERIMENTS

For a good many years the followers of Helmholtz have derived an important part of the support for their position from the stimulation deafness experiments, in which animals are exposed for a time to sounds of extraordinary intensity, and the effects upon the ear are then ascertained. The earliest use of the method seems to have been made by von Stein in 1894, but the first significant results are those of Wittmaack in 1907. In Wittmaack's and most of the experiments immediately following there were no tests of sensitivity, but the animals were examined histologically after the exposure and the effects on auditory function inferred from the lesions that were found. These experiments, carried out principally on guinea pigs, often revealed degenerations of the organ of Corti and sometimes of nerve fibers in the basal portions of the cochlea as a result of stimulation with high tones. Low tones gave generally uncertain or negative results.

The pathological changes resulting from stimulation by single tones were sometimes reported as limited to small areas, but more often they appeared to be rather extensive. Thus Yoshii, after stimulating with a tone of 4138 ~, observed cochlear changes through the middle portion of the basal turn and extending in lighter degree to the upper portion of that turn, and so covering one-half to two-thirds of a turn altogether. He could hardly claim that these were 'narrowly restricted regions,' but still he considered his evidence to be a verification of Helmholtz's hypothesis in a somewhat broadened interpretation.

The stimulation deafness experiment obviously gains in significance when hearing tests are included and a correlation is drawn up between the pathological changes and the effects on sensitivity. Marx, Röhr, and a few others tried to use the pinna reflex for this purpose, but encountered the uncertainties of this reaction already referred to. More recently the conditioned response method has been employed, notably by Upton, Horton, and Kemp. Tests by this method after exposure to loud sounds have generally revealed widespread rather than specific losses of sensitivity.

The electrical response of the cochlea provides a new means of determining the condition of the receptor, and its technique has been added to the others of the stimulation deafness experiment. Several studies in late years have made use of it. After an ear is stimulated by a tone of extreme intensity its cochlear potentials are impaired. If in the observation of an intensity function the stimulus is carried well beyond the point of the maximum the response falls off, usually rather suddenly, and the earlier function can no longer be observed. Figure 43 illustrates the change. The output from a stimulus of any given strength is now markedly less than before, and the maximum is well below that formerly attained. Note, however, that the curve is still linear over its lower course. Plainly the ear has suffered a general impairment of its electrical activity in response to sound.

The impairment is not just for the stimulating frequency, but for all frequencies. If the stimulating frequency is low the losses are about the same throughout the scale or if anything are more serious in the middle and upper regions of the scale. If this

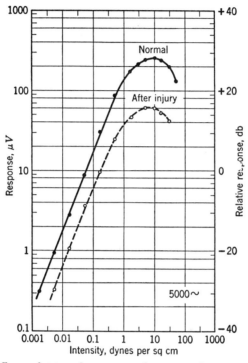

FIG. 43. Effects of injury by overstimulation, as shown in the cochlear potentials of the guinea pig. The solid line shows responses obtained to 5000 ∼ under normal conditions, and the broken line shows those obtained after injury with this tone.

frequency is high a clearly differential effect is found: the low tones are progressively less affected. The losses are never very specific even then; the curve changes only slowly with frequency. Results obtained by Smith and me on the guinea pig are illustrated in Fig. 44. For all these injury functions the stimulus had the same pressure of 1000 dynes per sq cm and was maintained for the same period, 4 min.

The histological study of these ears revealed striking differences, as Fig. 45 will show. The ears exposed to the low tones had extensive areas of damage to the organ of Corti, while those exposed to the high tones had only restricted damage. As indicated, the 300 ~ injury covers nearly the whole apical half of the cochlea, the 10,000 ~ injury is slight and covers less than a millimeter, and the injuries from 1000 and 5000 ~ fall between

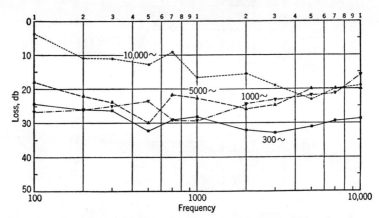

FIG. 44. Stimulation deafness as a function of the exposure frequency. The four curves represent different exposure frequencies as indicated, each presented for 4 min at a sound pressure of 1000 dynes per sq cm. Distances below the zero line represent impairments of sensitivity. From Smith and Wever [*Journal of Experimental Psychology*].

these two. At the same time the position of the damage along the cochlea changes systematically.

There is a lack of correspondence between the amounts of cochlear potential losses and of anatomical change. The loss of electrical response invariably is out of proportion to the observable damage. This lack of correspondence is even greater if the stimulation is more moderate and the potential losses are only 10 or 15 db, for then we usually see no anatomical changes at all: the cochlea appears histologically normal. A possible explanation is that the stimulation causes two kinds of alteration in the sense organ. One, of a milder sort, is an impairment of the capacity of the cells to generate electrical potentials. This is evidently not a permanent impairment but is slowly recovered

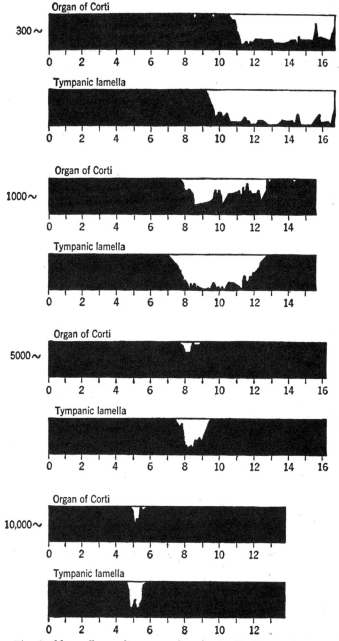

Fɪɢ. 45. Cochlear effects of overstimulation. Unfilled areas show regions of damage, measured in millimeters from the base of the cochlea. From K. R. Smith (2) and Smith and Wever [*Journal of Experimental Psychology*].

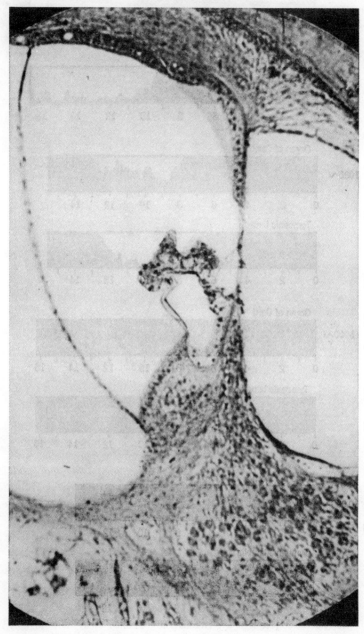

FIG. 46.   Grave cochlear injury produced by a 300 ∼ tone.   From K. R. Smith (2).

from, over a period of hours or days, depending on the severity of the stimulation. The other is an obvious mechanical damage, as pictured in Fig. 46, and from it little or no recovery can be expected. In fact, this kind of damage is followed in the course of a few days by a degeneration and disappearance of the nerve fibers and ganglion cells whose dendrites have been torn away in the sensory disruption.

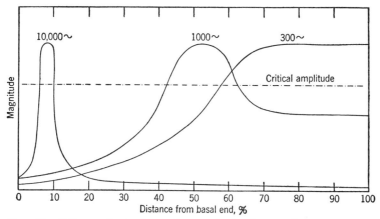

FIG. 47. Patterns of stimulus action on the basilar membrane, suggested by the stimulation deafness experiments, and also the results described later on maximum responses. The line marked 'critical amplitude' represents a stimulus level above which the ear suffers histological damage. Cf. Wever and Lawrence (2) [*Journal of the Acoustical Society of America*].

These results prove that for low tones the spread of action is very great when the stimuli are strong. For the high tones also the spread must be considerable, because the responses to these tones are impaired after overstimulation by other high tones, as well as by the low tones.

The question arises as to what feature of a sound determines its destructiveness to the sensory apparatus. Simple sound waves in a given medium may vary in four ways: in frequency, amplitude, particle velocity, and acceleration. Of these four dimensions the first two are independent; the third, particle velocity, varies as the product of frequency and amplitude; and the fourth, acceleration, varies as the product of amplitude and the square of the frequency. In this experiment the tones varied in frequency but were kept constant in particle velocity (which is directly proportional to sound pressure). Because the product of frequency and amplitude was held constant it follows that the amplitude varied inversely as the frequency: it was the greatest for 300 ~ and the least for 10,000 ~. The greater severity (as well as the scope) of the injury found for the low tones suggests strongly that it is the amplitude of a sound that measures its injurious character. In other words, the sensory apparatus is disrupted by being displaced too far from its normal position much as a stick is broken on being bent.

The results show further, and unmistakably, that the distribution of response over the basilar membrane varies as a function of frequency. For the low tones the action is most vigorous over the apical half of the cochlea, whereas for the high tones it is more concentrated in regions toward the base. Figure 47 shows pictorially this interpretation of the results. The critical amplitude as indicated represents the limit beyond which the sensory apparatus is damaged. The conclusions represented here are in harmony with those already mentioned as to the differences in the actions of high and low tones.

EMBRYOLOGICAL EVIDENCE

A study of the embryological development of the ear gives evidence that has been brought forward as pertinent to the problem of cochlear localization. Early students of the development of the ear (as, for example, Boettcher) remarked that the differentiation of cochlear structures begins in the basal region and then proceeds in an apical direction.

Kreidl and Yanase and later Wada observed this order of development for the rat and studied also the course of appearance of auditory function as indicated by reflex reactions to sounds. Wada reported that the organ of Corti first attains an essentially adult form in the basal regions of the cochlea on the tenth day after birth, or occasionally in a precocious animal on the ninth day, and it is then that the earliest reflex responses to sounds are elicited. These responses, which include reflex twitches of the pinna and general bodily movements, he claimed were aroused at first by high-pitched notes and only later, on the eleventh or twelfth day, by low-pitched sounds as well. It must be mentioned, however, that Wada's testing methods were crude, since as stimuli he used only three sounds: a clap of the hands, a whistle of a single pitch said to be about 2048 ~, and a sucking noise made with the mouth. His conclusion regarding the differential effect of high and low tones therefore is in need of further support. It seems clear, however, that sensitivity to sounds increases rapidly after it first makes its appearance about the tenth day and becomes well established two days later when cellular differentiation throughout the cochlea has approached its adult form. Wada regarded these relations between structure and function as supporting a place theory of hearing.

Recent studies carried out on the opossum have yielded more exact information both on the embryology of the ear and on early exhibitions of hearing. As is well known, this animal, a marsupial, is born in an extraordinarily immature condition, and its major senses develop slowly during its retention in the mother's pouch. Larsell, McCrady, and Zimmermann studied the growth of auditory structures in this animal and found the development of the cochlea to be the most advanced in the second half of the basal coil. A given stage of differentiation shows itself first in this region, and then in progressive fashion in regions toward the basal and apical ends.

These investigators obtained reflex responses first in pouch young of about 50 days of age in response to a tone of about 1305 ~. This first sign of hearing coincides with the stage in which the organ of Corti seems to have reached an adult form in the upper basal region. Later, as differentiation extends more widely, other tones of higher and lower pitch become effective.

These observations were continued by McCrady, Wever, and Bray by use of the electrical responses of the cochlea. Electrical potentials were first observed in pouch young of 48 days of age in response to intense tones between 2000 and 7000 ~. Older animals showed both an extension of range and a marked increase in sensitivity, and especially in sensitivity to high tones. Some of these results are reproduced in Fig. 48.

Larsell, McCrady, and Larsell carried out a histological study of some of these animals in which electrical tests had been made, and also of other pouch young of similar stages of development, and located more exactly than had been done formerly the zones of development of the organ of Corti for the different ages. For the 48-day animal, in which responses were obtained over the range from 2000 to 7000 ~, the organ of Corti was most advanced in differentiation at the uppermost end of the basal coil, and as in the opossum the basal coil is about twice as long as the remainder of the cochlea this observation

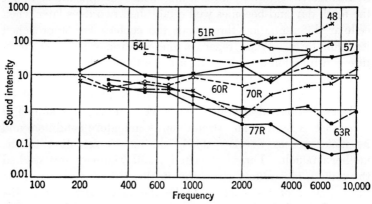

FIG. 48. The development of hearing in the opossum. Each curve shows, for a given animal, the intensity of sound required at various frequencies to produce a standard response of 3 microvolts. The varying ages of the animals are given in days by the numbers on the curves. Sound intensity is in dynes per sq cm. From McCrady, Wever, and Bray (1) [*Journal of Comparative Psychology*].

would seem to locate the range mentioned about two-thirds of the distance upward from the basal end of the cochlea. In later stages, as had been observed earlier, the differentiation proceeded both apically and basally until the entire organ of Corti took on an adult form.

These results were regarded by Larsell and his associates as pointing to a place theory of hearing. They are indeed consistent with that theory, but can hardly be accepted as evidence in their present state. We need to be cautious here because the observed extension of range could appear not only by the addition of new functional resonators, as a place theory will assume, but also by an over-all improvement in sensitivity. Any resonant system, and more noticeably one that is well damped, will extend its useful range when made more receptive or driven more vigorously. All elements of the ear could be tuned to a single frequency and still behave in the manner indicated. The crucial point is how close is the correlation between the appearance of particular tones and the differentiation of particular areas, and this point is still uncertain. The study will have to be continued with use of the graphic reconstruction method to give precise locations for the anatomical changes.

As the results now stand, they are more indicative of a localization of high tones than of low tones. This is so because after an acoustic response first appears it grows more rapidly in the direction of the high tones. An improvement of sensitivity alone ought to extend the range symmetrically. There is reason to believe, therefore, that continued study in this field will be productive for our better understanding of the problem at hand.

TOPOGRAPHICAL EVIDENCE

The electrical responses of the cochlea have been made use of in a more direct approach to the localization problem. Hallpike and Rawdon-Smith (1, 2) recorded these responses in the cat from two electrode positions, one near the basal end of the cochlear capsule and the other near the apical end. They first drilled small holes in the bone in these positions, deep enough that the fluid began to seep through but not so deep as to puncture the wall, and then placed the electrode wires in beads of mercury dropped into the holes. They found that the responses to a tone of 250 ~ when picked up from the apical electrode were about three times as great as when recorded from the basal electrode; and contrariwise the responses to 2050 ~ were greater when recorded from the basal position. This evidence they regarded as direct proof of the localization hypothesis.

Several others have repeated this experiment, mostly on the guinea pig whose cochlear capsule is thin and affords easy orientation. The most detailed study was reported by Culler and his associates. They did not drill holes in the bone but applied the electrode, a fine stiff wire, by hand to various points on the bony surface. They used numerous points and tested with several tones over the range from 60 to 7500 ~. At each point the tone was raised to the level necessary to produce an observable, small response. Now, on the localization hypothesis this stimulus level ought to be a minimum for some one tone at some given point, provided that it is possible to rule out inequalities in the sensitivity of the ear's conduction mechanism and inequalities also in the electrical impedance between the site of origin of the potentials and the point at which the electrode picks them up. These inequalities were handled by an elaborate statistical manipulation of the data, and finally a cochlear 'map' was drawn up in which a focal position was indicated for every stimulus frequency used.

Other experiments, but on a more limited scale, have been carried out by E. P. Johnson, Jr., and by me and my associates. All agree in showing that the magnitude of the recorded potentials varies systematically with frequency and position on the cochlear wall. These experiments thus join the others mentioned in supporting the principle of cochlear localization.

It is necessary to emphasize at this point, however, that these experiments do not give any further details on the character of the localization. They do not disclose, even in relative terms, the spread or sharpness of the response patterns. This fact is stressed because many persons have taken the results of Culler and his associates as indicative of a highly specific kind of localization. This impression probably has arisen on account of the particular statistical treatment of this study, which greatly emphasized the differences present in the observations. These writers in their reports made no claim for a high specificity of localization, and indeed pointed out that they had not explored this aspect of the problem. Perhaps in the future the topographical method can be extended to yield this sort of information.

CHAPTER 10

FURTHER EVIDENCE ON COCHLEAR LOCALIZATION: THE ACOUSTIC NEUROLOGY

Though Helmholtz and others after him rested the resonance theory on the form and expected behavior of the sensory structures, a particular conception of the nerve supply of the ear was always assumed or implied. Indeed, any place hypothesis in which the perception of a given pitch depends upon a specific sensory element necessarily supposes that the activity of this element is reported to the higher brain centers, and with the specificity of the action well preserved. Obviously an isolation of tones at the periphery is of no avail if this quality is lost in the nerve transmission process. Overlapping and interaction of nerve fibers in the course of conduction therefore must be held to a minimum, and ideally every cochlear element ought to have an individual line of communication upward.

On the other hand, the frequency theories do not demand such specific nervous representation, and in fact they often make assumptions rather to the contrary. Thus Rutherford, as we have seen, accounted for loudness by the increasing spread of excitation over the basilar membrane and its nerve fibers. The volley principle as outlined above falls in with the frequency theories here. In its operation it requires at least a moderate degree of spread of excitation or of innervation, or both, so that a single tone shall have available to it a number of nerve fibers sufficient to represent its frequency. Here, then, as a result of theoretical considerations, the projection of the cochlea in the acoustic nervous channels becomes a matter of crucial significance.

THE NEUROACOUSTIC MECHANISM

The nervous arrangement by which the ear's activities are reported to the cerebral cortex is one of great complexity, and its anatomical form is best considered in three stages, (1) the cochlear innervation and projection in the primary nuclei of the medulla oblongata, (2) the connections of these nuclei with others of the hind brain and their representation in the region of the thalamus, and (3) the projection on the acoustic cortex.

THE COCHLEAR INNERVATION AND PRIMARY PROJECTION

The auditory nerve fibers originate in bipolar ganglion cells that lie in rather irregular clusters in the bony spaces of the modiolus, as shown in the sectional view of Fig. 2, page 17. These cells send their dendritic processes outward to innervate the hair cells of the organ of Corti and their axons inward to the axis of the cochlear spiral where they unite to form the trunk of the cochlear nerve.

Out of the ganglionic clusters the dendrites wend their way, often a little tortuously, into the long, relatively narrow canals of the bony spiral lamina. These are the radial bundles, shown as 4, 5, 6, in Fig. 49. It appears, though the observations are incomplete on this point, that most of the fibers from a given ganglionic cluster stay fairly close together and form adjacent radial bundles that run out to supply a limited region of the organ of Corti. Ciocco's observation that the best correlation is obtained between local hearing losses and nerve atrophies if the results on the atrophies are taken in 1 mm steps is indicative of the rough boundaries within which the fibers ramify. There are some fibers, however, that escape this orderly arrangement. While still within the connected ganglionic spaces (which form Rosenthal's canal) they cross over the main, radial stream to take a spiral course and run for considerable distances toward the apex of the cochlea. These fibers (see 1, 2, Fig. 49) form the intraganglionic spiral bundles, discovered by Boettcher and verified by Kölliker (3). How far they run is not accurately known, though Held (2) and Lorente de Nó (3) reported them as extending at least a quarter of a cochlear turn. It has repeatedly been observed that each fiber in its upward course gives off several collaterals that turn outward to run with the radial bundles to the organ of Corti (see 2a, 3a, Fig. 49).

Let us trace the radial bundles farther. As Fig. 5, page 20, will show, the fibers that run outward in the radial canals bend

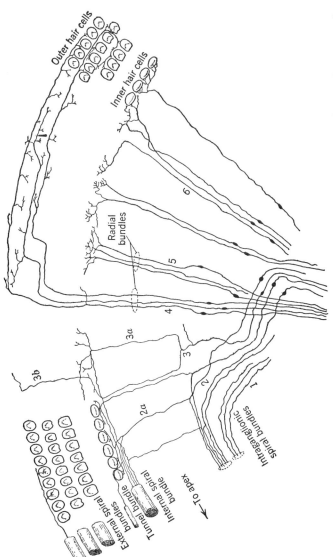

Fig. 49. The innervation of the cochlea. The diagram represents a narrow sector of the cochlea, oriented with its apical end to the left. The hair cells are indicated only in part, at the two ends of the figure. Given are examples of the principal types of fibers, their courses, and the neural bundles that they form. 1, 2, intraganglionic spiral fibers; 2a, 3a, internal spiral fibers; 4, external spiral fibers; 5, 6, radial fibers. Based on observations of Retzius (2, 3), Solovcov, and Lorente de Nó (3).

sharply as they approach the ends of these canals, lose their medullary sheaths, and pass through the tympanic lip in a region known as the habenula perforata. This brings them to the vestibular side of the basilar membrane, near the feet of the inner pillars of Corti and below the row of inner hair cells. A great many of these fibers, the *radial fibers* proper (5, 6, Fig. 49), reach upward to arborize about the bases of the inner hair cells. Each radial fiber comes in contact with several neighboring hair cells, and each hair cell is served by branches from several fibers; in other words, the innervation is both diffuse and overlapping.

Other fibers in these bundles, the *internal spiral fibers,* do not immediately terminate on issuing from the habenula perforata but form a spiral strand (the internal spiral bundle) lying just below the row of inner hair cells. According to Retzius (2), many of these fibers divide and send one branch apicalward and the other basalward, but from Lorente de Nó's observations this occurrence is at least uncommon; more often the fibers take only an apical course. In this course they repeatedly and rather irregularly send off collaterals, and though here the observations are uncertain it is probable that they end mainly on the inner hair cells, and only exceptionally (see 3b, Fig. 49) run out to the level of the outer hair cells. According to Lorente de Nó these internal spiral fibers are not independent fibers but are collaterals given off by the intraganglionic spiral fibers already mentioned.

Still to be described are the *external spiral fibers,* which take the most complicated courses of all (see 4, Fig. 49). They issue from the openings in the habenula perforata and pass below the inner hair cells, then out between the inner pillars of Corti. Most of them run across the tunnel space and through the openings between the outer pillars to the outer hair-cell region. Here they turn sharply and pass toward the base of the cochlea; some turn at once, below the first row of hair cells, others go farther before turning, to the second row or even the third. The rule is that they run basalward for a little way, passing three or four cells and sometimes more, and then swerve outward beyond another row of cells where they resume their basalward swing. Sometimes they continue in this fashion until they come to the last row of hair cells. In any event, they run along the rows of hair cells for varying distances, turn inward sharply, branch once or twice, and arborize around the adjacent hair cells. A fiber in this circumambient course repeatedly gives off fine collaterals to hair cells along the way. How far these fibers go is still to be established; Retzius found them to pass as many as 20 to 30 cells in their trajectory, and Lorente de Nó traced them even farther, over at least a third of a cochlear spiral (which would mean their passing some 1500 cells). These fibers in their courses basalward form small but well-defined strands, the external spiral bundles. There are as many of these bundles as there are rows of hair cells, which means that in the basal region of the cochlea there are three, and in the apical region (in man) four or five.

There is, besides, a tunnel bundle, formed by a few fibers that turn and take a spiral course just beyond the inner rods of Corti. According to Held (4), these tunnel fibers turn back and innervate the inner hair cells, and so are to be regarded functionally as belonging with the internal spiral bundles. There is the further possibility that some of these fibers on leaving the tunnel bundle go out to the outer hair cells.

These results show that any given point along the basilar membrane is represented by a good many nerve fibers. Some of these, the radial fibers, maintain a somewhat systematic relation to one another and the locality that they serve, but the others, the spiral fibers, are so widely distributed that no very specific locality can be represented by them.

The central or axon processes of the cochlear ganglion cells pass through fine holes in the modiolar wall and then bend rapidly into the cochlear axis to form the cochlear nerve. The accepted view, as Fig. 2, page 17, suggests, is that the most apical fibers take a central course through the nerve trunk, with the other fibers adding themselves from the periphery in regular order. This drawing shows also, as is more plainly indicated in Fig. 50, a twisting of the fibers on one another. This feature becomes understandable in a consideration of the embryological development of the ear. The nerve appears, evidently with all its fibers present and with its central connections with the medulla already formed, before the cochlea has developed. The first cochlear connections are made in the basal region—not, however, at what will be the extreme basal end, but a little way up from that point, in the region that is then the most advanced in differentiation. Thereafter as the cochlea grows in a spiral form the nervous elements are carried along, so that when development is complete the nerve fibers belong-

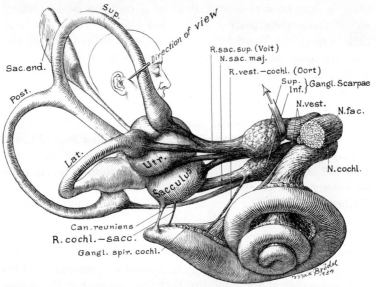

FIG. 50. The membranous labyrinth and its innervation. By Max Brödel, from Hardy (1) [*Anatomical Record*].

ing to each cochlear region are twisted in the same direction and through the same angle as is that region itself. In the right ear the apical fibers are twisted to the right, that is, clockwise; in the left ear they are twisted in the contrary direction. The most basal fibers are rather moderately twisted in a backward direction, opposite to that of the apical fibers, while those fibers whose connections are first formed—those at a point about a third of a turn from the basal end—remain untwisted. The result of these developments is that the completed nerve trunk assumes the general form of a twist of yarn, with the strands that serve the apex of the cochlea lying at the core and those that serve the remaining portions taking more peripheral positions in turn until at last we have the basal fibers on the very outermost layer.

In the internal auditory meatus the cochlear nerve is joined by the two divisions of the vestibular nerve, the whole constituting the eighth nerve; and also, for a little way, these trunks come in contact with the two parts of the facial nerve, the facial proper and the intermediate nerve. In this intimacy there is, however, little if any intermingling of fibers. As the cochlear and vestibular nerves pass out of the internal auditory meatus into the cranial cavity they rotate somewhat on one another, until (in man) the vestibular nerve takes an oral or anterior position with respect to the cochlear nerve; and it is in this relation that they enter the medulla.

The cochlear fibers run into the ventral cochlear nucleus and then divide into two branches, an ascending (or ventral) branch that continues toward the boundary of the ventral nucleus and a longer, descending (or dorsal) branch that goes to the other of the two primary nuclei, the tuberculum acusticum. As Ramon y Cajal indicated in a preliminary manner, and Lorente de Nó (1) showed in detail, the points of bifurcation of the fibers and also the paths taken by the ascending and descending branches have a remarkable arrangement, as pictured in Fig. 51. The fibers from the apical portion of the cochlea bifurcate soon after they enter the nucleus, but the more basal fibers penetrate farther before doing so, with the result that the branch fibers are arranged in a regular order in their progression through the nuclei.

In their courses within the primary nuclei the fibers give off numerous collaterals; and according to Lorente de Nó every fiber makes connections with each of thirteen distinct regions of the cochlear nuclei. The fibers have terminations of complex form, and of many kinds, and the neurons with which they make connections are of forty or fifty different types. Each cochlear fiber, it is estimated, establishes connections with many hundreds, and perhaps thousands, of cells.

According to Lewy and Kobrak's observations, the fibers from the apical region of the cochlea send their ascending branches to the ventral portion of the ventral cochlear nucleus and their descending branches to the ventral portions of the tuberculum acusticum. The fibers from the middle and upper basal regions of the cochlea send their branches to the more dorsal portions

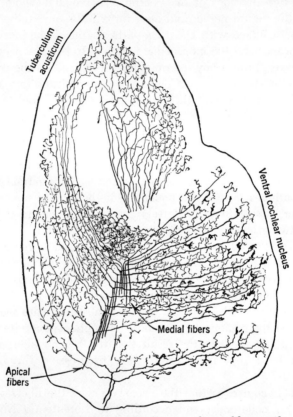

FIG. 51. Bifurcation of the acoustic fibers in the cochlear nucleus (cat). Fibers entering the nucleus from the apical part of the cochlea branch near the bottom of the figure, and fibers from the more basal parts near the middle of the figure. From Lorente de Nó (1) [*The Laryngoscope*] and altered according to his suggestions.

of these nuclei. Fibers from the lower basal end of the cochlea, however, fail to continue this pattern; they show a generally more diffuse distribution. Yet another peculiarity was claimed for the extreme basal fibers. Whereas the other fibers send a small number of branches out of the ventral nucleus and across the medulla through the trapezoid body to end in the trapezoid nucleus on the opposite side, this direct connection beyond the primary nucleus was not observed for the most basal cochlear fibers.

In the primary nuclei it is important to distinguish two types of ganglion cells with which connections are made. There are cells with long axons that carry impulses onward to secondary nuclei and hence are secondary neurons. Then there are cells with short axons that make connections only within the primary nuclei, and in fact form parallel paths between the primary fibers and the secondary fibers; hence Lorente de Nó designated them as 'regulator neurons' and postulated that their activities determine the conductivity of the synapses between primary and secondary neurons.

If we consider the synapses themselves, we find several kinds, according to the neurons involved and the nature of their endings. These are called 'terminal synapses' if the fiber terminates on the cell body or the central arborization of the dendrites and 'collateral synapses' if the fiber only sends one of its branches to a dendrite and continues on to form other connections. The collateral synapses far outnumber the others.

From these neurological observations it is clear that the primary nuclei are the seat of highly complicated operations. On the one hand there is a widespread distribution of the impulses from the cochlea to the thirteen nuclear areas referred to. In these areas the connections formed are sometimes fairly simple, but mostly they are extremely complex. Many synapses are made with the short-process cells, or 'regulator neurons,' which then form parallel chains extending in part to secondary neurons. Then there are multiple connections with certain of the secondary neurons. It is the view of Lorente de Nó that this multiplication of connections has the function of lowering the synaptic threshold; for if a given dendrite receives an impulse simultaneously from each of several axons it is more likely to become excited.

THE PROJECTIONS OF THE PRIMARY NUCLEI IN THE BRAIN STEM

Fibers running out to the primary cochlear nuclei take three principal courses, two of them dorsal and sometimes referred

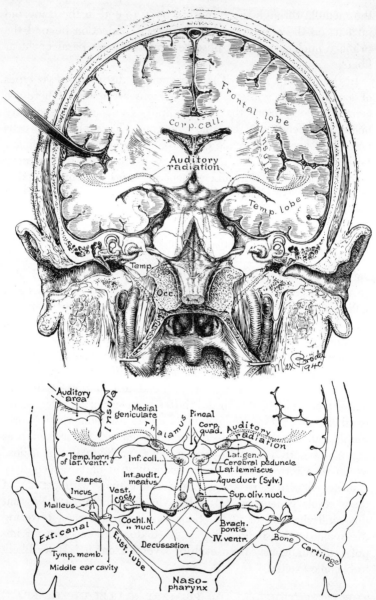

FIG. 52. The auditory pathways in the brain. Drawings by Max Brödel, from the *1940 Year Book of the Eye, Ear, Nose and Throat.*

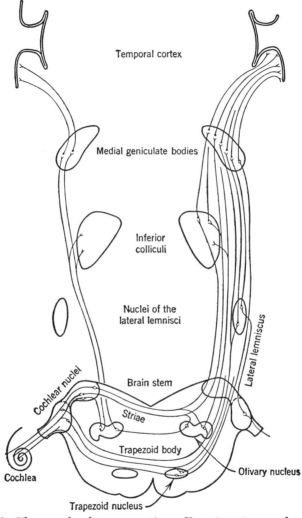

Temporal cortex

Medial geniculate bodies

Inferior
colliculi

Nuclei of the
lateral lemnisci

Lateral lemniscus

Cochlear nuclei

Brain stem

Striae

Trapezoid body

Olivary nucleus

Cochlea

Trapezoid nucleus

FIG. 53. The central auditory connections. For orientation, see the preceding figure; this diagram indicates the connections in greater detail.

to collectively as the dorsal acoustic tract, and one ventral, the ventral acoustic tract. The larger of the two dorsal tracts, known as the striae of Monakow, originates from cells in the tuberculum acusticum (or, more strictly, from its dorsal portion plus the nucleus centralis). The fibers run dorsally near the surface of the medulla and cross the midline in the floor of the fourth ventricle, then penetrate ventrally as far as the superior olivary nucleus, and finally course upward in the lateral lemniscus, which is the acoustic tract to the midbrain and thalamus. Collaterals are given off to the superior olivary nucleus in this trajectory.

The smaller dorsal tract, the striae of Held, arises from the more ventral portion of the tuberculum acusticum (the posterior nucleus) and sends its fibers to the ipselateral and contralateral superior olivary nuclei.

The ventral acoustic tract or trapezoid body arises from the ventral nucleus and the nucleus interstitialis and extends across the medulla. It includes two nuclei, the ipselateral and contralateral trapezoid nuclei. Some of the fibers in the trapezoid body run at once to the superior olivary nucleus of the same side, but most of them cross the midline, and then either end in the trapezoid nucleus or swing upward to enter the lateral lemniscus. On the way many send a branch to the contralateral superior olivary nucleus.

From this account it is plain that the cochlear nuclei provide connections mainly with crossed secondary neurons; in other words there is a heavy decussation of acoustic connections at the lower brain-stem level. There are some ipselateral connections, however, principally through the superior olivary nuclei. As already mentioned, the olivary nucleus is reached by ipselateral fibers from both the dorsal and ventral acoustic tracts; and this nucleus in its turn sends fibers into the lateral lemniscus and to its fellow, the superior olivary nucleus of the other side; and these multiple connections assure the representation of each cochlea on both sides of the brain.

The particular functions of these tracts and centers in the medulla are unknown. It is often suggested that Held's striae and the superior olivary nuclei have chiefly a reflex function. There is no question that acoustic reflex action is one of their roles, for the superior olives are intimately connected with motor nuclei, especially through the nucleus of the abducens nerve by which eye and head movements arise in response to sounds. However, the other portions of the system also are in close relation with motor pathways, and a special emphasis on the olivary complex in this regard may not be justified.

The lateral lemniscus, carrying fibers from all the acoustic nuclei, runs upward in the brain stem. In its path is a further nucleus of a diffuse type, the nucleus of the lateral lemniscus, in which some fibers end and where new fibers arise both to relay messages onward and to connect with other nuclei in this upper brain-stem region.

The lateral lemniscus ends in the inferior colliculus and the medial geniculate body. Some of its fibers go only to the inferior colliculus, but more of them send a branch to this nucleus and have their main ending in the medial geniculate body.

The inferior colliculus is regarded as a midbrain center for acoustic reflexes. It is closely connected with the motor areas of this region chiefly by way of the superior colliculi. Numerous fibers run from the inferior colliculus to the adjoining superior colliculus, which is a relay station for optic responses, and there connections are made with the tectothalamic and tectospinal tracts which control various motor activities. Other fibers from the inferior colliculus connect with the contralateral superior colliculus and thereby afford indirect cross connections between the two acoustic pathways. The inferior colliculus also sends fibers into the medial geniculate body.

The medial geniculate body is the thalamic auditory center. In it all incoming fibers end, and their impulses then are transmitted by way of the auditory radiations to the cerebral cortex.

THE CORTICAL PROJECTIONS OF THE ACOUSTIC SYSTEM

From the medial geniculate body the auditory fibers turn laterally and run through the ventral portion of the internal capsule outward to the superior temporal convolution of the cerebrum. Their arrangement in this course is fan-like, with the handle of the fan at the medial geniculate nucleus and its body lying in the horizontal plane. In the primates, the fibers end mostly on a part of the cortex that is hidden from external view:

on the dorsal, infolded lip of the superior temporal convolution, which forms the floor of the Sylvian fissure. Only a few fibers reach the free surface of the superior temporal convolution. In lower mammals the auditory area is in a corresponding position but is largely exposed to the outside, simply because there is less development of neighboring cortical tissue.

The auditory radiations observe a notable regularity of arrangement. They maintain a radial position, with their bundles distinct, not appreciably mixing with one another or with other fibers near which they pass. According to Poliak, the fibers from the dorsal part of the radiations reach the more dorsal end of the Sylvian fissure and those from the ventral part go to the oral end of this fissure, with other regions in order between.

Poliak obtained no evidence of communication between the two auditory radiations by way of the corpus callosum.

The orderly features of the cochlear innervation and the projection of the acoustic fibers in the primary nuclei, and, at the other end of the system, the simple arrangement of the cortical radiations, have prompted many to postulate a specific character for the acoustic connections as a whole, in which every cochlear element has its own exclusive representation on the cerebral cortex.

In this postulation the middle link of the acoustic chain, that from the primary nuclei to the medial geniculate body, is passed over lightly, for in this portion of the network a corresponding orderliness of pathways has not been demonstrated. Such orderliness may indeed exist here, and it is necessary, owing to our incomplete knowledge of the areas, to leave the matter undecided. On the other hand, as we have seen, the peripheral connections are orderly only in part: in the cochlea the systematic distribution of the radial fibers is cut across by the extensive and seemingly uncomposed arrangement of the spiral fibers. Then in the medulla where these fibers terminate the situation is still further complicated; there is evidence of a difference in the connections of basal and other cochlear fibers, which led Lewy and Kobrak to question the functional unity of the acoustic system. And everywhere—and this is the most compelling feature that our examination of the acoustic neurology discloses—there is an impressive, almost bewildering, degree of diffuseness and intertwining of connections. Though this complexity does not preclude a systematic spatial representation of cochlear activity, it undeniably must limit and encumber such a representation.

THE EFFECTS OF LOCAL LESIONS OF THE ACOUSTIC NERVOUS SYSTEM

For further information on the specificity of the acoustic nervous connections we turn to functional studies, in which measurements are made of hearing losses as a result of local lesions of the acoustic nervous system. If there is cochlear specificity and a point-to-point projection of cochlear endings, then the localized destruction of nervous elements at any level ought to impair hearing for particular tones.

CEREBRAL LESIONS

In consideration of this problem by far the greatest attention has been directed to the cerebral cortex, possibly because a demonstration of specific function here must necessarily prove its existence at all levels below.

Preliminary to an investigation of specificity it is necessary to demonstrate that the cortex is essential for hearing, or at least for some aspect of this function, and to identify the auditory area concerned.

That the cortex, and more particularly its temporal portion, is essential for hearing in man is shown through observation of a very rare condition known as cortical deafness. This form of deafness appears only after a loss of temporal cortex in both hemispheres. The loss of a single temporal lobe, or even an entire cerebral hemisphere, occasions no significant alteration of hearing in either ear. Threshold acuity, the differentiation of sounds, and comprehension of speech are retained without obvious departure from the normal. Figure 54 shows audiograms obtained in a patient after the right cerebral hemisphere had been removed in an operation for tumor; and considering the person's physical condition at the time of the tests the acuity is remarkable. This observation proves not only that each cochlea is represented in both hemispheres but that the representation is equal or practically so on the two sides.

Since the cochlear projection is bilateral, a cortical deafness can arise only from destruction of both right and left temporal areas; and as these two areas are well separated in the brain it is rare for both to be destroyed while enough of the surrounding cortex is left to support distinctive reactions or consciousness

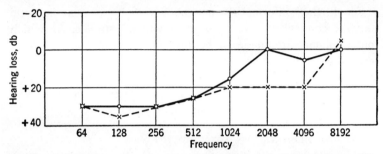

F𝚒𝚐. 54. Auditory acuity after loss of the right cerebral hemisphere. The solid line represents the right ear, and the broken line the left ear. The zero line shows the average normal acuity, but experience with tests on seriously ill persons proves that any score above the 20-db loss line represents good sensory function. This patient could not bear a firm pressure of the receiver on the ear, which perhaps accounts for the low-tone losses. From Bunch [*Journal of the American Medical Association*].

itself. A case of this type was described by Bramwell. A woman after two cerebral attacks became totally deaf, and later, after her death, an examination of the brain showed extensive disease of the left hemisphere including the temporal lobe, and a more restricted involvement of the right temporal area. A few other cases of like character have been reported (see Mills).

These observations show that the temporal region of the brain is essential for human hearing. In the animals below man, however, the brain is less specialized. Several experiments have demonstrated that simple acoustic reactions remain after bilateral destruction of the temporal areas or ablation of the entire cortex. Decorticate animals respond to sounds by pricking up the ears, erection of hairs, and general bodily movements. Cats prepared by Bard and Rioch, in which nearly all the cortex was removed, responded to even rather faint sounds by turning the ears and head and sometimes by walking toward the source. One of their animals was able on occasion to follow a person about a room, evidently guided by the sound of his footsteps.

In the experimental animals, learned reactions to sounds are lost as a result of removal of the temporal areas but can be re-acquired. Surprisingly enough, the relearning after operation is no more difficult than the original learning. Also, as Wiley showed for rats, animals deprived of the auditory areas before any training has taken place can acquire an auditory habit as readily as normal animals. If, however, the destruction extends beyond the temporal regions, and involves a considerable mass of the cortex, the learning then is impaired, and roughly in pro-portion to the magnitude of the destruction.

Immediately after the operation in which the temporal lobe lesions are made the animal usually is found to have suffered a loss of sensitivity, responding only to rather loud sounds, but as time passes the sensitivity is slowly regained until at last it is the same or nearly the same as before. Sometimes, as in French's experiment on monkeys, there is no loss at all. The suggestion is that a temporary dulling of responsiveness can arise from surgical shock or other incidental effects of the operation.

From these results it is clear that in the animals below man simple reflex and conditioned reactions to sounds can be handled by subcortical centers. Less is known regarding the more com-plicated acoustic functions. Studies by Rosenzweig and by Raab and Ades showed that cats deprived of the temporal cortex can respond to a change of intensity level in an intermittent tone. Just as is true for simple sound reactions, the training required to set up a motor response to this intensity change is no greater for operated than for normal animals, and though trained ani-mals lose the habit as a result of operation they can be retrained as easily as before.

As regards pitch discrimination, the serviceability of the lower centers is more in doubt. Some of the early experiments like those of Kalischer seemed to demonstrate a capacity for fre-quency discrimination in dogs without the auditory cortex, but later tests have indicated that these animals probably were receiving unintentional visual or other cues from the experimenter. Johnson's decorticate dogs, which were handled so as to exclude secondary cues, failed to discriminate pitches, though they still oriented to noises.

The investigation of more specific functions of the auditory cortex can be carried out in two ways, by the removal of corresponding local areas in the two hemispheres or by the complete removal of one temporal lobe and specific injuries in the other. Munk used the latter procedure on dogs and reported that injuries to the anterior part caused losses for high tones. Larionow repeated this work and obtained what he thought was evidence of finer localization. These older studies are subject to the uncertainties regarding secondary cues already referred to.

Girden in a modern study employed the method of bilateral extirpations. He removed restricted portions of the acoustic areas in nine dogs and observed the effects upon both threshold acuity and the localization of sounds. He tested with six tones at octave intervals from 256 to 8192 $\sim$ and found that acuity was seriously impaired immediately after the operation but returned progressively (without requirement of further training) until at the end of the tests it was essentially normal or but moderately dulled. However, these changes were unequal for the different frequencies. In one animal, for example, the first test after operation showed an absence of response to 256 $\sim$, a 39 db loss for 512 $\sim$, and losses of the order of 61 to 73 db for the higher tones. On the following day this picture had radically changed; responses to the 256 $\sim$ tone were still absent, but now acuity to the 512 $\sim$ tone had fallen to 52 db below the normal, while the higher tones had recovered markedly to levels 20 to 36 db below normal. In the further process of recovery this striking alteration of pattern continued to appear.

The animal's ability to localize tones was unaffected by some of the operations and abolished by others; here all the test tones gave the same result, so that no differential effect in respect to frequency was revealed.

Because the losses of acuity observed on any given occasion varied from tone to tone, Girden concluded that the cortex functions specifically for different frequencies. It may be so; but in view of the wide variations that he found both in absolute and relative acuity this evidence is hardly compelling.

LESIONS IN SUBCORTICAL CENTERS

The evidence on the functional effects of localized lesions in the auditory nervous system just below the cortex deserves only passing reference. Ades, Mettler, and Culler worked on the medial geniculate bodies and reported rather specific effects from localized bilateral lesions. Kryter and Ades, however, in a later paper gave slight credence to these findings because insufficient attention had been directed to progressive improvements in sensitivity after the injuries. They cut the fibers to the medial geniculate bodies on both sides and found no significant alterations of conditioned acoustic responses; hence it appears that simple reactions to sound are adequately served by centers below the inferior colliculi.

Bilateral removal of the inferior colliculi, in Kryter and Ades' study, produced a loss of sensitivity of 15 db on the average. This loss was often greater for some frequencies than for others, and they suggested that accidental variations in the operation may have caused differential damage to fibers passing upward to the medial geniculate bodies. When the lateral lemnisci were cut just below the inferior colliculi, thereby eliminating all centers above the nuclei of the lateral lemniscus, the responses were seriously altered in character and the thresholds elevated sharply. It appears that the inferior colliculus is the primary subcortical center for simple motor reactions to sounds.

In the course of a variety of these operations, in several combinations both unilateral and bilateral, there were occasional instances of frequency difference like that just mentioned for the inferior colliculi, and the authors considered such results as evidence for a theory of specific projection. It is obvious, however, that much more must be learned before we are able to draw a clear picture of acoustic representation in the subcortical areas.

AUDITORY NERVE LESIONS

In clinical experience there are occasional lesions of the auditory nerve, or tumors in the tissues near by that cause pressure on the nerve and thereby impair its function. Generally, such diseases cause a total loss of hearing or, because they include the adjacent tissues of the cerebellum and brain stem, produce such broad effects that they throw no light on our problem. Occasionally, however, the effects are more specific. A case of interest was reported by Crowe (1). A man whose hearing was limited to only the lowest tones, up to 128 ~, showed after his death a carcinoma in the internal auditory meatus that had obliterated all but a few of the auditory fibers, those supplying the apical portion of the cochlea. This evidence, as Crowe pointed out, indicates that the apical part of the cochlea can serve for the perception of low tones. It does not prove, though, that low-tone perception is localized exclusively there; and Crowe suggested on a basis of these and other results that high tones are fairly well localized both in the cochlea and the nerve, but that low tones are diffusely represented and hence can be transmitted by any undamaged fibers.

Our most valuable information on the effects of auditory nerve lesions in man comes as an incidental product of the surgical treatment of Ménière's disease, in which a partial section of the cochlear nerve is carried out. Ménière's disease is a distressing disorder characterized by periodic attacks of vertigo, often extreme in character, with sensations of whirling of the person or his environment, nystagmus, nausea and vomiting, and sometimes postural disturbances and falling. Commonly, though not invariably, there are auditory symptoms as well, generally referred to one ear: tinnitus, often of a roaring or rushing, noisy type, sometimes hissing or ringing; and an impairment of sensitivity, consisting usually of a general, progressive deafness and noticeable fluctuations of acuity from day to day. The vertiginous symptoms seem plainly the result of an 'explosion' of labyrinthine function; and the auditory manifestations have much the same character. One theory of this disorder is that it results from an overaccumulation of endolymph, which by its pressure excites the labyrinthine and cochlear endings (see Crowe, 2; Hallpike and Cairns; Hallpike and Wright).

In extreme cases of this disease the attacks are so frequent and disabling that operative measures are resorted to. Dandy (2, 4–7) in recent years, following a sagacious suggestion of Charcot made before the days of aseptic surgery, proved that the symptoms cease after division of the eighth nerve on the affected side.

At first, in Dandy's surgical treatment, the entire eighth nerve was severed, causing a complete loss of auditory as well as labyrinthine function on the one side. In many instances, where hearing on this side has already deteriorated greatly and the opposite ear is sound, the surgical elimination of this last vestige of auditory function on the one side occasions no deep concern. In others, however, where serviceable hearing is present on the afflicted side, and especially when the other ear for some reason has suffered a hearing loss, this surgical treatment becomes a serious matter. Then, too, there are cases in which the auditory symptoms are lacking and there is nothing in the clinical picture to indicate which is the affected side (the labyrinthine symptoms are not definitive here). In these cases a selection of the proper side for surgical intervention is a hazardous affair, and it sometimes becomes necessary to operate on both sides. There is a possibility also of true bilateral Ménière's disease. Consequently, Dandy refined his technique so as to sever only the vestibular portion of the nerve and leave the cochlear fibers largely intact.

There is (except in rare instances) no visible demarcation between vestibular and cochlear branches in the short course of the nerve from internal auditory meatus to medulla where the surgical approach is made, but the vestibular fibers lie on the anterior side and make up approximately half the total bulk of the bundle. An incision of the anterior aspect of the trunk therefore was tried and found successful. In this treatment the aim has been to err in the direction of cutting some cochlear fibers rather than to miss labyrinthine fibers that might allow the disease symptoms to continue; and therefore by intention the incision is carried a little farther than halfway through the nerve trunk, and so presumably it includes some fraction of the cochlear fibers. Especially in the early, experimental stage of the partial sectioning technique a very considerable portion of the cochlear fibers was sacrificed. The effects on hearing were learned from careful audiometric tests carried out before and after the operation.

In one patient the section, as judged at the time of the operation, included the greater part of the cochlear fibers. As Fig. 55 shows, the loss of hearing was profound. Whereas before the operation tones from 64 to 5796 ~ were heard, after the operation all the high tones were lost, throughout more than 4½ octaves, and hearing remained only for tones up to 256 ~, and that somewhat dulled in sensitivity.

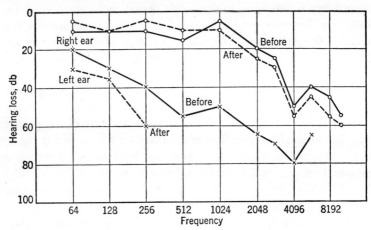

Fig. 55. Effects of eighth-nerve sectioning for Ménière's disease. Audiograms are shown for each ear before and after a partial section of the left nerve. It was estimated that most of the cochlear fibers were severed. After Crowe (2).

In another instance it was estimated that half the cochlear fibers had been cut. Tests made soon after the operation showed a loss of a little over an octave at the upper end of the patient's range, and other tests made four months later indicated a loss of somewhat less than an octave. The highest tone heard before operation was 13,004 ~, and afterward was 8192 ~, but this last tone had suffered a drop of sensitivity of 50 db.

Yet another case is illustrated in Fig. 56. According to the surgical report, about one-fourth of the cochlear fibers were cut. As the audiograms show, acuity was unaffected for the principal range of tones, but tones of the upper octave, above 4096 ~, were no longer audible.

In still other instances no notable changes appeared in the audiograms following the operation. But invariably, when there was change, it consisted in an impairment of the highest tones. Never was there a selective loss of low tones.

An extension of these results has come from animal experiments. Wever and Bray (5), working on cats, studied the effects

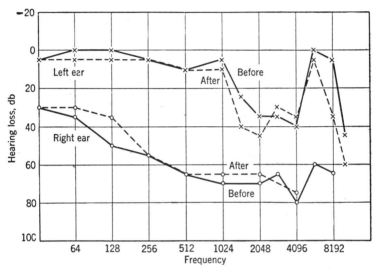

FIG. 56. Effects of eighth-nerve sectioning for Ménière's disease. Results before and after a partial section of the right nerve, which destroyed about one-fourth of the cochlear fibers. After Dandy (4).

of partial sections of the auditory nerve on the audioelectric responses of the medulla. One cochlea was destroyed and an electrode placed in the trapezoid body on that side. Limited lesions were then made in the nerve to the cochlea that remained. Some of these lesions caused no change in the nerve potentials evoked by sounds; others produced a loss of responses to high tones. More drastic lesions led to a general loss of responses. There was never a selective loss for low tones.

More thoroughgoing studies, also on cats, were carried out by Neff. The animals, 11 in number, first had one cochlea destroyed and then were trained by a conditioning method to respond to tones over a wide range of frequencies. These tones were presented at various intensities to obtain a normal acuity curve. Thereupon a partial lesion was made in the nerve supplying the intact ear, and a new test of hearing was carried out. Five animals showed no significant change, while two suffered a complete loss of hearing. The four remaining animals were normal for the low tones but were seriously affected for the high tones, just as was true for some of Dandy's human subjects

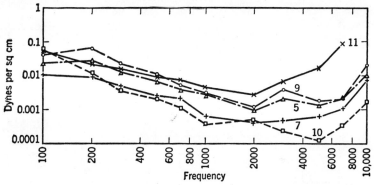

FIG. 57. Cochlear potentials after partial sectioning of the eighth nerve in cats. Curves for five animals are shown, and represent the stimulus intensity required at various frequencies to produce a standard response of 1 microvolt. All these functions are normal in form except No. 11, which shows a loss of sensitivity in the high-frequency region. From Wever and Neff [*Journal of Comparative and Physiological Psychology*].

already reported. The ears of some of these cats were studied further by recording the electrical responses of the cochleas and finally by histological examination (Wever and Neff). The results of the electrical study are shown in Fig. 57. With one exception, the cochlear responses were normal, as was to be expected because the sensory structures were intact. The histological study revealed a considerable variation of neural atrophy, from about ⅖ to nearly complete, in correlation with the hearing loss demonstrated in the conditioning tests. The smaller atrophies, involving up to about half the neural elements, occasioned no loss of threshold acuity; the more profound atrophies, up to ⁹⁄₁₀ or more, gave complete deafness; and the intermediate atrophies gave good low-tone hearing but a high-tone loss.

Figures 58 and 59 illustrate these correlations. Cat 4, as the first of these figures shows, was unchanged in acuity after the operation, yet, as the chart of Fig. 59 indicates, the nerve fibers were absent or seriously reduced through the lower half of the cochlea. Evidently the apical half of the cochlea serves adequately for threshold response over the range tested, which extended from 125 to 8000 ~.

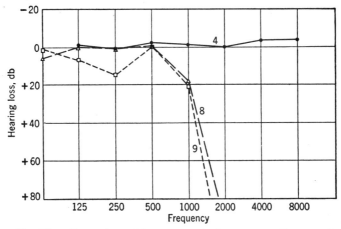

FIG. 58. The effects of partial nerve sectioning upon auditory acuity in cats. The hearing was tested by a conditioned response method before and after the sectioning, and the graphs represent the differences between the two tests. Cat 4 remained normal; cats 8 and 9 lost acuity for the high tones. After Neff.

Cat 8 retained good hearing for the low tones, up to 1000 ~, but was altogether deaf to tones above about 1750 ~. This animal had only slight amounts of neural elements in the basal and middle portions of the cochlea and only a moderate supply in the apical region. The deficiency is especially striking for the ganglion cells. Cat 9 was similar; it possessed hearing only up to about 1500 ~ and showed a corresponding lack of neural elements over the lower portion of the cochlea. Evidently a nerve supply at the apex of the cochlea can serve adequately for a number of octaves of low-tone hearing.

An animal with extreme atrophies throughout the cochlea, like cat 10 of Fig. 59, showed no evidence of hearing.

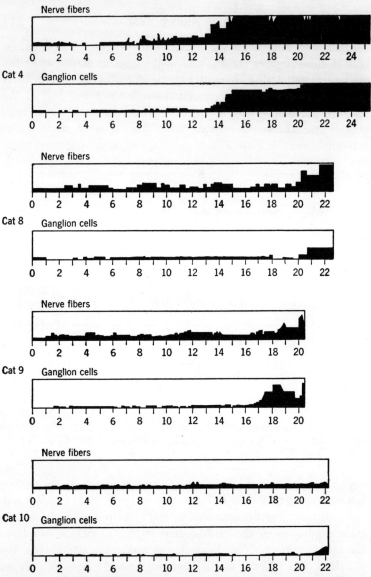

FIG. 59. Histological effects of partial sectioning of the eighth nerve in cats. Results are shown for four ears, the ones whose acuity is represented in the preceding figure and another (cat 10) that was completely deaf. The degree of black filling of the ribbons represents the amount of normal structure present. The scales show distances along the cochlea in millimeters from the basal end. No records are shown for the organ of Corti because in all these ears this structure was normal. From Wever and Neff.

These results are in agreement with the view that there is cochlear localization for the high tones, though not of a highly restricted character. They do not reveal a corresponding specificity of representation for the low tones, but rather indicate that any considerable remnant of nerve can serve for the reception of these tones, at least at threshold intensity.

Further results incidental to this experiment add weight to this conclusion. As mentioned above, and illustrated in Fig. 57, there was one exceptional animal in the group. Cat 11, unlike the others, exhibited an abnormal pattern of cochlear potentials after the sectioning operation. Whether this abnormality was related to the operation or had some other cause is unknown; but in any case the results are pertinent to our problem.

As the figure shows, the cochlear potentials when taken at the 1-microvolt level reflect about the same sensitivity as that shown in the other animals at the low frequencies, but they are impaired at the high frequencies. Beginning at 700 ~ this curve lies above the others, indicating poorer sensitivity; and above 3000 ~ the difference grows increasingly significant. Beyond 7000 ~ the potentials were absent for any stimulus intensity that was considered safe to apply.

Further study disclosed the basis of this abnormality. Whereas in the other ears the sensory structures were normal, in this ear they showed a partial atrophy in the basal region. For a little over 1 mm at the extreme basal end there were no hair cells. Then for about 5 mm farther the inner hair cells were present, except for small gaps, but the outer hair cells were absent. Thereafter appeared a few patchy atrophies involving one or more outer hair cells, but in general the condition was normal, as the diagram of Fig. 60 shows.

These observations reveal that in this ear the cochlear responses for the high frequencies are mainly dependent upon the extreme basal end of the cochlea. More specifically it seems that the first 6 mm (lower 30 per cent) is essential for the tones above 7000 ~, and has a share in the responses to all tones above 700 ~.

We can enlarge this picture of localization by a study of the intensity functions in this ear. In the first place, the impairments found at low levels of response became even more obvious when the level was raised by increasing the stimulus intensity. The abnormality already apparent in the high-tone responses as a reduction in sensitivity was emphasized, because the potentials failed to rise as high as usual: they quickly became overloaded. Thus at 7000 ~ the maximum response observed was only 0.9 microvolts in comparison with the usual maximum of 500 to 700 microvolts.

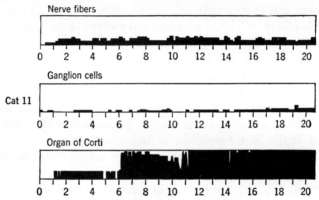

FIG. 60. Histological observations after partial nerve sectioning. Shown here is an exceptional animal, in which the organ of Corti suffered hair-cell atrophies, mainly at the basal end. From Wever and Neff.

In the second place, this situation extended to the low tones. Though at low response levels (as Fig. 57 shows) this ear seemed normal in low-tone sensitivity, it was no longer so at high levels. The intensity functions for these tones, like the ones for the high tones, exhibited overloading relatively early, and the maximum responses were below normal. These facts are clearly brought out by comparing the maximums for this ear with those for another ear of the group (one whose responses are typical of the normal cat), as is done in Fig. 61. The lower curve of this figure expresses the differences in decibels, and they are clearly significant over the whole range, even for the low tones. It is evident that the low tones when strong spread fully into the extreme basal region.

Also included in this figure (in the upper curve) is a representation in decibels of the differences between the two ears at the 1-microvolt level (results already expressed in another form in Fig. 57). Consider now the varying separation of these two curves, which discloses the changing patterns of response for various tones as a function of the response level. The separation is greater for the medium tones than for the high tones; and the reason is that the high tones have response areas that are more sharply peaked, and even at high levels they depend mainly on the basal regions, whereas the medium tones have flatter curves

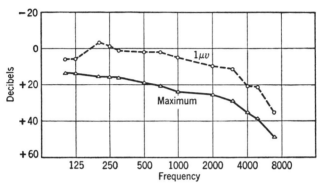

Fig. 61. Comparisons of cochlear responses in a normal ear (cat 5) and in one with partial hair-cell atrophy in the basal region of the cochlea (cat 11). The curves show differences between the two ears. The upper curve represents a comparison made at the 1-microvolt level and gives (in decibels) the differences in sound pressure required to obtain this amount of response. The lower curve represents differences in the maximum responses obtained in the two ears, regardless of the stimulus intensity.

that at low levels mainly occupy the middle and apical regions but at high levels extend all the way to the basal end.

Acoustic Nervous Connections as Shown by Electrical Recording

The problem of the projection of cochlear elements upon the nervous system has lately been approached by electrophysiological methods. Again, as in the study of local lesions, we begin with the more inclusive problem of cortical representation.

LOCALIZATION IN THE CEREBRAL CORTEX

A novel method of exploring the cochlear projection to the cortex was devised by Woolsey and Walzl. They exposed the auditory nerve fibers in the spiral lamina to local stimulation and determined the cortical areas over which electrical potentials could be observed. The experiments were carried out on cats under anesthesia deep enough to depress the spontaneous activity of the cerebrum. The bony capsule of the cochlea was

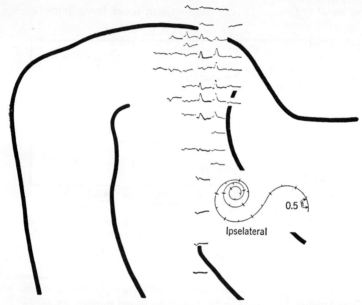

FIG. 62. The cortical projection of auditory nerve fibers (cat). The wavelets represent positions on the cerebral cortex at which potentials were observed on electrical stimulation of the auditory nerve fibers at a point 0.5 mm from the basal end of the cochlea. See Fig. 64 for orientation. From Woolsey and Walzl [*Bulletin of the Johns Hopkins Hospital*].

dissected away, and stimulation at selected spots was effected with a brief electric current applied through a pair of fine wires placed on the edge of the bony spiral lamina. In all, 31 points of stimulation were used. The temporal cortex was explored in millimeter steps with the recording electrode, and the results were mapped on a sketch of the cortical surface.

The record of one series of tests is given in Fig. 62. Here the point of stimulation was 0.5 mm from the basal end of the cochlea. The wavelets shown in the figure represent cortical positions at which responses were obtained, and the size of the wavelets is representative of the magnitude of the potentials. Figure 63 shows similarly the results of apical stimulation, at a position 19 mm from the basal end.

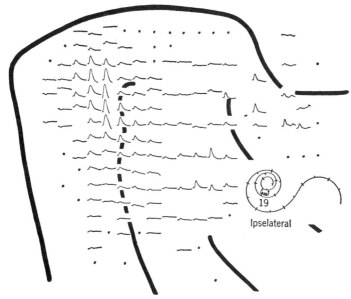

Fɪɢ. 63.   As in Fig. 62, on electrical stimulation at a point 19 mm from the basal end of the cochlea.   From Woolsey and Walzl [*Bulletin of the Johns Hopkins Hospital*].

As will be seen in an examination of these records, the cortical potentials appeared over a rather extensive area.   They show a general focus of activity, and dwindling amplitudes in the surrounding region.   The diffuseness is particularly marked for apical stimulation.   Also, in the latter case, there is a secondary response area to the right and below the primary one.   In some of the trials, especially when fairly strong stimulation was used, a secondary area appeared for basal positions also.

Figure 64 is a composite representation of the results of numerous experiments.   The circles indicate the primary focal areas observed for points of stimulation designated by the enclosed numbers, which express the distance in millimeters from the basal end of the cochlea. Secondary areas are not indicated in detail, but are represented by the cross-hatched region of the figure. The primary projection area extends across the upper ends of the anterior and posterior ectosylvian sulci, with the basal end of the cochlea most strongly represented anteriorly

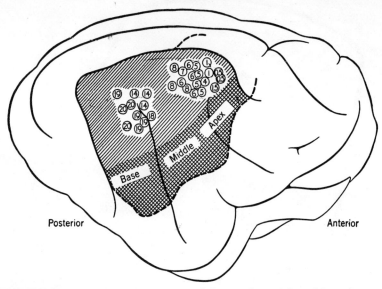

FIG. 64. A composite representation of the Woolsey and Walzl results on the cortical projection of auditory nerve fibers in the cat. The brain is seen from the left side, with its frontal pole pointing to the right. The numbered circles represent the centers of strongest responses as a result of stimulation at points whose distances from the basal end of the cochlea are given in millimeters by the numbers. These circles occupy the primary auditory area. Below, distinguished by cross hatching, is a secondary area. [From the *Bulletin of the Johns Hopkins Hospital.*]

and the apical end posteriorly. The secondary projection area lies below, with this order of representation reversed. It is suggested that this dual representation probably follows a similar duplication of connections in the medial geniculate body.

Clear evidence was obtained that cochlear projection is bilateral, for the same response patterns appeared in either hemisphere on stimulation of one cochlea.

According to the evidence, the diffuseness of cortical projection is only to a minor extent the result of a spread of excitation at the electrodes. The electrode tips were only 0.7 mm apart, and the current ordinarily was kept only slightly above threshold. Moreover, a reversal of polarity of the excitatory shock altered the cerebral pattern. Hence it appears that the areal character of the cortical representation of a single cochlear position arises in a diffuseness of neural connections, and is the result both of divergence in the paths of neural elements initially together and a multiplication of connections by branching and synaptic junctions.

Another electrophysiological method, which has had more extensive use, is to record potentials of the cortex aroused by stimulation with sounds. Most studies of this kind have employed only noises as stimuli, and though they reveal more precisely than any other method of exploration the limits of the acoustic cortical area, they do not appreciably extend our knowledge of specific localization.

The use of tones as stimuli offers greater possibilities. Licklider, in an experiment yet unpublished, observed cortical potentials in the temporal area of the cat in response to tones and reported some evidence of differential activity. A similar experiment on the monkey, by Licklider and Kryter, gave still more definite localization. According to their results the major effects of low tones appear in the anterolateral part of the auditory area and those of high tones in the posteromedial part. Lipman reported similar results on the dog.

More extensive evidence on localization was reported by Tunturi, whose experiments on the dog included stimulation over the range from 100 to 20,000 $\sim$. He found any point within the auditory area to respond to a wide range of frequencies, especially when the stimuli were strong. For weak stimuli—barely sufficient to yield observable potentials—he found areas of activity that overlapped only in part. Figure 65 presents the results. Here two general regions of response are exhibited, one dorsal and the other ventral. The dorsal region, which occupies the middle ectosylvian gyrus, has the focal areas for high tones disposed anteriorly and those for the low tones posteriorly. The ventral region is made up of an anterior portion in the anterior ectosylvian gyrus where the low-tone areas are concentrated, and a corresponding posterior portion in the posterior ectosylvian gyrus for the high tones, with intermediate tones rather sparsely distributed between. The responses to some of the intermediate frequencies appeared to spread into the depths of the ectosylvian sulcus, a region not easily explored. Responses were observed in the ventral region only for stimuli somewhat stronger than those necessary to evoke activity in the dorsal area. Further experiments revealed (in some specimens at

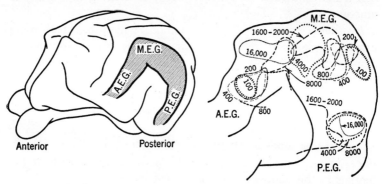

FIG. 65. The localization of cortical responses to tonal stimulation (dog). The outlines show regions within which cortical potentials were recorded on stimulating the ear with short bursts of tones of the frequencies indicated. A.E.G., M.E.G., P.E.G. designate the anterior, middle, and posterior ectosylvian gyri. From Tunturi (1) [*American Journal of Physiology*].

least) a third region at the extreme ventral end of the anterior ectosylvian gyrus where it joins the coronal gyrus. This region, like the ventral region, showed within its boundaries little differentiation with frequency.

LOCALIZATION IN SUBCORTICAL CENTERS

Only a beginning has been made in the electrophysiological exploration of acoustic tracts and centers of the brain stem. Kemp, Coppée, and Robinson recorded from the trapezoid body and inferior colliculus of the cat, and observed that a click stimulus produces a response wave of complex form and that the form of the wave varies somewhat according to the position of the electrode. This form varies also when, with the electrode in the inferior colliculus, some of the fibers of the lateral lemniscus are severed. These observations are interpreted as signifying that the complex wave produced by the click is made up of several components carried in different fibers.

Further evidence for specific response in the inferior colliculus comes from tests in which a pure tone was introduced along with the click. Such a tone produces a modification of the click wave by the reduction or 'occlusion' of one or more of its component parts, and the nature of the modification varies with the tonal frequency. Moreover, the occluding effects vary according to electrode position. An electrode in the superior portion of this nucleus gives a click wave that is most affected by high tones, whereas deeper positions give a wave affected by low tones. It is suggested that fibers representing the various frequencies all run into the posterior portion of the inferior colliculus and that those representing the low frequencies terminate there, whereas others representing the high frequencies pass forward to end in the medial and superior portion.

SPECIFIC RECORDING FROM THE AUDITORY NERVE OR ITS NUCLEUS

We turn now to the earlier stage of neural activity. Here we refer once more to the experiments of Galambos and Davis, in which they recorded from the root of the cat's auditory nerve by means of a microscopic electrode and obtained simple patterns of response which evidently represented single elements. As already suggested, these may have been primary elements, from the cochlear nerve itself, or, rather more likely, they were secondary elements, lying in the cochlear nucleus. In either case the results probably represent the initial pattern of nervous activity caused by a sound.

The stimulation of an element was found to follow a certain preferential pattern. Each element is most readily excitable by some one tone, and when the stimulus intensity is minimal the element may be said to belong exclusively to that tone. But as the intensity is raised other frequencies above and below the nominal one become effective also; and therefore at a high level the element is responsive to a broad frequency band. It follows, as we look at these relations in a converse sense, that a given tone arouses a response in a limited number of elements when its intensity is low and gives an ever more massive and distributed discharge as its intensity is raised.

It is significant that the preferential kind of action described here seems to be limited to the intermediate and high frequencies: no element was ever found that in this sense 'belonged' to the low frequencies. In 43 trials the lowest characteristic frequency observed was 420 ~. Only 4 elements were encountered with characteristic frequencies below 1000 ~, but from that frequency up to about 22,000 ~ the distribution was fairly uniform. If we can assume that the sampling was adequate, and the results representative of the whole population of elements, then here again we have a significant difference in the representation of high and low tones. It is of course possible that the sampling was biased, as perhaps by a spatial distribution of the elements that made it improbable for the electrode to come in contact with a low-frequency element.

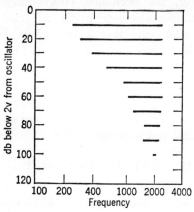

FIG. 66. Range of excitability of auditory nerve elements. A certain element, most sensitive to 2000 ~, was tested at various levels of intensity, and at each level it was responsive to tones over the range indicated by the horizontal line. Note that the spread as intensity rises is mainly toward the low frequencies. From Galambos and Davis (1) [*Journal of Neurophysiology*, courtesy of Charles C Thomas, publisher].

Taking the results at their face value, it appears that the low tones do not have the exclusive use of any elements. They must force the excitation of elements that properly belong to the other frequencies. This they do when their intensities are raised. Figure 66 illustrates the principle. An element most easily excitable by 2000 ~ was responsive to tones over a wider and wider range as the intensity was raised, until at last, at a very high intensity level, it was excited by all tones over a range from 250 to 2500 ~, or about 3½ octaves. Note, however, the asymmetry in the distribution of this range: the extension is about 3 octaves below the characteristic frequency and only ½ octave above it. Plainly, a tone below the characteristic frequency of an element is more favorably situated than one an equal distance above it. The result is that a low tone will readily gather into its response the many neural elements whose characteristic frequencies are in the middle range and above; whereas a high tone will not easily excite elements outside its own frequency region. This is the same difference in the degree of spread of high and low tones that has been indicated in many other experimental situations.

A Review of the Foregoing Evidence

The functional evidence on the problem of cochlear localization shows a consistency that is remarkable in view of the va-

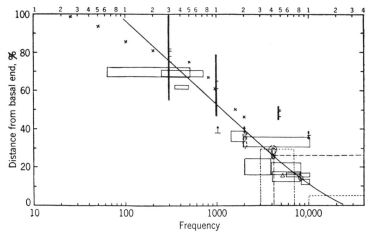

FIG. 67. The localization of tones in the cochlea: composite graph of observations from various sources. Results are included for the guinea pig, cat, and man. For the guinea pig: triangular point (Held and Kleinknecht) and heavy vertical stripes (Wever and Smith). For the cat: solid rectangles (Walzl and Bordley) and short dashed rectangles (Wever and Neff). For man: long dashed rectangles and bar with arrow (Crowe, Guild, and Polvogt), solid circle and oval (Ciocco), and crosses (Békésy, 12).

riety of experimental approaches and the technical difficulties encountered in all of them. Figure 67 brings together the results that are sufficiently quantitative for graphing. Data from work on the cat, the guinea pig, and man are grouped together here, and since the lengths of the basilar membranes vary greatly in these animals the positional scale is in relative terms: in percentage of the total length of the basilar membrane concerned. The data lend themselves variously to representation. Some yield points or small areas whose precision is inversely indicated by their size; others give only general limits, and they are represented by rectangles, or more vaguely still by a boundary line on one side connected with an arrow pointing to the undisclosed boundary on the other side. The four stripes show the results of stimulation deafness experiments.

The general trend of the data is evident, and a simple line is drawn to fit. It is plain that the high tones have their loci in the basal region and the low tones are more diffusely represented toward the apex. The intermediate tones fall naturally between.

The stimulation deafness results, especially for the higher tones, do not fit in well with the others. We must recall that they differ in that they represent the action of tones at maximum intensities, and disclose not the whole area of stimulation but only where it is of destructive amplitude. We may account for the difference in localization by supposing either of two things; either the maximum of response shifts toward the apex of the cochlea as the stimulus intensity is raised, or, perhaps more reasonably, the sensory structures are progressively more fragile toward the apex, and therefore the more apical portion of the heavily stimulated region suffers the greatest damage.

THE RANGE OF COCHLEAR ACTIVITY

It is evident from the above results, and the others of a less concrete character, that cochlear localization is a relative matter, varying in degree in a systematic way from one end of the cochlea to the other. More strictly, we ought to think of the form of the response curve: the relative amount of the action from point to point throughout the cochlea, or the degree of concentration of the stimulus energy; this we must picture rather than the range in a strict sense which we have found (on a basis of the nature of the intensity function for the cochlear potentials) to be always maximal. This aspect of the problem of localization has had far less attention than the primary one of whether localization exists. Certainly there are fewer indications of its character.

There are a few experiments, however, that will serve at least as a basis for an estimate. First to be considered are the observations of Galambos and Davis on the range of excitability of single nerve elements, and the stimulation deafness experiments.

Galambos and Davis found in the studies already described that though a given element responds most readily to a certain frequency it is stimulable also by other tones over a considerable range. The observations are few, but as far as they go they indicate that this range is less the higher the element's characteristic frequency (less, that is, as measured on a logarithmic scale, which is appropriate for the high-frequency range). Thus, three elements were studied in the medium high-tone region and found to have characteristic frequencies of 2000, 2600, and 3700 ~, or an average of 2767 ~, and they responded, at a level 30 db above threshold, to other tones over a range of 1.0, 1.7, and 1.6 octaves, respectively, or an average of 1.4 octaves. Another element, most sensitive to 7000 ~, was responsive at this same level over a range of 0.7 octaves, and still another, with a characteristic frequency of 17,100 ~, responded over a range of but 0.4 octaves.

Further indications on this matter come from the stimulation deafness experiments in which both the stimuli and their effects upon the ear were dealt with quantitatively. The results obtained on guinea pigs by Smith and me, already illustrated in Figs. 45 and 67, are now summarized in Table II on page 260.

This table gives the limits of cochlear injury as shown histologically in the hair cells of the organ of Corti after exposure to the tones indicated, when all the tones had the same sound pressure of 1000 dynes per sq cm. For each of 10 ears these limits are expressed as a percentage of the distance from the basal end, which as usual makes the figures comparable for cochleas of different lengths. As will be seen, the range and locus of the histological changes varied characteristically for the four exposure frequencies. The effects of the 300 ~ tone extended, on the average, from just beyond the middle of the coch-

lea practically to the apical end, or more exactly from the 55.6
per cent to the 99.5 per cent points. Similarly, the average
effects of the 1000 ~ tone extended from the 47.1 per cent to the
79.1 per cent points, and those of the 5000 ~ tone from the 45.9
per cent to the 52.8 per cent points. The one ear mapped after
stimulation with 10,000 ~ showed a small lesion about the 37
per cent point. It is notable that the lower limit of the injury
varies less than the other, yet it as well as the upper limit is
consistently displaced toward the base as the frequency is
raised.

TABLE II. THE EXTENT OF COCHLEAR INJURY IN STIMULATION
DEAFNESS EXPERIMENTS

Exposure Frequency	Guinea Pig	Lower Limit	Upper Limit	Range
300 ~	465 L	47.2	100	52.8
	475 L	62.2	100	37.8
	481 R	54.4	98.7	44.3
	481 L	58.5	99.4	40.9
1,000	441 L	44.5	74.2	29.7
	452 L	49.7	84.0	34.3
5,000	459 R	43.8	50.5	6.7
	459 L	47.2	55.2	8.0
	462 R	46.8	52.6	5.8
10,000	509 L	34.7	39.1	4.4

These results and those of Galambos and Davis are combined
in Fig. 68. The construction of this figure was as follows. The
four points for the stimulation deafness data were first plotted
and a connecting curve drawn. Then the 2767 ~ point from
the Galambos and Davis observations was placed on this curve,
and the points for 7000 and 17,100 ~ were allowed to fall as
shown.

The assembly in this figure of data from the guinea pig and
cat is justified only if these animals have reasonably similar
peripheral mechanisms. There is reason to believe that they
do. Their cochlear response curves are fairly close, though by
no means identical, in form and range of sensitivity. They differ most notably at the extreme low-frequency end, where the
cat is much the less sensitive.

Another approach to this problem is by use of the intensity functions for the cochlear response, functions like the one shown in Fig. 29. The following study was carried out on the guinea pig ear (see Wever and Lawrence, 2). With an electrode on the round window membrane, the functions were determined for a number of tones over the frequency scale, with special attention to the region of distortion. The measurements included only

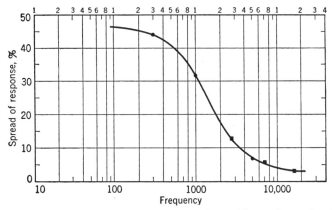

Fig. 68. The relative spread of response in the cochlea. The circles show the width of regions of histological damage after stimulation deafness, and the squares show the relative ranges of excitability of certain neural elements.

the fundamental component and excluded the overtones which appear as a result of distortion. In these functions are two points of special interest in this connection, the point of initial departure from linearity and the point of the maximum. When these points are plotted for a number of stimulus frequencies the results are as shown in Fig. 69.

Consider first the lower curve of this figure, which represents for various tones the magnitude reached by the cochlear response when this response first begins to depart from a linear form. The general function as shown is flat at its lower end and then slants downward, at first rapidly and then more slowly, at its upper end. For the low tones, from 100 to 700 ~, distortion enters at a magnitude of response that is relatively great, around 350 microvolts, and is constant within the error of measurement. Then for all the higher tones this level is significantly reduced, until at 15,000 ~ it is only about 12 per cent of its value for the low tones.

The general function for the maximum responses, shown as the upper curve of Fig. 69, presents much the same form as the other. The maximum responses have a uniform value, around

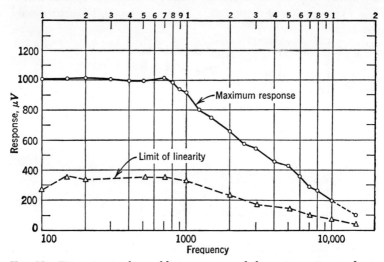

Fig. 69. Distortion in the cochlear responses of the guinea pig as a function of frequency. The upper curve shows the maximum responses and the lower curve the responses at the point of initial departure from linearity, both plotted as a function of frequency. Note that the response scale is linear. The 15,000 ~ point in the upper curve does not represent a true maximum but only the response reached when the series was broken off to prevent damage to the ear.

1000 microvolts, for all the low tones from 100 to 700 ~, and then rather sharply become less and continue to fall as the frequency is raised. At 10,000 ~ the maximum varies in different ears from a sixth to a tenth of what it is for the low tones. In some of the ears the break between the flat part of the curve and the falling portion appeared around 1000 ~ instead of 700 ~ as shown here.

In carrying out this experiment it was found that a determination of a maximum of response for the higher tones is a particularly hazardous undertaking; unless more than usual care is exercised the ear will be damaged. It is necessary to approach the maximum by small steps, and to apply the stimuli only as long as needed to make the observations, and to stop the procedure as soon as the first diminution of response has shown the maximum to have been passed. Some ears will not withstand the tests even with these precautions, but are damaged, and thereafter (though they may recover if left unstimulated for a few minutes) they give unstable results. For the highest tones, beyond 10,000 ~, a true maximum cannot ordinarily be found, for the ear suffers injury while the response curve is still rising.

These results plainly reveal a systematic variation in the pattern of cochlear stimulation as a function of frequency. Let us attempt their further interpretation.

Consider first the problem of the initial departure from linearity. Because we consider the cochlear response as representing the combined activity of many hair cells, we can picture the function of the individual cell as generally similar to the observed function: as linear over the principal range of intensities and then bending at the extreme intensities. However, as the stimulus energy is distributed unevenly over the cochlea, at any given intensity some cells will be stimulated strongly and others only moderately. The cells will be operating at different points along their individual response curves. For a strong stimulus the cells so situated as to receive the most vigorous activation will be operating in the region of distortion, while the others are still operating linearly. It follows that the individual function must bend more sharply in the distortion region as compared with the observed function; the latter is a composite of both bending and linear curves.

The point of departure from linearity reflects the action of the most strongly stimulated elements, those occupying the peak of the curve of action on the basilar membrane. It is the point where the reduced contribution of these elements to the total response first becomes noticeable. It is reasonable to suppose that this reduction grows noticeable when it comes to be some fairly constant fraction of the total response.

Now let us make the assumption that the distortion processes are similar for all regions of the cochlea, and that the individual function for any hair cell shows bending when the local stimulation has reached some particular level. In making this assumption we have to presume a uniformity of elastic properties for the basilar membrane and its structures, including the hair cells, about which serious doubts may be raised; but let us make the assumption provisionally, subject to modification a bit later on.

If we make this assumption and say that every tone at its point of departure from linearity produces the same peak value of mechanical action on the basilar membrane, then we can infer the general form of the action pattern from the magnitudes of the cochlear response. We can do this because up to the critical point with which we are dealing the response in every cell is linear, and the magnitude of the cochlear response represents faithfully the pattern of mechanical activity. So for the low tones, whose responses at this point are large, the mechanical patterns must be broad and flat, with a great many elements in vigorous action. For the high tones, on the other hand, these patterns must be sharply peaked, with relatively few elements in vigorous action. These pattern differences are evident in Fig. 47, which was drawn to represent simultaneously the results of these and of the stimulation deafness experiments mentioned earlier.

As the stimulus intensity is raised further the elements occupying the peak areas of the mechanical patterns will distort more and more and finally will pass their individual maximums. Thereafter an increase in the stimulus intensity will cause these elements to diminish their responses: their further contributions to the total potential are now negative. As the intensity is raised further, other elements near by will be raised high in the distortion function likewise and also will show negative increments. When the negative increments of all these elements just balance the positive ones contributed by the more outlying elements the composite response function will have reached its maximum. Then any further increase of intensity will make the negative contributions paramount, on which the function bends downward. At this point the central elements, exposed the most drastically to the stimulus action, will be in danger of serious injury.

It is clear that the magnitude of the maximum response attained for a given tone will depend upon the form of its mechanical pattern. For a large maximum it is necessary to have a broad and reasonably uniform action, in which many elements reach high levels in their individual response curves before overloading sets in for any considerable number of elements. The low tones evidently produce this kind of pattern. The high tones, on the contrary, have more highly peaked patterns, in which a certain few elements are much more strongly stimulated than the outlying ones. These central elements rise to overloading and bend the response curve over before the outlying elements have become much involved, and so the maximum has a relatively low value.

From the uniform values of the maximums obtained for the low tones it appears that these tones have mechanical patterns of similar nature. These patterns are not necessarily of identical shape, but they are alike in the areal distribution of stimulus action. The curves for 300 and 1000 ~ in Fig. 47 illustrate this relationship; they differ in shape but are alike in the distribution of amplitude that is important here. The higher tones have curves in which the action is progressively more concentrated.

The absence of a true maximum for the highest tones, those beyond 10,000 ~, indicates that for them the area on the basilar membrane occupied by the peak portion of the pattern is particularly small in relation to the outlying area. It appears that for these tones at every condition of intensity the contributions made by elements away from the peak outweigh those of elements at the peak itself; and this relation indicates some peculiarity in the form of the mechanical pattern. The facts suggest, though they do not finally prove, that here we have passed the limit of tuning of the ear, and the mechanical pattern is only the 'tail' of a resonance curve, such as represented in Fig. 21.

The results on maximum responses and on initial departures from linearity give similar indications of the patterning of action in the cochlea, despite the fact that they require somewhat different assumptions in their interpretation. Yet now we have to consider some limiting conditions.

It may be that the actual variation in the mechanical patterns is somewhat greater than these results directly indicate. Two conditions, one in the experimental situation and the other in our interpretations, may operate to make this true. The experimental condition is the place of application of the electrode, which is the round window membrane, a place that favors the recording of the activity of the more basal elements. Because these basal elements principally serve the high tones, the high-tone responses are favored and appear relatively larger than they should. This condition is perhaps more serious for the comparison of points of departure from linearity than for the comparison of maximums, because at the high intensity levels the low tones strongly involve the basal regions as well as the others. But if in either case the high-tone responses have been exaggerated, then we must suppose their patterns to be even more sharply peaked than the results directly show.

The second condition has to do with the assumption of a uniformity of distortion characteristics over the basilar membrane. Let us examine the alternative: that these characteristics vary. A consideration of the cochlear anatomy shows without much doubt that if they vary they do so in such a way as to favor the attainment of relatively large peak responses for the more basal elements. The argument is that the basal portions of the membrane are narrower, thicker, and seemingly more rigid than the others and ought to sustain greater vibratory forces before becoming non-linear. If the basal elements, serving the high tones, are individually producing greater responses at the distortion point than the other elements, then again we must infer that the high-tone patterns are more peaked than the results directly indicate.

These results on distortion, when taken at their face value, indicate that the response patterns for the low tones are 6 to 10 times broader than the ones for the high tones. The data from other sources given in Fig. 68 represent this differentiation as about 12-fold. Here is fair agreement, with some room for the operation of the two conditions just discussed. The distortion data lend general support to our conception of the cochlear patterns, even though their precise quantitative indications remain in some doubt.

These results are for the guinea pig and cat, and it is only with a certain hesitation that we make use of them in a consideration of human hearing. The general similarities in the structure of these ears and ours, and the functional similarities also, give comfort to this extension of the data. Hearing tests on cats and guinea pigs show fairly close resemblances to man, except for a little greater sensitivity to the higher tones and a range of perhaps half an octave more than we have at the upper end.

Perhaps further experimentation will add more definition to this picture of the spread of localization in these animal ears and in man's. The obvious importance for auditory theory calls for such a clarification. Still, the results as they stand probably are not too far from the true ones, and they will be referred to repeatedly in the discussions that follow.

Chapter 11

SENSITIVITY

The volley theory has been set forth in relation to the physical, clinical, and neurological evidence, and up to now its value has been adjudged principally by its consistency in respect to this evidence. Another area of evaluation remains: its performance on the psychological side. Indeed, the ultimate worth of the theory—its very reason for being—derives from its ability to account for the facts of auditory experience. The substance of the following chapters, therefore, will be a consideration of the theory in relation to the phenomena of hearing.

The most basic attribute of the ear is its sensitivity: its ability to make effective use of the minimal amount of vibratory energy. The curve of threshold sensitivity has already been exhibited in Fig. 39. As plotted, on double logarithmic scales, its form is crater-like, depressed most deeply (for the greatest sensitivity) in the region from 400 to 5000 ~ and ascending with great rapidity on either side.

This function is contributed to by each of three sets of conditions, two peripheral and one central. The peripheral conditions are *mechanical*, including the resonances of all the receptive structures from the external meatus to the inner ear, and *electrophysiological*, including the excitatory actions of the sensory cells together with the nervous processes within the cochlea. The *central* conditions include all the processes beyond the ear that lead finally to our perceptions of sounds. These last we know the least about; but the assumption will be made, as already incorporated in the volley theory, that our appreciation of loudness at the threshold as well as beyond depends upon the magnitude of the nervous discharge. More specifically it is assumed that there is a central process through which the series of impulses in many fibers is summated as a quantity of energy to which the loudness is directly proportional.

THE MECHANICAL CONDITIONS

THE ACOUSTIC RESONANCE OF THE EAR

The ear, anatomically considered, is a very complicated device, in that many parts are involved in its vibratory actions, and yet there is reason to believe that these parts are closely coupled one to another so that when driven by a sound they execute the same movements with only minor variations. If any considerable part of the system were able to take up relatively independent motions, in accordance with resonance properties of its own, the result would be a serious dissipation of vibratory energy and also a distortion of wave form. The evidence is to the contrary. Throughout the middle range the ear is almost incredibly sensitive: only a few quanta of energy suffice to excite it. In this range at least there can be little lost motion. Moreover, throughout the frequency range and even for large intensities the fidelity of representation of wave form by the peripheral portion of the ear is remarkable (Wever, Bray, and Lawrence, 1, 2). Accordingly, for the conditions obtaining at the threshold and immediately above, it is reasonable to treat the ear as though it were acoustically simple.

Now, as we know, the behavior of a mechanical vibratory system of simple form is governed by three of its dimensions: by the mass of the moving parts, their elasticity, and the frictional resistance to which they are exposed.

If the ear is such a simple system, then we can express its mechanical actions in terms of just three values, one for each of these dimensions. This means that we are lumping the properties of all members of the vibratory system: drum membrane, ossicles, ligaments, muscles, cochlear fluids, and the basilar membrane with all its parts, each in so far as it enters into the movements. The assumption involved here, that all these properties are invariable with frequency, is no doubt justified except for the last-named part, the basilar membrane. As we have good reason to believe, this structure behaves somewhat differently in response to different frequencies; but it is most convenient at this point to neglect its variations and to come back to their effects a little later on.

A method is available—at least in theory—for ascertaining the purely physical properties of the acoustic mechanism. It consists of coupling the ear, treated as a passive object, to some acoustic system whose characteristics can be determined and measuring the changes reflected upon that system due to the ear's presence. This method was first used by Wegel and Lane in 1923 (Wegel, 2); and they found that at low frequencies, below perhaps 500 ~, the impedance of the ear is predominantly elastic. Thuras and also Tröger verified this observation and obtained further data indicating the mechanical resonance frequency of the ear to be in the neighborhood of 800 ~. Several others * have attempted such measurements, but unfortunately the results so far are incomplete and rather discordant, and fail to delineate in full a mechanical function for the ear. The errors of measurement are large, especially at frequencies away from the resonance point, and certain variations of method are hard to evaluate. The best measurements of this kind were made by Metz, and will be described presently.

If the ear is properly regarded in the simple manner indicated, its behavior will be determined largely by its stiffness at low frequencies (i.e., frequencies well below its resonance frequency), and correspondingly by its mass at high frequencies. If we stimulate with various tones whose velocities are equal in the auditory meatus, the mechanical vibrations which they set up at the hair cells will have a velocity that in the low range varies directly with frequency and in the high range varies inversely with frequency. The stimuli thus will have a maximum effect at the resonant frequency and a progressively smaller effect above and below. An assumed function of this sort, drawn as a 'mechanical resonance curve' is shown as ab in Fig. 70. This is an equal-response curve. It represents the relative amounts of sound required at various frequencies to produce the same response. It is arbitrarily assumed that unit sound pressure (say, 1 dyne per sq cm) produces a standard response (which is any constant, observable velocity of movement) at a frequency of 300 ~; and then according to the function the same response

---

* See Inglis, Gray, and Jenkins; Geffcken; Békésy (7); Waetzmann (2); Kurtz; and especially the review by Metz.

will be elicited at other frequencies by the pressures indicated. The changes of velocity with frequency were taken as uniform except within an octave on each side of the resonance frequency of 800 ~. In this resonant region, where mass and stiffness reactances cancel one another, a considerable amount of frictional resistance is assumed, so that a smooth transition is made

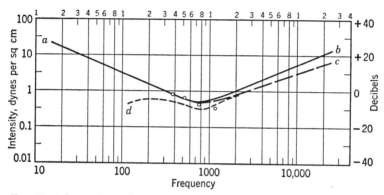

FIG. 70. The mechanical resonance curve of the ear (hypothetical). Curve *ab* represents the simple, uncorrected function, and *ac* represents this function after allowing for variations of mass at the high frequencies. The circles indicate empirical measurements by Metz, and the short-dashed curve (curve *d*) indicates measurements by Békésy. For Békésy's results the left-hand ordinate is to be read in absolute terms, but for the other curves the ordinate values are only relative.

between the right and left branches of the curve and no sharp peak of response appears.

The assumption made in the foregoing discussion, that the mechanical characteristics of the responsive system are constant and do not vary with frequency, is of course contrary to the place hypothesis. Inasmuch as this hypothesis in a modified form is accepted by the volley theory it is now necessary to add a correction to the mechanical resonance curve.

Although according to the volley theory all parts of the basilar membrane respond to every tone, they do not all respond with equal vigor. Most strikingly is this true for the high tones, and the concentration of their action in certain places makes them reflect the local conditions in a significant way. More specifically, the action of these tones will reflect the variations in the mass of the moving structures, and, because as the frequency rises the tonal patterns grow progressively narrower, the mass contributed by the inner ear must grow correspondingly less. The effect of this variation will be to lower the curve of mechanical response somewhat—that is, to improve the sensitivity—but how much is a little difficult to determine. For the present we shall have to be content with an estimate based upon such data as are available.

We have to determine for various tones the mass of the sensory structures in most active movement, and also the mass of the fluid that moves along with these sensory structures. The effect of this variable mass is then assessed in relation to the total mass of the vibratory system.

A comment ought to be interjected at this point, for to include the mass of the fluid in the loading of the ear may seem to follow Lux's theory of loading by fluid columns, already examined and discredited. There is an important difference here, however. The loading is now regarded as a consequence and not a cause of differential tuning. As I have already contended, fluid loading cannot operate to produce a differentiation; yet after it is produced by the differentiation it is reflected in the sensitivity of response.

The data utilized for an estimate of the variations in mass are those of Figs. 67 and 68 on the locus and spread of cochlear action, together with measurements of the dimensions of sensory structures and fluid canals. The calculations are carried out in two stages, the first of which gives the volume and thereby the mass of the sensory apparatus in most vigorous movement and the second of which deals similarly with the fluid columns. Table III shows the successive steps. For the various tones the principal locus, or center of the active region, is obtained from Fig. 67 and is expressed in terms of the percentage of distance from the basal end. The low tones are treated just like the others here, by extrapolating downward the curve of Fig. 67, even though, as has become abundantly clear, any precise localization for them is unwarranted. The procedure serves merely to indicate a general region for them.

TABLE III

Frequency 15 ~	Principal Locus (%)	Spread (%)	Lower Limit of Spread	Upper Limit of Spread	Sensory Structures (cu mm)	Fluid Columns (cu mm)	Total Variable Mass (mg)	Total Mass (Variable + Constant) (mg)	Ratio to Mass at 300 ~	Decibels
15 ~	100	50.5	49.5	100.0	0.331	96.8	97.13	177.13	1.004	0.04
30	100	49.0	51.0	100.0	0.322	96.8	97.12	177.12	1.004	0.04
100	97	46.0	54.0	100.0	0.303	96.8	97.10	177.10	1.003	0.03
200	84	45.0	55.0	100.0	0.296	96.8	97.10	177.10	1.003	0.03
300	76	44.0	54.0	98.0	0.297	96.1	96.39	176.39	1.000	0.00
400	73	43.0	51.5	94.5	0.301	94.6	94.90	174.90	0.99	0.09
500	66	41.5	45.2	86.7	0.286	90.4	90.69	170.69	0.97	0.29
700	59.5	37.5	40.8	78.3	0.247	85.0	85.25	165.25	0.94	0.57
1,000	53	31.5	37.3	68.8	0.195	76.8	76.99	156.99	0.89	0.99
2,000	39	17.5	30.3	47.8	0.085	59.0	59.08	139.08	0.79	2.06
3,000	32	12.0	26.0	38.0	0.049	50.9	50.95	130.95	0.74	2.61
5,000	22	7.0	18.5	25.5	0.021	40.8	40.82	120.82	0.68	3.29
7,000	15.5	5.0	13.0	18.0	0.015	34.7	34.72	114.72	0.65	3.75
10,000	8.0	4.3	5.9	10.2	0.012	26.3	26.31	106.31	0.60	4.14
15,000	3.5	4.0	1.5	5.5	0.010	14.3	14.31	94.31	0.53	5.44
20,000	1.5	3.7	0.0	3.7	0.009	10.0	10.01	90.01	0.51	5.85
24,000	0.0	3.5	0.0	3.5	0.008	9.2	9.21	89.21	0.50	5.93

The next step is to determine the effective spread, also in percentage, as shown in Fig. 68. It is assumed that the spread is equal on either side of the principal locus, except at the two ends of the scale, where it is obviously asymmetrical and has to be measured from one end. So for the low tones, below 300 ~, the apex is taken as the upper limit and the lower limit then determined simply by the indicated distance of spread. At the

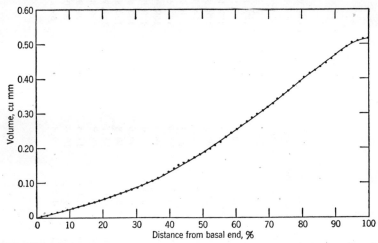

FIG. 71. Volume of the sensory structures, measured from the basal end of the cochlea. Included are all the parts above and below the basilar membrane that seem to be involved in its vibrations. This curve was obtained by a graphic integration of curve *a* of Fig. 19.

other end of the scale the basal end is taken as the lower limit, and the upper limit is found similarly. The limits so derived are shown in columns 4 and 5 of the table.

Now we make use of measurements of the cross-sectional area of the basilar membrane and its associated structures. The area measured includes those portions of the organ of Corti and its supporting cells that lie over the mobile part of the membrane, and also the tympanic lamella below, as indicated in Fig. 5. Such measurements have been carried out in three human ears, but here we shall use but one set, those for ear *a* in Fig. 19. This curve of varying areas was integrated by a graphic method to give Fig. 71, which now expresses the volume of the sensory structures from the basal end to any given point along the membrane. From this graph we read, for each tone, the volume up to the lower limit of effective spread and likewise the volume up to the upper limit, and take the difference of these two values as the volume of sensory structures in most active motion (column 6). The mass in milligrams is equal to this volume in cubic millimeters (assuming a density of 1). This mass evidently varies about 41-fold from 15 to 24,000 ~.

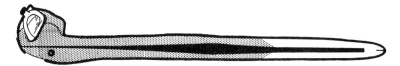

FIG. 72. The cochlea unrolled, to illustrate the idea of fluid masses. The stapes is shown at the vestibular end, and below is the round window. The basilar membrane, thickened to suggest its vibratory motion, separates the scala vestibuli and cochlear duct above from the scala tympani below, except at the helicotrema at the extreme right (apical end). That part of the fluid conceived to be in most energetic motion is shown as dotted. (The little circle in the vicinity of the round window represents the opening of the cochlear aqueduct, which is a communicating tubule between the perilymph of the cochlea and the cerebrospinal fluid.)

Next we determine the fluid masses. Figure 72 will clarify the mechanical situation that is conceived here. The cochlea, unrolled, is drawn to scale, with the basilar partition indicated as in motion in response to a middle frequency. The cochlear fluid is naturally set in motion all the way from the basal end to the place where the basilar membrane is most active, and this motion is indicated by dotting. There will of course be some fluid disturbance farther on, and indeed to the very apex of the cochlea, but its amount is considered negligible in relation to the other.

For this calculation we use the upper limit of principal action as already determined, and for each tone we find the volume of the fluid columns to that point. This calculation is based upon measurements of the cross-sectional areas of scala vestibuli, scala tympani, and cochlear duct, made on the same ears referred to above, and shown in Figs. 73, 74, and 75. Here again we use only ear *a*, for which these areal measurements have been combined and integrated in Fig. 76. From this graph the values of volume for the double fluid column are found and entered in Table III. Again the mass in milligrams is taken as equal to these values of volume in cubic millimeters. These

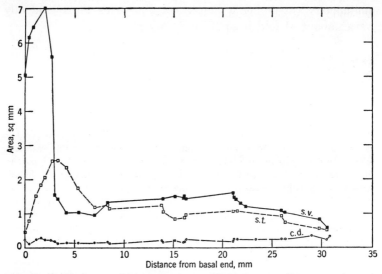

Fig. 73. Cross-sectional areas of the cochlear passages (human ear). *s.v.*, scala vestibuli; *s.t.*, scala tympani; *c.d.*, cochlear duct. This figure represents ear *a*, already employed in other measurements in Figs. 18 and 19.

values vary about tenfold and are so much larger than those for the organ of Corti as to make the latter negligible. Column 8 of the table gives the sums of the two sets of mass values, which now represent the total variable masses.

The effect of this variation in mass for different tones obviously depends upon the total mass of the vibratory system. The drum and ossicles have a mass of about 77 mg, and if we add 3 mg as an estimate of the mass contributed by ligaments and tympanic muscles we have 80 mg as the invariable mass. Column 9 of the table shows the totals after adding on this amount. Now the range of variation has been reduced to about twofold.

The ratios are shown in column 10 with respect to the value for 300 ~. We can translate these variations into sensitivity changes on the assumption that the velocity of motion is inversely proportional to the mass. The variations in decibels are those indicated in the last column of the table and graphed in the broken curve of Fig. 70. The gain in sensitivity from the variation in mass becomes significant only for the very high frequencies, amounting finally to about 6 db.

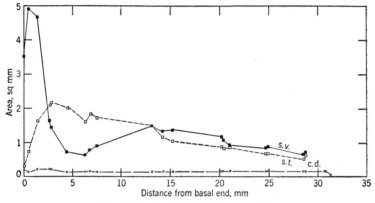

FIG. 74. As in Fig. 73, for ear *b*.

Now, two sets of empirical measurements have been added to the theoretical graph of Fig. 70. The four circular points represent measurements of the ear's impedance made at four frequencies by Metz. As the ordinate values here are only relative, Metz's observation at his lowest frequency, 384 ~, was set on the theoretical curve, and then the other points were allowed to fall as indicated. The agreement is good for the two middle frequencies but poor for the highest frequency; and it is pertinent to mention that Metz pointed out that his results were not very reliable above the resonance frequency.

The short-dashed curve gives the results of two experiments made on specimens of the human ear by Békésy (9, 12) and combined in a manner suggested by Munson (2). Békésy first measured the transmission characteristics of the middle ear apparatus. After dissecting away parts of the inner ear he placed a measuring instrument (a capacitative probe of his own devising) opposite the footplate of the stapes and observed the stapedial movements during stimulation at the drum membrane with sounds. The resulting function showed a diminishing sensitivity as frequency increased, with the most rapid changes beyond 1000 ~. It should be noted that this method required

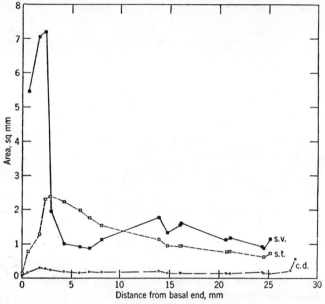

Fig. 75.   As in Fig. 73, for ear c.

the draining of the cochlear fluids, and the natural impedance of the moving parts was altered by this change as well as by any post-mortem variations in the tissues.

In a second experiment Békésy exposed portions of the cochlea, and under suitable magnification observed the movements of the basilar membrane as a result of driving the stapes at various vibration frequencies. The peak amplitudes of basilar membrane movement found for the different frequencies gave a function in which there was a fairly regular improvement of sensitivity with frequency. Again it is necessary to bear in mind the possibility of post-mortem changes.

When these two sets of results are combined they give a general mechanical response curve over the range of 120 to 2000 ~ as shown in the figure. These results are in absolute terms and are so plotted against the left-hand ordinate. The main part of this curve has practically the same form as the

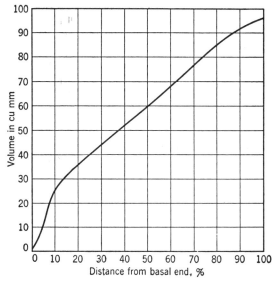

FIG. 76. The volume of the cochlear fluids (contents of scala vestibuli, scala tympani, and cochlear duct), as measured progressively from the basal end. Obtained as an integration of the curve of Fig. 73 (for ear *a*). (To obtain distances along the cochlea in millimeters, multiply the abscissa figures by 0.315.)

middle portion of the theoretical curve, and if it were raised about 2 db it would give good coincidence with that curve. The lower end, below 300 ~, exhibits a downward curl away from the theoretical curve; but this variation perhaps can be attributed to the removal of the cochlear fluid in the first experiment, which by relieving the middle ear mechanism of a part of its normal stiffness may have caused an artificial raising of the low-tone sensitivity.

In general, the empirical data give a satisfactory agreement with the theoretical function. This function, representing a relatively simple conception of the ear's mechanical properties, will serve as a basis for discussion until we can gain more extensive information.

ENERGY DENSITY

The mechanical conditions enter into the determination of sensitivity in yet another way. A sound attains threshold loudness, we suppose, when it excites some minimum number of nerve impulses, and its success in doing so depends not only on the amount of energy applied but on the distribution of that energy. Because nerve fibers have a threshold below which excitation is wholly ineffective it is more advantageous, when the quantity of excitatory energy is small, to focus it on only a few elements rather than to spread it over a great many. The high tones, for which the stimulus action is relatively concentrated, secure an advantage on this account.

TABLE IV. EFFECTS OF ENERGY DENSITY

Frequency	Spread (%)	Ratio to 300 $\sim$	Decibels
15 $\sim$	50.5	1.15	0.61
30	49.0	1.11	0.45
100	46.0	1.05	0.21
200	45.0	1.02	0.09
300	44.0	1.00	0.00
400	43.0	0.98	−0.17
500	41.5	0.94	−0.25
700	37.5	0.85	−0.66
1,000	31.5	0.72	−1.46
2,000	17.5	0.40	−4.00
3,000	12.0	0.27	−5.64
5,000	7.0	0.16	−7.99
7,000	5.0	0.11	−9.44
10,000	4.3	0.10	−10.09
15,000	4.0	0.09	−10.41
20,000	3.7	0.08	−10.75
24,000	3.5	0.08	−11.00

The magnitude of this effect can be determined if we assume that at threshold the variations of stimulus pattern have the same general form as indicated for strong tones in Fig. 68. We then

can assume further that the effectiveness of a quantity of energy
at threshold varies inversely with the spread.

The calculations of this effect made use of the data on spread
already given in the third column of Table III. These data are
repeated in Table IV (column 2) and are converted first into
ratios (column 3) and then into decibels, again with respect to
300 ~. The results are plotted in Fig. 77 as the relative amount
of energy that has to be introduced into the ear to give threshold

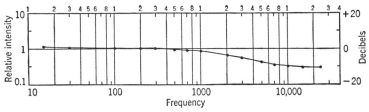

FIG. 77. Effects of energy density. The curve shows the effectiveness
of various tones as determined by the relative concentration of their energy
on the basilar membrane. The function is plotted as the relative intensity
required for threshold response, with the intensity at 300 ~ as the reference
intensity.

excitation, other conditions being equal. It is easily seen that
there is little effect of this condition up to the middle range but
that the high tones gain an advantage that finally amounts to
11 db.

ELECTROPHYSIOLOGICAL CONDITIONS

NEURAL EXCITABILITY

Earlier the hypothesis was advanced that the transmitted vibrations in acting upon the hair cells distort their form so as to
produce the electrical effects that we record from the vicinity
and call the cochlear potentials. As is now well known these
potentials correspond closely to the applied sounds, reproducing
their wave form with great fidelity (except for harmonic distortion at high levels).* It is assumed further that it is these potentials that constitute the excitatory agency for the auditory nerve
terminations. Our next step is to review what is known in the
field of electrophysiology on the stimulation of nerves by intermittent electric currents.

In nerve studies, several kinds of intermittent currents have been used. The most extensive work has been done with square waves and condenser discharges, usually delivered singly but occasionally in a series of several pulses. Some study has been made with alternating waves of sinusoidal form. Very little has been done with pulsating direct currents. It is these last two forms of current, whose effects are least known, that are our chief concern. As has been indicated, the hair cells when stimulated probably establish in their vicinity a pulsating direct field, or, more specifically, a positive field that undergoes sinusoidal variations of magnitude (see page 147 ff.). On the other hand, since the nerve fiber continually lies in the field of polarization it becomes accommodated to the steady component, and its behavior toward the pulsations occasioned by an acoustic stimulus will closely resemble that of an isolated nerve exposed to simple alternating current. Therefore in this situation we can apply rather generally the results obtained with alternating currents, with a particular modification to be considered later on.

According to the classical theory of nerve stimulation by electric currents, a fiber is excited at the cathode when a current is applied, and again at the anode on its withdrawal. Hence with alternating currents we should expect excitation at both the negative and positive halves of each cycle. It has been shown with simple nerve preparations that at low frequencies and fairly high intensity levels this is indeed the case (Schaefer and Göpfert). However, the cathodic excitatory effects are larger than the anodic, and as the current intensity is reduced the anodic response is the first to disappear. With threshold stimulation therefore only cathodic excitations will arise.

The excitatory effects of alternating currents vary with frequency. One of the two primary conditions is the rate of rise of the current. Du Bois Reymond long ago pointed out that any stimulus to be effective must exceed a certain minimum rate of rise. The reason is that the fiber accommodates to the impressed charge, and if the rate of application is slow the fiber compensates fully and no depolarization results. A very low frequency of sinusoidal current therefore will be ineffective unless the amplitude is markedly raised to give the required slope in the current curve. In other words, it is the velocity of the current that is important here.

A second condition of excitation is the duration of the cathodic half-cycle. Work is done upon the fiber membrane in the process of depolarizing it, and an appreciable time is required to carry the process through to the critical stage where excitation occurs. If the duration of the cathodic half-cycle is very brief (as it is for high-frequency stimuli), the strength of the current must be

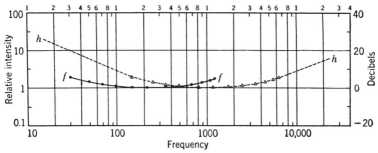

FIG. 78. The excitability of nerves by alternating currents. Curve f, excitability of frog's sciatic nerve at various frequencies, from measurements by Hill, Katz, and Solandt. Curve h, estimated function for human auditory nerve. For each curve the intensity necessary to excite is plotted relative to the intensity needed at the frequency at which the sensitivity is a maximum (220 ∼ for frog's nerve, 1100 ∼ for human nerve).

correspondingly great. The rule is, in fact, that the duration multiplied by the current strength is a constant.

As frequency varies, these two conditions of rate of current change and period of excitation obviously operate in contrary directions in their effect upon sensitivity: the requirement of rate tells against the low frequencies, while the requirement of period tells against the high frequencies. As a result there is an optimum frequency for alternating current excitation.

Curve f in Fig. 78 shows how this excitability varies with frequency for a particular nerve (frog's sciatic nerve) studied by Hill, Katz, and Solandt. An optimum is shown around 220 ∼. In this region the curve is rather flat: the necessary value of current for threshold excitation does not vary greatly here. Well above the optimum this value rises linearly with frequency, and well below the optimum it rises linearly as the reciprocal of the frequency. Hill developed a formula that expresses these relations.

The value of the optimum frequency varies with the nature of the nerve and other conditions, especially the temperature. The optimum of 220 ~ as shown for frog's sciatic nerve was obtained at a temperature of 28° C. The optimum rises with temperature at a rate of about 2.5-fold for every 10° C; hence at man's body temperature this same nerve should have an optimum around 550 ~. For a fast type of nerve like the auditory nerve the optimum might well be higher still. Yet, as Coppée (1) showed, such shifts in the optimum frequency occasion no alteration of form in the excitability function; the curve remains symmetrical about the optimum (as drawn on a logarithmic scale).

Curve *h* of Fig. 78 represents a guess as to this function for human auditory nerve; this curve is simply curve *f* shifted upward in frequency until the optimum falls at 1100 ~—double the calculated optimum for the frog's nerve at the same temperature. The doubling is arbitrary but seems justified in view of the general time differences between frog's sciatic and fast mammalian fibers. The end portions of the curve represent an extrapolation to the upper and lower frequencies made according to Hill's formula.

CATHODIC SUMMATION

Now, the data of Fig. 78 and Hill's formula are based upon the condition that excitation occurs once for every cycle. Therefore the function represented in *h* of this figure requires modification for the upper frequencies where complete synchronism fails and skipping occurs. The modification is in the direction of a lowering of the threshold.

When in repetitive stimulation of a nerve fiber a given cathodic pulse fails to excite, it nevertheless leaves an effect behind (see Hodgkin). This effect, according to Katz, often is twofold. It consists in part of a 'local potential'—simply the lingering depolarization produced directly by the stimulus pulse. It includes also, if the pulse was within about 50 per cent of threshold, a 'local response'—a further depolarization contributed by the nerve itself, and evidently much the same sort of thing as an action potential except that it is not propagated. Both these local changes tend to die away in time, roughly following an exponential curve as shown in Fig. 79.

If now a second cathodic pulse follows this one, it is more efficacious than it would be by itself: its own effects are added to those remaining from the preceding. Such effects can summate over several pulses, until excitation finally occurs.

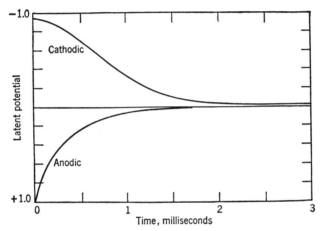

FIG. 79. Temporal course of the local after-effects of electric pulses applied to nerve fibers. The cathodic effects are negative (facilitating further excitation) and the anodic effects are positive (depressive). Data from Katz (1) [*Proceedings of the Royal Society of London*].

An anodic pulse, on the other hand, leaves behind a local potential that represents an addition to the polarization normally present, and hence it is depressive in its effects. This anodic potential, however, is not contributed to by a local response as is the cathodic action.

From these conditions it follows that alternating currents, as they are raised in frequency until skipping begins, will become more effective in threshold stimulation than if they excited in every cycle. The anodic effects only partially counteract the cathodic, and so the response curve falls away from the curve of Fig. 78 and the predictions of Hill's formula in the direction of increased sensitivity.

How much sensitivity can be gained in this summational process is not very clearly shown by direct observations. Some study was made by Hill, Katz, and Solandt with alternating condenser discharges as stimuli. They found only slight improvements of sensitivity as skipping appeared for frequencies up to 2000 ~. However, their stimuli were too brief to permit optimal summation.

Katz (2, 3) later investigated this question more fully, with the use of alternating currents of fluctuating intensities, and obtained gains of sensitivity for all frequencies from about 500 ~ up to the highest studied, which was 10,000 ~. The gains were small at the low frequencies and then progressively larger as the frequency was raised, up to a maximum in the region of 5000 to 6000 ~. Beyond 6000 ~ the sensitivity showed a decline, though only just appreciable in amount. At times, depending upon the preparation and its treatment, the enhancement was as much as 2.5-fold (8 db), but the usual amount was around 2-fold (6 db).

This experiment is fraught with technical difficulties, and Katz was careful to point out that his results are not to be taken too seriously in their quantitative aspects. He worked with frog's sciatic nerve and used the attached gastrocnemius muscle as an indicator of the nerve's activity. It seems likely that this method demanded more continuity of action of the nerve than would be needed for a bare (sensory) threshold. Therefore his indications for summation are probably conservative.

Perhaps a better indication of the possibilities of summation can be obtained indirectly from the after-effects of positive and negative pulses as given in Fig. 79. Calculations made on the basis of these data involved the assumption that the maximum frequency for a single auditory nerve fiber under minimum excitation is 400 ~, and hence that firing occurs on the average at every second cycle from 400 to 800 ~, at every third cycle from 800 to 1200 ~, and so on. Although it matters little in the outcome, it was further assumed that there are no significant effects during the absolute refractory period. In the calculations for the upper curve (curve c − a) of Fig. 80, account was taken of the anodic as well as the cathodic effects, whereas in those for the lower curve (curve c) only the cathodic effects were considered. In either case, as will be seen, there is a marked improvement of sensitivity over the base curve.

It is now necessary to recall that according to the theory presented earlier the hair cells set up a pulsating direct current, and not a simple alternating current. For sensitivity, this kind of current has an important advantage over the other. There are no anodic depressive effects; the residual changes are wholly cathodic. Hence they accumulate at a rapid rate. Curve c of

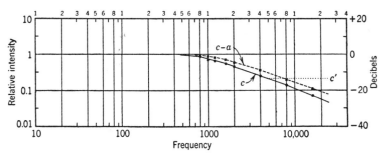

FIG. 80. Effects of neural summation, calculated from the data of Fig. 79. Curve c, cathodic effects only; curve $c - a$, cathodic less anodic. Branch c' shows the course that curve c will take if the summational effect ceases to increase beyond 5000 ∽. The curves show the intensity necessary to stimulate when summation is present, relative to the intensity needed at 300 ∽ and at other low frequencies where summation is absent.

Fig. 80 therefore seems the better indication of the summation.

How high in the frequency scale these summational effects will continue is uncertain. Hill, Katz, and Solandt suggested that a departure from theory is to be expected at the extreme high frequencies on account of capacitative effects, alterations of the condition of the fiber, and the like. Those who have used the highest sonic and the ultrasonic frequencies of current in nerve stimulation have not often had any clear indications of the current strengths, but evidently these have been relatively enormous. We have seen that Katz's function leveled off in the moderately high frequencies and attained a maximum around 5000 or 6000 ∽. It seems reasonable therefore to accept the indications of Fig. 80 only up to this point and to look for a leveling thereafter. The dotted branch, labeled c', represents this expectation. There may even be a turning upward, such as Katz observed in slight degree, but no attempt has been made to indicate it here.

Sensitivity, at the threshold and elsewhere, is a function of two further variables in the nerve response. These are the rate of impulses in the individual fibers and the number of fibers in action. The threshold represents the lower practical limit for these variables; it is probably a discharge of some small number of impulses integrated both over the group of nerve fibers acting and over a brief interval of time. We need to discover how stimulus intensity must vary for different tones to give this threshold discharge. We consider first the variation in the individual fiber.

RATE OF NERVE IMPULSES

In the low-frequency range, where limitations on account of refractory phase do not appear, every nerve fiber is capable of responding at every wave of sound. The rate of nerve impulses will rise regularly in proportion to the stimulus frequency.

As the frequency is raised beyond about 400 ~ the impulses will begin to fall into the relative refractory periods of their predecessors, and then, after a transition period as already described, the response rate in each fiber will fall to one-half the stimulus frequency.

The average rate in an entire group of fibers will show a gradual transition from that at full synchronism, where all fibers carry the stimulus frequency, to the lower rate where each fiber is in fractional synchronism. The transition is gradual because no one fiber makes the change abruptly and especially because the fibers differ somewhat in refractory periods and not all make the change at the same point in the frequency scale. Some fibers will continue to maintain full synchronism when others have stepped down to the lower rate. As the frequency continues to rise there are further drops to lesser submultiple rates, as the volley principle describes. The necessity for a fiber to maintain synchronism even though it skips many waves will lead to some slight fluctuations in the average rate of impulses at the higher frequencies; a frequency near the limit of one submultiple rate is relatively better represented than a frequency a little higher that requires a lower submultiple rate. Apart from these irregularities the rate at the higher frequencies has a fairly constant value determined by the relative refractory period. These relations are shown in Fig. 81. The function is plotted to show that (when other conditions are equal) the sensitivity varies directly as the impulse rate: the higher the rate the less the intensity required to establish a threshold discharge. Through

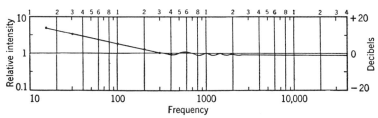

Fig. 81. Sensitivity as a function of rate of nerve impulses. The curve indicates in a relative fashion the intensity required to reach the auditory threshold, on the assumption that the rate of nerve impulses increases with the frequency up to 400 per second and then stabilizes at that rate.

the low-frequency range where full synchronism prevails the rate per fiber increases in proportion to the stimulus frequency, and then, as skipping begins, there are a few minor fluctuations and a final stabilization at the maximum rate.

It is possible that at the threshold these rules are not obeyed rigidly. Doubtless the fibers skip many waves on account of irregularities in the stimulus intensity and variations in excitatory states. However, the relative picture will be as shown.

NUMBER OF ACTIVE NERVE FIBERS

The function just outlined represents the average rate of impulses per fiber, but not the magnitude of the entire nerve discharge. We have still to consider the number of fibers entering into the action.

When the stimulus intensity is held constant the number of active fibers varies with frequency for two reasons: because the different tones vary in their ranges of effective action and because the density of innervation varies in different regions of the cochlea.

The ranges of effective action have already been considered in Fig. 68 and Table III. In the low-frequency region the range is broad and does not vary greatly. Then as the frequency is raised the range narrows, slowly at first and then rapidly, until at the high frequencies it is fairly restricted. These results come from studies of tones of high intensity, but it is reasonable to assume that as the intensity falls the range is narrowed for all tones proportionately, and the relations shown continue to hold at all levels, even at the threshold. We shall proceed on this assumption.

We have now to consider the density of innervation of the cochlea. This problem was investigated in the human ear by Guild, Crowe, Bunch, and Polvogt. They used serially sectioned material and counted the ganglion cells in every fifth section throughout the length of the cochlea. The results were reported as the average number of cells per millimeter for four divisions of the cochlea: the lower basal, upper basal, and lower middle half-turns, and the remaining apical portion. Their averages for 10 ears of normal hearing are as follows: lower basal, 983 cells per millimeter; upper basal, 1215; lower middle, 1144; and upper middle plus apical, 608. The average total number of ganglion cells was 29,024. Similar counts were made in additional ears by these and other members of the Hopkins group, especially by Dr. Mary Hardy, but have not yet been published. Through the kindness of Dr. Stacy R. Guild the original records on 23 ears were placed at my disposal, and the following is an analysis of them.

Before proceeding with this analysis it is necessary to consider certain matters that are basic to this problem. It is desirable to have a more detailed indication of the innervation than by general regions only. Such an indication, however, must rest upon an assumption that there is a close correspondence between the number of ganglion cells at a given level and the number of nerve fibers supplying the organ of Corti at the same level. This means that the ganglion cells at a given level largely send their fibers out to the organ of Corti at that level. There is anatomic evidence that generally bears out this assumption, as given in detail earlier. Most of the ganglion cells send their fibers directly through the radial bundles to end on the adjacent hair cells. The ones that form the intraganglionic spiral fibers, which cross over the radial lines and move apically, are relatively few. So also are the others whose fibers pass through the radial bundles and then take a spiral course, or send off branches that run spirally, largely in a basal direction. Because some of these fibers are dispersed apically and others basally their effects upon the pattern of innervation are somewhat counteractive, and their net influence is largely to broaden the area of diffusion without seriously shifting its locus. The diffusion itself need not be a serious matter, for if it is fairly uniform throughout the cochlea the pattern at the hair-cell level will not depart very far in form from that exhibited by the ganglion cells themselves.

Evidence that the pattern at the level of the radial bundles conforms well to that of the ganglion cells was obtained in the study already referred to on a partial cutting of the eighth nerve in cats (Wever and Neff). An examination of the microscopic sections of these ears, and especially the ones in which the nerve damage was severe, showed a close correspondence in the distributions of the remnants of ganglion cells and of nerve fibers in the radial channels. An example of these results has already been given in Fig. 59.

We now proceed with the treatment of the Hopkins data. On a spiral chart representing to scale the form of each individual cochlea a number of radial lines were drawn connecting the various points along the ganglion with points on the spiral of the basilar membrane, and each count of ganglion cells was assigned to its position on the membrane as so determined. There is no difficulty in doing this for the first three half-turns of the cochlea, but from there on the allocation grows increasingly doubtful. The reason is that the ganglion cells that supply the apical end appear in a cluster in the upper part of the modiolus, and it is not easy to make out their final distribution in detail.

The fact (which is portrayed in Fig. 50) that the ganglion cells are not uniformly distributed in Rosenthal's canal, but have a nodular arrangement, adds only a minor complication. Doubtless this irregularity is fully smoothed out in the diffusion of the innervation already described. The procedure used to handle it here was to sum up the numbers of cells step by step beginning at the basal end and to plot this integrated curve. Such a curve is not very sensitive to local variations.

The points along the membrane where the counts were made were identified in terms of their distances in millimeters from the basal end. Then, since the individual basilar membranes

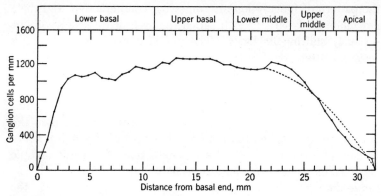

FIG. 82. The density of innervation of the human cochlea. The graph shows the number of ganglion cells per millimeter of length of the basilar membrane. The solid line represents the observations, treated as described in the text; the broken line is possibly a truer representation of the pattern at the upper end. Based on observations on 23 ears by members of the Otological Research Laboratory, Johns Hopkins University.

varied in length, these distances were expressed in percentages of the total length in each instance. Steps of 2 per cent were used, and the data for the 23 ears were averaged. The distances were then reconverted into millimeters, now representing the average length of the cochlea.

The results are given in Fig. 82. This curve indicates that the density of innervation rises sharply in the first three millimeters from the basal end, then ascends gradually to a maximum near the middle of the cochlea. Thereafter there is a slight decline, and then a rapid one over the final third (last 10 mm) of the cochlea. The actual figures, as shown, indicate a slight rise around the 22 mm point, but this is probably an artifact arising out of the difficulty of properly dealing with the apical end, as already mentioned. It is likely, as suggested by the broken line, that the decline is continuous over this apical third of the cochlea.

The maximum density, reached in the 40 to 50 per cent region, is about 1250 cells per millimeter of length. The mean density is about 970 per millimeter.

We now proceed to use these results along with those on the spread and locus of cochlear response to determine the number of active fibers available to various tones over the frequency scale. We use the data on the principal locus of action in Fig. 67 and then by reference to Fig. 82 we find for each tone the density of neural elements at its central position; the results are given in column 3 of Table V.

TABLE V.   AVAILABILITY OF NERVE FIBERS

Frequency	Spread (%)	Density (Ganglion Cells per mm)	Score (Spread × Density)	Ratio to 300 ∼ Score	Decibels
15 ∼	50.5	56.7	2,863	0.063	11.96
30	49.0	116	5,684	0.125	8.92
100	46.0	173	7,958	0.176	7.52
200	45.0	787	35,415	0.785	1.04
300	44.0	1,025	45,100	1.000	0.00
400	43.0	1,100	47,300	1.05	−0.21
500	41.5	1,150	47,725	1.06	−0.25
700	37.5	1,160	43,500	0.96	0.13
1,000	31.5	1,225	38,587	0.86	1.04
2,000	17.5	1,210	21,175	0.47	3.26
3,000	12.0	1,140	13,680	0.30	5.17
5,000	7.0	1,025	7,175	0.16	7.99
7,000	5.0	1,085	5,425	0.12	9.19
10,000	4.3	975	4,192	0.09	10.30
15,000	4.0	432	1,728	0.04	14.15
20,000	3.7	179	662	0.015	18.32
24,000	3.5	15.7	55	0.0012	29.24

If, now, for each of these tones we multiply the figures for innervation density by the spread data we obtain numbers indicating in relative terms the nerve fibers available in the central region of each response position. These numbers bear a direct relation to the sensitivity, because, in line with the assumptions already made, a stimulus must be raised in intensity until it brings forth some minimum number of nerve impulses, and the more plentiful the elements at its peak position the less the intensity required. Again with 300 ~ as the reference frequency these data are expressed as ratios (column 5) and finally in decibels (column 6). They are plotted in Fig. 83.

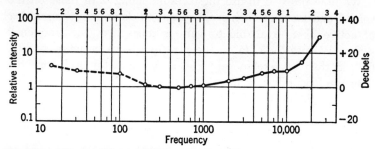

FIG. 83. Effects of the availability of nerve fibers. The curve shows the effects on sensitivity of the relative number of nerve fibers available to stimuli of various frequencies. The threshold intensity rises at the extreme frequencies because the relative number of fibers is reduced.

It will be noted that the factors of energy density and number of active fibers are in part contrary to one another in their effects upon sensitivity. Consider the highest tones, for example. Because the sensory actions of these tones are relatively restricted and the threshold energy is concentrated upon a limited number of sensory and neural elements, these tones are favored in sensitivity. Yet at the same time just because the number of neural elements is small the summation that represents their perceptual effects is correspondingly limited. The first effect represents a gain in sensitivity, the second a loss. That the two do not fully cancel one another in their effects is due to the fact just brought out that innervation density enters into the second and introduces its own regional peculiarities.

THE COMBINED FUNCTION: A THEORETICAL SENSITIVITY CURVE

We have now before us six particular functions that enter into the over-all sensitivity response of the ear: the functions of me-

TABLE VI. SUMMARY OF THE SENSITIVITY FACTORS

Frequency	Mechanical Resonance	Energy Density	Neural Excitability	Cathodic Summation	Rate of Nerve Impulses	Availability of Nerve Fibers	Sums
15 ∼	26.5	0.61	23.8	0	14.3	11.96	77.17
30	20.5	0.45	17.6	0	11.3	8.92	58.77
100	9.7	0.21	7.0	0	6.0	7.52	30.43
200	3.5	0.09	1.5	0	3.0	1.04	9.13
300	0	0	0	0	1.2	0	1.20
400	−2.4	−0.17	−0.7	0	0	−0.21	−3.48
500	−4.5	−0.25	−1.2	−0.5	0.8	−0.25	−5.90
700	−7.0	−0.66	−1.4	−1.0	0.4	0.13	−9.53
1,000	−7.0	−1.46	−2.0	−2.9	0.6	1.04	−11.72
2,000	−1.9	−4.00	−2.0	−7.1	0	3.26	−11.74
3,000	1.0	−5.64	−1.0	−9.9	0	5.17	−10.37
5,000	5.0	−7.99	1.1	−15.2	0	7.99	−9.10
7,000	7.5	−9.44	3.4	−15.2	0	9.19	−4.55
10,000	9.8	−10.09	6.0	−15.2	0	10.30	0.81
15,000	12.0	−10.41	9.4	−15.2	0	14.15	9.94
20,000	14.0	−10.75	11.7	−15.2	0	18.32	18.07
24,000	15.0	−11.00	13.0	−15.2	0	29.24	31.04

chanical resonance, energy density, neural excitability, cathodic summation, rate of nerve impulses, and availability of nerve fibers. They are brought together in Table VI. The data of column 2 come from curve *ac* of Fig. 70, those of column 3 from Table IV, those of column 4 from curve *h* of Fig. 78, those of

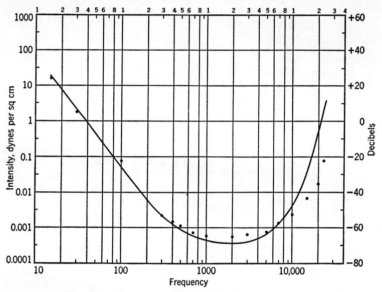

Fig. 84. A theoretical sensitivity function. The points in this graph were obtained from Table VI as the sums of the six factors considered as determining the ear's threshold sensitivity. The curve represents the observed sensitivity, taken from Fig. 39.

column 5 from curve *cc'* of Fig. 80, those of column 6 from Fig. 81, and those of column 7 from Table V. All these numbers are in decibels with respect to an arbitrary base line, and positive values mean a relative raising of the threshold (a reduction of sensitivity), whereas negative values mean a lowering of the threshold. The last column of this table shows the result of combining these data into a single function.

The combined function is represented graphically by the points in Fig. 84. The solid line in this figure is the actual sensitivity curve, already given in Fig. 39. The vertical location of the theoretical function is quite arbitrary; it has been made to coincide with the actual sensitivity curve at 300 ~.

The correspondence with the sensitivity curve is surprisingly good at low and intermediate frequencies but becomes poor at the high frequencies. Possibly there are two reasons for this divergence at the upper end. The data on the spread of response, on which some of the calculations have depended, are derived altogether from work with cats and guinea pigs, and these animals have somewhat better high-tone sensitivity than man. It should be noted that the divergence on this account might be even worse were it not that the spread data enter into both the functions for energy density and the number of available fibers, but in contrary ways, so that the effects cancel in part.

Probably the main divergence arises in the function developed for cathodic summation. As already suggested, this function is most uncertain for the highest frequencies. The calculations made use of the assumption, represented by the dotted curve of Fig. 80, that beyond about 5000 ~ the gain in sensitivity contributed by cathodic summation reaches a maximum which is thereafter maintained steadily. At the same time it was pointed out that this maintenance of summation is not expected to exist in fact; the function was represented so only because there were no clear indications of its further course. For various reasons we must expect that at some high frequency the summational effect will reach a maximum and then decline. We found that Katz in his experiments obtained this form of function, though the decline that he observed (up to 10,000 ~) was only slight. A very considerable loss at the extreme frequencies may well exist. It is reasonable to suppose further that this reversal of the summation function is associated with the other irregularities of neural function whereby the discharge loses its last vestiges of synchronism and becomes altogether random.

The correspondence shown between the derived function and the sensitivity data is enough to give a measure of confidence to the theoretical structure on which the function is based, and to stimulate further investigations of the component variables.

According to this analysis, the character of the sensitivity function is determined quite as much by neural as by mechanical conditions. Especially the great degree of acuity to high-frequency sounds seems to be bestowed by the nervous processes. Wegel (2) on other grounds reached this same conclusion, with the comment, from the standpoint of the acoustical engineer, that "the mechanism of the ear does not have the appearance of a high frequency device."

Because in all the higher mammals the nervous processes can be expected to be much the same, the view developed here accords well with the fact that notable high-frequency sensitivity characterizes the other mammalian ears as well as man's. We do not have many measurements on animals, but we know that in guinea pigs, cats, monkeys, and chimpanzees there is rather close similarity to human hearing, with perhaps half an octave greater range on the high-frequency end. Some others like opossums and bats show even greater high-tone acuity.

We must not of course diminish unduly the role of the mechanical factors, which are obviously essential. To them we may ascribe many of the individual variations of normal human ears: the numerous ups and downs shown in a detailed mapping of sensitivity. To them also we can attribute many of the differences found among the various mammalian species.

CHAPTER 12

LOUDNESS AND FATIGUE

LOUDNESS

From the conditions that govern the intensities of sounds at the threshold we turn to those that operate through the range of practical hearing and determine the phenomena of loudness. The topics to be considered are the loudness function, the variation of loudness with frequency, loudness discrimination, and the relation of loudness to duration.

THE LOUDNESS FUNCTION

That the loudness of a sound grows with intensity is obvious; from weakly audible it passes to uncomfortably loud, and at last to distractingly blaring. It is easy to make rough, general references like these as to how loud a sound is, but it is difficult to discover just what the variation is with physical intensity. The problem has occupied psychophysicists for a good many years, for there are difficulties both of observation and method. The observer must do more than merely judge that one sound is louder than another; he must judge how much louder. This quantitative task is troublesome, and the performance shows wide variations. It is even more serious that different experimental procedures arouse different attitudes, and these may give rather divergent results.

A number of procedures have been tried. One, for example, is the estimation method, in which an observer is given a tone at two different levels and is asked to make a quantitative comparison of the two loudnesses: to say what numerical relation one loudness bears to the other. A second is the fractionation method, in which a tone is delivered at some chosen level and the observer operates a control so as to vary the loudness by some designated amount, as by setting it to one-half its original value. Still other methods have different characteristics and often require special assumptions in their use; one calls for the indication of the midpoint of loudness between two tones, another for the balancing of one tone against two or more in combination, and a third for the equating of a tone in one ear to the same tone in both ears.

All these procedures when carried out systematically show how the loudness changes in relation to stimulus magnitude. Certain manipulations on the basis of such data will yield a scale of loudness. What amounted to such a scale was derived by Fletcher and Munson (1) in the course of development of a method for computing the loudness of complex sounds. Churcher derived one explicitly. He took data that had been obtained by several of the above methods and that he considered consistent enough to be thrown together, and from them constructed a loudness scale.

The method of constructing such a scale is most easily explained by referring at first only to the fractionation data. Suppose we decide, as Churcher did, to designate a reference tone at 100 db above threshold as having a loudness of 100 units. Then we find what level (in decibels above threshold) this tone must have to be judged half as loud as it was before, and designate this loudness as 50 units. Then we find the next lower level, judged half as loud as this second one, and designate it as having 25 units, and so on. Actually, Churcher, Fletcher and Munson, and others who have worked on these scales have used not only the fractionation data but also those available from the other methods and have made the scales to fit all of them as closely as possible. The result of this sort of procedure, if the data hang together consistently enough, is a scale in which the loudness numbers by which any two tones are represented bear the same ratio to one another as their subjective loudnesses.

The loudness scales developed by Fletcher and Munson and by Churcher are given in Fig. 85. These curves show (because they rise progressively in steepness) that a given logarithmic change of intensity is more effective the higher the level of intensity. A rise of 1 db in a strong tone adds more to its loudness than a similar rise in a weak tone. It is apparent that Fechner's law, according to which sensory magnitude is said to rise in proportion to the logarithm of stimulus intensity, does not hold in audition, for if it did the curves of Fig. 85 would be straight lines. The relation shown is in a sense intermediate in form between the linear and the logarithmic: a linear curve that fits well at low intensities will rise too rapidly at high intensities,

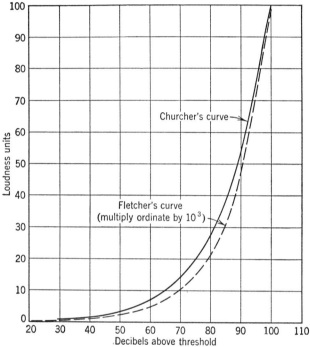

Fig. 85. Loudness scales. The loudness units assigned to a tone at a given level above threshold are designed to be proportional to its subjective loudness. Solid line, Churcher's function; broken line, the Fletcher and Munson function as revised by Fletcher (4).

whereas a logarithmic curve that fits at low intensities will not rise rapidly enough at high intensities.

The figure just shown is a semi-logarithmic graph. A clearer conception of the relations of loudness and intensity can be gained from a plot of both these quantities on linear scales, as in Fig. 86. Now it is seen that in terms of stimulus pressure the loudness of a sound rises rapidly at first and then progressively more slowly.

To discover the physiological basis of this function we must look for a stage of activity in the ear in which a transformation appears from the linear form as existing in the stimulus to a decelerated form as exhibited in the loudness curve. No such transformation appears at the cochlear level. As already shown in Fig. 29, page 147, the intensity function for the

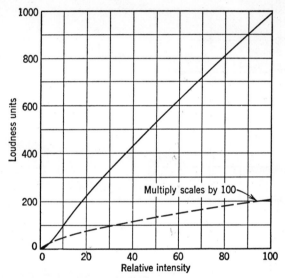

FIG. 86. Fletcher's loudness function from Fig. 85 plotted on linear scales. The portion of the function for the fainter sounds is shown by the solid line, and its extension to the louder sounds is shown by the broken line. A decline in steepness with intensity is just discernible in the solid line, and becomes obvious in the other.

cochlear response is linear at low intensities and remains linear for a considerable range, up to the region of overloading. It is evident that the change of form must arise in the acoustic nerve activity.

According to the volley theory, loudness depends upon the number of nerve fibers acting and their individual rates of firing. It is not necessary to assume that these two factors have equal status, but it is simpler to do so, for then, as already suggested, they combine to determine the composite rate: the total number of impulses carried in the nerve discharge per unit of time.

The variation of firing rate with intensity is indicated by the results of Galambos and Davis on the activity of elements in the root of the cat's auditory nerve. Some of their results are given in Fig. 87. Here are shown curves for four elements, one each

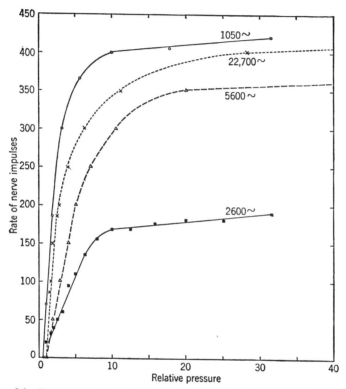

FIG. 87. Frequency of impulses in auditory neural elements, as a function of the intensity of acoustic stimulation. The element stimulated with 2600 ∼ was adapted, the others were unadapted. Data from Galambos and Davis (1).

under stimulation with a tone of 1050, 2600, 5600, and 22,700 ∼. The conditions varied somewhat: the element stimulated with 2600 ∼ was adapted, while the others were unadapted. The curves differ in the level of impulse rate attained, which as expected is greatest in the unadapted elements, and they differ also in their slopes; but the feature of chief interest here is that all are linear for a short distance, and then bend rather rapidly to approach a limiting rate.

A combination of curves of this type, from a number of neural elements acting simultaneously, could readily produce the form of the loudness function. It is only necessary that at each step of intensity, and increasingly so as the intensity mounts, there be a fair degree of dispersion in the activity of the elements, in the sense that they operate at different places along the rate curve. Some must be working in the linear part, and others in the region of bending. Such dispersion of action is just what is expected if the stimulus spreads widely and excites some elements more vigorously than others.

There is more palpable evidence that the dispersion exists. Kemp, Coppée, and Robinson, in recording from the lateral lemniscus of the cat, found different electrode placements to give different intensity ranges: in a sense certain of the elements took up the action where others had left off.

What obviously is needed here is a response curve that represents the combined action of all the neural elements involved in the response to a given tone. Though there is doubt that any electrode placement can record faithfully from all such elements, it is evident that the use of large electrodes, rather than microscopic ones, will approach the complete picture.

Unfortunately, the data available from the use of such an electrode are none too plentiful. There are two sources. Derbyshire and Davis, in recording from the auditory nerve of the cat, used a concentric needle electrode which though small was not microscopic, and while the results were rather irregular they showed in general a decelerated form of intensity function. The same is true of measurements made by Kemp, Coppée, and Robinson with a similar electrode in the lateral lemniscus. Some of the more uniform curves of these investigators are reproduced in Fig. 88.

These curves, it should be noted, show the amplitude of the nerve potential rather than the composite rate. The two are related, but not in a simple way, as the amplitude of discharge of a group of neural elements is determined by the size of the impulses as well as their number. This feature is not necessarily a limitation to the application of the results to our problem, however; it may even be a virtue. It may be that total discharge magnitude rather than the composite rate is the important thing; this point we cannot decide now because we do not know the nature of the final summational process that takes place presumably in the cerebral cortex.

It is plain that these curves approach more closely the form of the loudness function than do the curves for single neural units

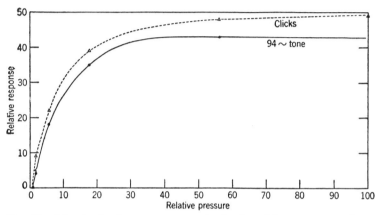

FIG. 88. Magnitude of nerve responses in the lateral lemniscus as a function of acoustic stimulation. Data from Kemp, Coppée, and Robinson.

and that increasing the number of elements recorded from has led us in the right direction. It remains to be seen whether the true nerve function (the function representing all the active elements) has the same form as the loudness curve; if it does, then loudness is fully accounted for, but if not we must look for other processes farther along in the acoustic nervous system.

The loudness functions shown do not extend to the extreme intensities, and the reason is that the very loud sounds are disagreeable to work with. There are some results on very powerful low tones, on which Békésy (8) made observations despite their unpleasant character. He found that their loudness rises to a maximum and then falls away as the intensity is increased. It is probable that the same will be found for all tones, if subjects can be prevailed upon to endure them long enough to make the necessary judgments. This character of the loudness function can be accounted for by the behavior of the cochlear response at extreme intensities, for as previously described this response passes through a maximum and then decreases as the intensity mounts to extreme values.

THE VARIATION OF LOUDNESS WITH FREQUENCY

The loudness function reproduced above was based upon observations on several tones in the middle frequency region, but as variations of loudness with frequency are small in this region the results could be thrown together and taken as a single function, assigned to 1000 ~. It would be possible to work out functions in other regions of frequency in the same manner, yet it is in some way simpler to use a different approach, a method of comparison. If the function given can be taken as the true one for 1000 ~, then the others can be obtained by making loudness balances between this tone and the other tones in turn.

Fletcher and Munson made loudness balances between a 1000 ~ reference tone and various tones over the range from 62 to 16,000 ~, each at several intensities. The results are given in one form (as equal-loudness contours) in Fig. 89, and again in another form in Fig. 90. The graph of Fig. 89 gives a better over-all picture of the results, but that of Fig. 90 is more useful for our present purposes. In Fig. 90 the reference tone is taken as linear, and the other curves represent departures from this form. It is evident that the low-tone curves have a relatively steep slope over most of their courses and then bend somewhat at high intensity levels. The high-tone curves, on the other hand, are straight at first and then at the extreme levels swing upward slightly.

This peculiar behavior of the high-tone curves raises the question whether it may be in a sense an artifact, a product of the choice of a reference tone. For if the 1000 ~ tone and its neighbors really behave like the lower tones and bend over—although to a lesser degree—the higher tones by comparison must seem to swing upward. It is plain that if the results were replotted with one of the high tones (say, 8000 ~) as the reference, then all the high-tone functions would be straight, and the low-tone functions, including 1000 ~, would be relatively steep at first and then bend at their upper ends.

This consideration shows that we need to account for only two features in this set of curves, the differences of slope in the main part of the function and the differences in the bending over at the upper ends. And it is probable that if the observations were extended to the extreme intensities all the curves would show the

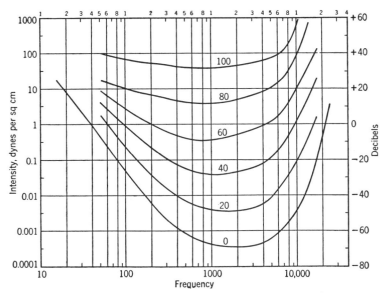

Fig. 89.   Equal-loudness contours.   Each curve represents the intensity required to produce a tone judged equal in loudness to a 1000 ∼ tone whose level above threshold is indicated on the curve.   Data from Fletcher and Munson (1).

bending.   Certainly the cochlear response functions bend at extreme levels for high tones as well as low.

Let us now take up the systematic variations in slope.   Three conditions can be found that operate so as to bring about a relatively more rapid growth in loudness for the low tones, while a fourth condition works in the contrary direction.

1. It will be recalled that low-tone sensitivity at threshold suffers a penalty from the fact that the available energy is spread out over a considerable number of sensory cells, and all but a few of these cells are unable to excite their nerve fibers.   As the stimulus intensity is raised above threshold this loss is recovered,

since for these outlying cells only a little more energy is needed to be effective. Accordingly, for these tones, a stimulus that is carried a little above the threshold will add nerve fibers at a rapid pace compared with what happens for the high tones for which the energy at threshold is more concentrated.

An idea of the magnitude of this effect can be obtained from Fig. 77, now considered in an inverse sense.

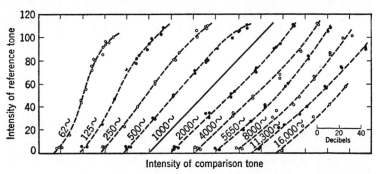

FIG. 90. Loudness functions. Loudness balances were made between various tones and a reference tone, and the results are shown here. The curve for 1000 ∼ is straight because it was the reference tone. The ordinate scale is in decibels above the 1000 ∼ threshold. Each comparison tone is measured in decibels with respect to its own threshold, and the scale shown on the right ought to be placed for each tone with its zero point lined up with the mark near the foot of its curve. The curves have been arranged along the abscissa without regard to absolute sensitivity. These are the data on which Fig. 89 is based.

2. A second condition derives from the patterns of spread and innervation. As the stimulus intensity rises the low tones spread more and more effectively into the basal region of the cochlea where the density of innervation is relatively great. The high tones, on the other hand, do not spread so far and (except at the very upper end of the scale) are in a region of great density to begin with. Hence a given rise of intensity brings in nerve fibers more rapidly for the low tones than for the high tones.

It is possible to obtain a quantitative indication of this second condition from data already given. In Figs. 67 and 68, and the fourth and fifth columns of Table III, we have results on the locus and spread of response of different tones at high levels of stimulation, and from the innervation pattern we can determine, at least relatively, the numbers of neural elements involved. To do so it is convenient first to draw up an integrated curve of

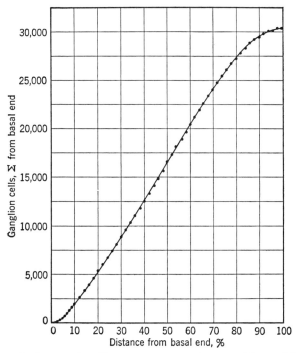

FIG. 91. The density of cochlear innervation, in integrated form. The curve of Fig. 82 was integrated to show the total number of ganglion cells from the basal end of the cochlea to any given point. The percentage distances may be converted to actual distances in millimeters for the average cochlea by multiplying these numbers by 0.3152.

innervation as shown in Fig. 91. This curve indicates the total number of ganglion cells from the basal end of the cochlea to any given point (with the distances expressed in percentage of the total length). Now it is easy to determine the number of ganglion cells up to the lower border of the principal response area of a given tone, and then the number up to the upper border; and the difference is the number contained within the area. This has been done for several tones in Table VII, and the differences are plotted in Fig. 92.

For the tones above 300 ~ this curve closely resembles the one shown in Fig. 83 for the innervation patterns at threshold. The differences below this point represent the gain in loudness accruing to the low tones when a rise of intensity above threshold alters their patterns on the basilar membrane.

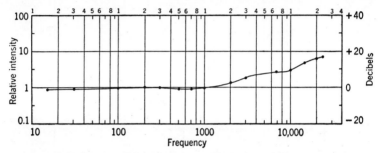

FIG. 92. Innervation patterns for tones well above threshold, and the effects upon loudness. Results on cochlear localization and relative spread have been combined with innervation data to show the effects of the relative number of neural elements available to different tones. The curve is plotted as the relative intensity required to produce a given loudness, other conditions being equal. Compare with Fig. 83; the differences for the low tones represent a relative gain of loudness as these tones are raised above threshold.

3. A third condition is harmonic distortion. Distortion occurs in the cochlea for all tones as intensity rises, but it is more important for the low tones for two reasons. In the first place, these tones (as Fig. 39 illustrates) are already strong in a physical sense when they are barely audible, and this is more true the lower they are. Therefore the amount of distortion—the amount of energy converted into overtones—is relatively large for them. In the second place (and this is the more important circumstance) the greater frequency possessed by their overtones adds correspondingly to the number of nerve impulses excited. Thereby the loudness mounts. This extra steepness in the loudness function that is imparted by the overtones must diminish progressively as frequency rises because beyond some rate the nerve fibers are no longer able to respond at every wave.

The first of these conditions, the bringing in of nerve fibers that are already stimulated near their thresholds, is probably most important over the range immediately above threshold. Thereafter the second and third conditions gain sway and increase their effects as intensity rises until eventually a maximum is reached.

TABLE VII

Frequency	Number of Ganglion Cells	Ratio to 300 ∼	Decibels
15 ∼	14,300	1.15	−0.6
30	13,620	1.10	−0.4
100	12,450	1.01	−0.1
200	12,000	0.97	0.1
300	12,360	1.00	0.0
400	13,190	1.17	−0.7
500	14,620	1.18	−0.7
700	14,020	1.13	−0.5
1,000	12,230	0.99	0.1
2,000	6,800	0.55	2.6
3,000	4,490	0.36	4.5
5,000	2,400	0.19	7.2
7,000	1,660	0.13	8.8
10,000	1,235	0.10	10.0
15,000	490	0.04	14.0
20,000	255	0.021	16.7
24,000	210	0.017	17.7

4. A fourth condition favors the high tones. It is the stepping up of the rate of impulses in a nerve fiber as intensity rises, by virtue of the fact that a stronger excitation can be effective earlier in the relative refractory period. This condition does not operate significantly below about 400 ∼ except for 'marginal' fibers —ones barely above threshold—but above that frequency it grows increasingly more important.

With so many conditions entering into the loudness function it is no wonder that this function is complex in form.

LOUDNESS DISCRIMINATION

Our ability to tell one loudness from another when the difference is small has been investigated many times in the past, yet only two modern experiments have been carried out with adequate equipment and large enough ranges of both frequency and intensity to give a good over-all picture. Knudsen (1) worked with tones over a range from 100 to 4000 ~, and Riesz with a still wider range, from 35 to 10,000 ~.

Unfortunately, both these experimenters used methods of presenting their stimuli that are rather special, and their results are a little difficult to interpret in this relation. Instead of presenting a tone at one intensity and then at another and asking the sub-

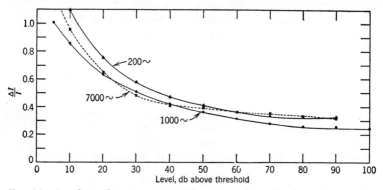

FIG. 93. Loudness discrimination. The curves show, for three frequencies, the values of the relative jnd ($\Delta I/I$) as a function of the level above threshold. Data from Riesz.

ject to indicate the louder tone, which is the conventional procedure, they gave continuously fluctuating tones and had the subjects say whether they perceived the fluctuations or not. Knudsen made the fluctuations sudden, while Riesz made them gradual, and both varied the amount of fluctuation until it became barely appreciable in order to obtain a measure of discrimination. The complication in this method is that, theoretically at least, it involves changes of pitch as well as of loudness, and so possibly provides cues that are extraneous to our present interest (see Kock). Still, for want of any others, these results will be used in the discussion that follows.

Results on loudness discrimination may be presented as the absolute amount of change (ΔI) that is just appreciable, expressed in either acoustic energy or pressure units; or as the relative change ($\Delta I/I$), also expressed in either energy or pressure

units. The first is called the absolute jnd (just noticeable difference) and the second the relative jnd. Riesz gave his data
in the relative form, in energy units. In Fig. 93 some of them,
for 200, 1000, and 7000 ~, are reproduced in the relative form,
but in pressure units. It is seen that as the intensity rises the
relative jnd grows smaller. Beyond a comfortable level of about
40 db the further decline is rather gradual, but it continues to
the very end of the intensity range studied. These results plainly

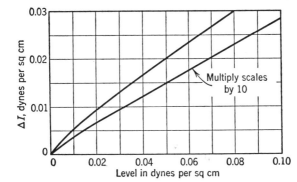

FIG. 94. Loudness discrimination for 1000 ~, expressed as the absolute
jnd (ΔI) and on linear scales. The upper curve shows the early part of
the function, and the lower curve its continuation to higher levels. Data
from Riesz.

deny Weber's law, according to which discrimination as expressed in the relative manner ($\Delta I/I$) ought to be constant.

A better conception of how loudness sensitivity changes can be
gained from Fig. 94, where the results for 1000 ~ are given in
absolute terms, and on a linear scale of pressure. Here it is
shown that the amount of pressure that must be added to a
given sound to be just noticeable is small at low levels and rises
steadily as the level is raised. The rise is a little more rapid at
first than it is later.

Figure 93 already shows that loudness discrimination varies for
different frequencies. The complete picture is presented in Fig.
95, where it is seen that discrimination is poor at the low end
of the frequency scale, then improves steadily as the frequency
rises until the region of 2500 ~ is reached, after which it be-

comes poorer once more. It will be recognized that this region of best loudness discrimination is also the region of the ear's greatest absolute sensitivity.

Why is discrimination the poorest for the low tones? It may be that for these tones, once the threshold is well past, an increase of intensity can affect the nervous discharge in a relatively limited way, apart from distortion effects which are to be

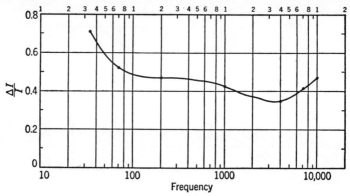

FIG. 95. Loudness discrimination as a function of frequency. The curve shows the value of the relative jnd, $\Delta I/I$, expressed in pressure units. Data from Riesz.

discounted as far as discrimination is concerned. The fibers carrying the fundamental frequency are already operating at the maximum rate—the frequency of the stimulus itself—and increasing the intensity can not change this rate. Increasing the intensity can be effective essentially by bringing in new fibers, and even this process encounters some limitations. The number of fibers is large only a little above threshold, and a good many more need to be added to be appreciable. Then, too, the spread is mainly effective in only one direction, toward the basal end of the cochlea, since it is fair to assume that these tones, especially the very lowest ones, even at moderate intensities fully occupy the apical end. For these same reasons the number of discriminable steps for the low tones is comparatively small.

The extreme high tones, like the low tones, can spread in only one direction, toward the middle of the cochlea, but the other high tones, localized a little distance from the basal end, will not suffer from this restriction. For physical reasons their effective range is relatively small, and there is room for this range to be extended in both directions. Principally these tones encounter a restriction in the variation of nerve impulse rate, just as the low tones do, but for a different reason. For the high tones the fibers are called upon, even at threshold, to respond at very high rates. An increase in intensity can raise this rate, but only slowly because the fibers are working in their relative refractory periods. Some limited measurements by Galambos and Davis are of some relevance to this point. As Fig. 87 shows, they measured the rate of rise of nerve impulses with intensity for three elements under similar conditions of adaptation; the rate was highest for the element stimulated at 1050 ~ and lower for elements stimulated at 22,700 ~ and 5600 ~, in that order. The sampling was too small for firm conclusions, however.

The middle tones encounter fewer restrictions. They are free for effective spread of nerve excitation both up and down the cochlea. They do not so soon, or so seriously, suffer the limitation of refractory phase.

A question that Fechner raised and that has long claimed attention is whether all differences that are just discriminable are subjectively equal. The question turns out to be complicated because there are various ways of defining subjective equality; but one way, which will concern us here, is to say that adding a just discriminable step ought always to raise the loudness of a tone the same amount, no matter how loud the tone was to begin with. Fechner's question when put in this fashion can be tested with the data now at hand. If we begin at threshold and add on one just discriminable step after another, taking account of the fact as Fig. 94 shows that we shall have to vary the physical size of the steps as we go along, we shall be building up a kind of loudness function. This is of course a process of integration. If Fechner's assumption is true, the integrated function ought to look like the psychological loudness function of Fig. 85. Figure 96 shows the result of the integration for 1000 ~, when plotted in semi-logarithmic fashion. Note that over its main course this curve rises less rapidly than the loudness function of Fig. 85. If plotted on linear scales like Fig. 86 this would be a decelerated curve, just as the loudness function is, yet decelerated to a considerably greater degree. The relatively greater steepness of the loudness curve means that loudness grows more rapidly than the number of just discriminable steps. To put the matter another way, a step added to a strong tone raises it more in loudness than a step added to a weak tone. By our definition, therefore, the steps are not subjectively equal, as Fechner thought, but grow larger with the level of loudness.

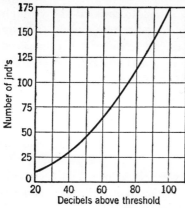

FIG. 96. Integrated jnd's of loudness, for 1000 ~. Beginning at the threshold, the jnd's have been stepped off, taking account of their varying sizes, so as to show the number passed over in reaching any desired level. Compare this function with the loudness function of Fig. 85.

This conclusion of course is no more secure than the results we have on both the loudness function and loudness discrimination. If, for example, Riesz's experiment really contained an extraneous cue like a pitch change, and this cue grew more important as the intensity was raised (as we would expect it to do), then his values for the just noticeable differences are too small, and the more so the higher the intensity level. The integrated function worked up from his data then must show a lower rate of ascent than it should. The disparity with the loudness function could arise as simply as that.

If the loudness function and the integrated jnd curve had turned out to be identical—or if future experimentation establishes their identity—then a theory of loudness discrimination would be merely an extension of our theory of subjective loudness. We could suppose that there is a transformation of the cochlear activity to a decelerated function, and as has been suggested this transformation would probably occur in the process of nerve excitation, and the decelerated function would represent the magnitude of nerve discharge. Then loudness discrimination would be the appreciation of some constant change in this magnitude. If the two functions are actually different then this theory must be made more complex, by assuming that the central processes by which discrimination and loudness arise do not make use of the changes in discharge magnitude in the same way, or utilize different aspects of those changes. The volley theory permits the working out of this sort of possibility because it recognizes two processes, the number of nerve fibers and their rates of firing, as entering into the representation of stimulus intensity, and these two processes can be made use of differently in the central activities. But before we make special assumptions of this kind to complicate the theory we need to be certain that the facts demand them.

One more point is to be mentioned in this connection. As distortion occurs, the resulting overtones undoubtedly add greatly to the loudness, as already suggested, but they probably do not contribute in the same degree to discrimination. Here is a problem that ought to be studied further.

LOUDNESS AND DURATION

Several studies have shown that loudness depends upon duration. A sound is heard but faintly if it lasts only a very short time. Kucharski (2) observed a systematic relation between the duration of a 1000 ~ tone and its threshold intensity: the shorter the duration (up to a limit that he placed at 0.125 sec) the stronger it must be made to become barely audible. Later he worked with other tones of lower frequencies and found this same principle to hold. For these tones, however, the period during which the loudness continued to mount was still more prolonged. This period evidently bears a systematic relation to frequency: the lower the frequency the longer the period of summation.

Békésy (2) worked with tones well above threshold and made loudness comparisons while varying the duration. He found similarly that the effectiveness of a tone grows with its duration, up to a limit that he placed at 0.17 sec, for an 800 ~ tone. The loudness rises rapidly up to the maximum and then undergoes a slight decline as the duration is extended. Békésy's observations agreed with Kucharski's that the high tones reach their limits of summation relatively early.

Buytendijk and Meesters, working with click sounds, observed a development of loudness up to a maximum around 0.2 sec, which agrees well with Békésy's time, and found thereafter a rapid and then a slow fading of the sensory effect over a period of 0.35 to 0.40 sec.

Munson used a 1000 ~ tone presented at durations up to 0.2 sec and found likewise a systematic building up of loudness. Contrary to expectations from the earlier results, however, his function failed to reach a maximum within this span of time, and from its trend it gave evidence that an extension of the observations would show a continuing gradual rise for perhaps as long as a second.

Other studies have dealt with the effects of duration on pitch discrimination (Békésy, 3) and loudness discrimination (Garner and Miller) and with the relation of intensity to the perception of duration itself (Lifshitz). The results are generally consistent with expectations on the basis of the dependence of loudness on duration, and they show that within the range of the interval of summation the factors of intensity and time carry out similar roles.

The more precise nature of the durational effect now claims our attention. The question is whether time, within the period of summation, is simply interchangeable with intensity, or whether a more complex relation holds. The pertinent results are those of Békésy (2, 3), Lifshitz, and Munson (1). Békésy's statements are obscure, but his observations during a limited period seem to be in agreement with Lifshitz, who chose the first of the above alternatives and said that time operates just as intensity does in the determination of loudness. This means, more concretely, that the acoustic power is directly integrated over the time, and the loudness represents a further operation performed on the product so obtained. Munson on the other hand found that his results, and those of Békésy as well, were better fitted by adding two further conditions, one a dissipation factor and the other an adaptation factor. The dissipation factor represents the supposition that whatever physiological product appears through the action of a quantity of intensity does not linger indefinitely but fades away in time in a characteristic fashion (described by a simple exponential). The adaptation factor comes from Galambos and Davis' observations of the dwindling frequency of impulses given off by a neural element during the ear's exposure to a steady stimulus. Munson's formula incorporating these assumptions gives good agreement with his observations.

It is well attested that the integration of acoustic power that we are dealing with here is a neural and not a sensory process. In the first place, as Munson pointed out, the length of the summational period is too great for any mechanical process to continue in the receptor. Furthermore, we have the positive evidence that the integration is not to be seen in the cochlear potentials.

On the other hand this kind of summation is well known in the action of nervous elements. It is easily observed in the excitation of nerve fibers and especially of neuronic chains involving synapses. The longer summational periods are characteristic of the synapses.

We cannot positively identify the process either in the nerve fibers proper or their synapses by which an accumulation of excitatory effect takes place. Current theory speaks of the accumulation of ions at membrane surfaces, or a concentration of chemical substances, or a combination of such processes. Yet, whatever the process, we may be sure that somewhere in the auditory nervous system the impulses aroused by a sound have a cumulative effect, within the span of a second or less, and the loudness we perceive depends on the magnitude of the effect so built up.

AUDITORY FATIGUE

For a long time the problem of auditory fatigue has been vexed with uncertainty and controversy; some investigators denied its existence altogether, and others were able to observe it only fleetingly and in slight degree. Certainly in casual observations, as on listening to a continuing, constant sound, we are not conscious of any fatigue effect. Nevertheless by suitable procedures an effect can be demonstrated. It can be shown either as an elevation of the threshold or as a reduction in the loudness of a sound in the fatigued ear as compared with the other ear that has been left unexposed.*

The important conditions are the frequency, intensity, and duration of the fatiguing tone, and the particular susceptibility of the ear under test. As expected, the amount of fatigue in-

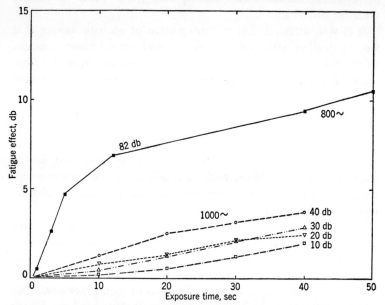

FIG. 97. Fatigue of the ear as a function of tonal duration. The intensity in decibels above threshold is indicated on each curve. The fatigue effect, in decibels, is the elevation of the threshold resulting from the exposure. Data for 1000 ~ from Caussé and Chavasse, and for 800 ~ from Békésy (2).

creases with the intensity and duration of exposure. For a moderate intensity of stimulation, up to 40 db above threshold for a 1000 ~ tone as Caussé and Chavasse observed, the increase is approximately an exponential function of time—the function gives a simple line when plotted in decibels, as shown in the four lower curves of Fig. 97. Békésy (2) used 800 ~ and an intensity about 40 db higher (10 dynes per sq cm) and obtained

---

* Some in dealing with changes of sensitivity resulting from stimulation prefer to speak of 'adaptation,' but 'auditory fatigue' is the traditional designation.

a different form of function; his curve, shown in the upper part of this same figure, rises much more rapidly during the first 15 sec and then settles down to about the same slope.

It is notable that clear fatigue effects arise with levels of stimulation only a little above threshold, as shown by Caussé and Chavasse. These authors were of the opinion that many of the

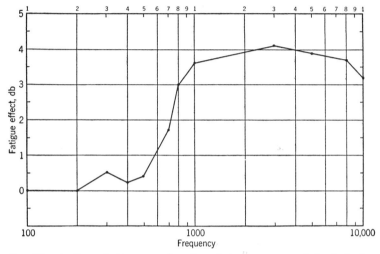

Fig. 98. Auditory fatigue as a function of the frequency of the fatiguing tone. Only the high tones, above about 600 ∼, are clearly effective. The effect is measured as an elevation of the threshold. Data from Caussé and Chavasse.

discrepancies that appeared in the earlier experiments came from the use of sounds of unduly great magnitude. Such sounds, they pointed out, bring in the early stages of stimulation deafness, and therewith give changes not truly ascribable to fatigue.

When the stimuli are moderate a significant relation to frequency is revealed. Figure 98 shows the results obtained by Caussé and Chavasse for various tones presented at 30 db above threshold and for equal periods of time (probably 30 sec). The lowest tones are quite ineffective, and all up to 500 ∼ give only dubious and unreliable indications of fatigue. At 640 ∼ a marked effect is found, and the curve rises swiftly with the frequency to an amount of 3 or 4 db for all tones over 1000 ∼. The curve rises further to a maximum at 3000 ‿, but it is doubtful if the variations in the high-frequency range are significant.

Also of interest are the numbers of persons who suffered any fatigue at all in the different regions of frequency. The numbers rise from none at 100 ‿ to 29 per cent at 500 ‿ and then suddenly to 84 per cent and more for the higher frequencies. The largest individual differences in fatigability appear for the frequencies just below 500 ‿.

Other experiments, like those of Rawdon-Smith, Pearce, and Davis and his associates (Davis, Morgan, et al.), likewise indicate prominent fatigue effects for the high tones, but they sometimes show low-tone fatigue as well. To do so, however, they employ very strong stimuli, and it is at least likely, aside from the possibility of entrance of trauma, that in such cases it is the overtones both in the stimuli and generated in the ear that are responsible for the effects.

Recovery from fatigue seems fairly rapid under usual conditions. After stimulation is at an end, if only moderate intensities were used, the ear returns to its normal state of sensitivity in about a minute. The period is lengthened when the stimuli are made more burdensome.

Of particular theoretical interest is the specificity of the fatigue effect, which is studied by exposing the ear to one tone and then testing with various other tones above and below. Again the level of stimulation is important: at low levels the effects are fairly specific, whereas at high levels they are more general. The results of Caussé and Chavasse, obtained at three frequencies, 1000, 3000, and 8000 ‿, are given in Fig. 99. The over-all ranges of these curves, in absolute terms, are 220, 450, and 450 ‿, respectively. Because the end points of the curves are not very precisely determined a better comparative measure is a reduced range, as, for example, the range within which the curve exceeds 37 per cent of its maximum value, and this range is 108, 234, and 264 ‿, respectively, for the three frequencies. Though these values as expressed in cycles show a rise with the frequency, the distances that they span on a logarithmic scale grow progressively smaller, as the figure shows.

Békésy fatigued with 800 ‿ at the much higher level of 10 dynes per sq cm for 2 min, and observed effects over a wide range, from 200 to 4000 ~. Similarly, Rawdon-Smith with 2000 ~ and similar conditions of intensity and duration obtained effects well beyond the fatiguing tone itself, and especially at the octave above. Davis and his associates, using still more

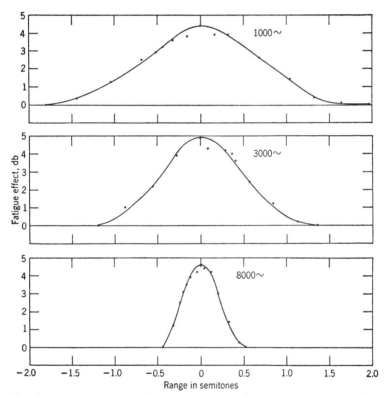

FIG. 99. The specificity of the fatigue effect. The curves show, for three different fatiguing tones, the range of frequencies over which a dulling of sensitivity results. The scales are logarithmic. Data from Caussé and Chavasse.

intense stimuli, as high as 135 db above threshold and for periods up to 64 min, observed a general impairment of acuity that amounted to as much as 60 db and extended over several octaves. Though these probably are not simple fatigue effects but a combination of fatigue and injury, they prove how extensive is the action of a powerful stimulus.

The fatigued ear resembles an ear that is suffering from nerve deafness, in that it manifests the behavior called 'loudness recruitment' (see page 366). The impairment of its acuity is prominent when tests are made with stimuli at threshold and levels immediately above, but it is noticeably less as the level is raised. Both Békésy and Davis and his associates, on making loudness balances between the two ears after fatiguing one of them, found that the impairment that is obvious at the lower stimulation levels largely vanishes at the higher levels. Just as in nerve deafness, the fatigued ear catches up with the normal ear as the stimulus intensity is raised, so that strong stimuli sound almost equally loud in both. At the high levels the equal-loudness contours for the fatigued ear are nearly flat and only moderately displaced above the normal contours.

We now come to the question of the nature and locus of the fatigue process. There is no doubt that the process is peripheral, at least in a general sense. It is confined to the stimulated ear and its particular neural elements. This fact is shown by experiments in which one ear was exposed and tests of sensitivity carried out on the opposite ear. The work of both Békésy and Caussé and Chavasse gave no evidence of contralateral effects. A dissenting opinion was voiced by Rawdon-Smith, who obtained some changes in the contrary ear, but it seems likely that under his conditions sound leakage caused a direct fatiguing of the opposite ear.

Pattie added further evidence that the fatigue is peripheral, or at any rate is not due to such central processes as attention. He stimulated both ears equally, but adjusted the phase of the stimulating tone so that to the subject the sound seemed to be present in only one ear; and under these conditions he found no difference in the fatigue effect in the two ears. From this experiment and a number of others that showed a displacement of localization after one ear was fatigued we have a fair indication that the site of the fatigue process lies peripheral to the binaural localization process.

We know on the other hand that the fatigue process is not in the extreme periphery. It is not due to contractions of the tympanic muscles, as some have supposed. These muscles indeed have the power of reducing the sensitivity, but in a very different fashion. Their effects are not confined to the region of the stimulating tones. Also when they contract they affect the sensitivity in both ears, not just in the ear stimulated; this is true because their reflex control is bilateral. Finally, their contractions are not smoothly sustained but diminish as the stimulation continues because the muscles themselves grow fatigued.

That fatigue does not enter anywhere in the middle ear or early cochlear processes is shown by its absence in the cochlear potentials. When in an experimental animal the action of the tympanic muscles is excluded by the use of curare, and adequate precautions are taken to maintain good physiological condition, the potentials produced by a sustained tone do not fall off in magnitude. It is of course necessary in this experiment to avoid stimuli of an extreme intensity, for these indeed will overtax the ear and either temporarily or permanently impair its electrical responses. Such stimuli evidently were used by Hughson and Witting to produce what they called auditory fatigue; but theirs is not the effect under consideration here. Even after an animal's death, though the cochlear potentials decline progressively, their rate of decline is not accelerated by stimulation (Wever, Bray, and Lawrence, 6). Hence we conclude that up to the cochlea, and indeed to the place within it where the cochlear potentials are generated, there appears no process that is subject to exhaustion by normal stimulation. The fatigue process lies somewhere beyond.

We have indicated the site of fatigue as between the electrocochlear activity and the binaural localization process. Fatigue therefore seems to be an early neural process. The resemblance found between an ear under fatigue and one suffering nerve deafness lends strength to this conclusion. The other features of fatigue—its temporal course in growth and recovery, its intensity relations, and the prominence of individual differences—are all consistent with its nervous origin.

A theoretical explanation of the fatigue process can now be formulated. As envisaged in the volley hypothesis, the rate of impulses conveyed by a nerve fiber is determined by three conditions: the frequency of the excitations, their magnitude, and the excitability of the fiber. In the problem before us we are concerned primarily with progressive changes in this third condition. We know that if a fiber is called upon to respond early in its relative refractory period its subsequent activity is affected: its refractory period is somewhat prolonged, and, more important still, its excitability is impaired. Moreover, these effects are cumulative over a period of time. Therefore as the fiber is overcrowded its impulses continually diminish in rate. Galambos and Davis observed this change in their single-unit recordings. The whole volley of discharge, in which many fibers are undergoing this same decline, accordingly suffers a shrinkage in magnitude.

It is now clear why the low tones are not subject to fatigue, or only when presented at extraordinary levels of intensity. Their excitations come so well separated in time that the nerve fibers recover fully after every impulse and the train of activity is undiminished. Fatigue enters only beyond that critical frequency where the fibers begin to be pushed into their relative refractory periods. This frequency will vary somewhat with the intensity level prevailing. The evidence cited shows that for tones of an intensity level of 30 db the critical frequency is in the region of 500 ~. Tones below that frequency occasion little or no fatigue. As the frequency is raised above that point the fatigue effect mounts rapidly, because the responses of the fibers are being forced earlier and earlier into their relative refractory periods. The rapid rise is ended as the absolute refractory period is reached and skipping of impulses begins, which at this intensity evidently occurs around 1000 ~. Thereafter the fatigue effect remains on a high level, no longer subject to any systematic frequency variation because all the fibers now are in rotational activity. Some minor variations in individual fibers may be expected with changes in ratio between the periods of stimulus and refractory phase, but in the aggregate activity of large groups of fibers these will largely be ironed out.

In the upper frequency range where volley action prevails, just as in the region immediately below, the fatigue increases with intensity because the fibers are brought into action more often and so are more frequently subjected to the depressing effects of forcing.

CHAPTER 13

PITCH AND PITCH DISCRIMINATION

Pitch is formally defined as the qualitative aspect of auditory experience which extends in a continuum from the lowest audible to the highest audible tones. Though it is indeed a continuum, in that no interruptions or critical changes appear, it is easy to observe certain qualitative differences along the range. The low pitches are undulating or vibrant: a periodic character is a matter of direct experience. The middle pitches, on the contrary, are smooth and continuous; perceptually they carry no hint of periodicity. The high tones have still a different quality, best described as shrill and piercing. It seems likely that these qualitative variations arise in the different modes of representation of tones in the auditory nerve response: frequency for the low tones, place for the high tones, and both for tones of the middle range, as already described.

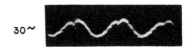

FIG. 100. Auditory nerve responses for low tones (guinea pig). The figure shows the cochlear potential curve for 30 ~, with the nerve potential in the form of sharp spikes superimposed upon it. From Wever, Bray, and Willey.

More specifically, the representation is thought of as follows. For the low tones the stimulation is practically in phase for all parts of the basilar membrane, and the nerve fibers are stimulated almost simultaneously. Also, differences in latency of the fibers are of little consequence in relation to the periods of the waves. The result is that the volley is an abrupt one and occupies only a fraction of the total period, as may be seen in Fig. 100. Discontinuity is then a neural characteristic. As the stimulus frequency is raised the volleys come to scatter relatively and to occupy more and more of the period of the wave, and then the perception smooths out. Still later, with the high frequencies, the dispersion extends over more than a period, and the pitch

327

must depend altogether upon another condition, the particular nerve fibers acting.

THE LIMITS OF PITCH PERCEPTION

It is first necessary to make a clear distinction between a lower limit of pitch and a lower limit of frequency sensitivity; they are by no means the same. The statement that the pitch scale ends around 15 ~ does not mean that for lower frequencies nothing is heard. The lower frequencies give rise to auditory sensations of a complex, noisy character, much resembling the chugging of a reciprocating pump heard from a long way off (Wever and Bray, 5). The sound is made up of numerous components, of rather high frequencies estimated as well over 1000 ~. Curiously enough, as the stimulus frequency is varied downward from the region of 15 ~, the pitch of the noise pattern seems to rise. Audibility extends at least to 5 ~, and Békésy (8) has reported observations down to 1 ~. It is evident that the perception of noise when the ear is stimulated with sinusoidal waves below 15 ~ depends upon distortion: a transformation within the ear of a portion of the stimulus energy into higher components.

The low-frequency sensitivity functions obtained for both pitch and noise are indicated in Fig. 101. The branch labeled 'noise' is taken from Békésy's study in which the 'auditory threshold' was determined over the range from 1 to 100 ~. The branch labeled 'tone' is based on observations made by Vance and Brecher and is not very precisely determined.

If the sensitivity function given in Fig. 39 were included here it would run between the two curves shown. The tone curve at first follows its direction and then curls upward to approach a limit around 15 ~. The noise curve gradually pulls away in the direction of greater sensitivity. The tone curve suffers from a withdrawal of energy from the fundamental component and a swamping of this component by the overtones. By the same token the noise curve benefits from the ear's greater sensitivity to these distortion products.

The rapid change in the form of the tone curve at its low-frequency end determines rather critically the lower limit of pitch perception. Let us consider further the evidence that this change results from the entrance and rapid rise of distortion in the ear. Distortion is more nearly related to the absolute intensity of a tone than its level above threshold. More exactly, the distortion depends upon the intensity prevailing at the site of the distortion

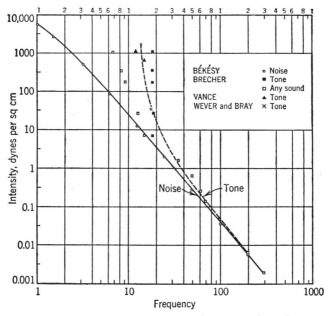

Fig. 101. Sensitivity to low frequencies. The curves show the intensities required to give thresholds of tone and noise. Data from various sources as indicated.

process, and so it represents the stimulus intensity after modification by the mechanical resonance of the ear. Sensitivity on the other hand reflects other processes, mainly neural, as we know. Hence it follows that as the stimulus frequency is lowered and the intensity is raised to compensate for the falling sensitivity the distortion level rises relatively rapidly, and a point finally is reached where distortion is present in appreciable amount when the tone is barely audible. As the intensity is raised further the distortion increases rapidly. Each overtone component rises more rapidly than the fundamental does; in fact, such a component rises as a power function of the sound pressure with an exponent equal to the order of the component: the second harmonic increases as the square of the pressure, the third harmonic as the cube, and so on (Wever, Bray, and Lawrence, 3). At the same time this emphasizing of the distortion products is carried still further on account of the ear's changing sensitivity function, which favors the higher components.

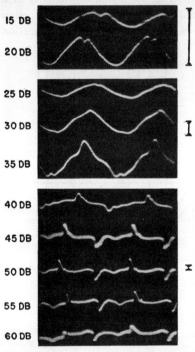

These effects may be seen in the cochlear potentials. For low tones the responses show appreciable distortion even at moderate levels of stimulation—levels of the order of the human threshold (Fig. 102).

Complications in the action of low tones appear also in the neural responses. When the imposed stimuli are strong these responses may contain more than one volley of impulses per cycle. In the simplest case there are two discharges in a cycle, one larger than the other, one near a peak and the other near a trough, as shown in Fig. 103. No doubt the double frequency represents the first overtone which has arisen through distortion in the ear.

FIG. 102. Low-tone distortion. Cochlear responses to a 15 ~ tone at various intensities. For each curve the intensity is indicated in db above 1 dyne per sq cm by the number to the left. The amplification varied for the three blocks of curves, and is indicated by the vertical lines to the right; each of these lines represents the deflection produced by a response of 250 microvolts. Nerve spikes may be seen in the uppermost traces. (The human threshold for this tone is around 60 db—1000 dynes—according to the indications of Fig. 101.) From Wever, Bray, and Willey.

The upper limit of hearing, as previously mentioned, lies in the region of 24,000 ~ for young persons of unimpaired hearing.

Like the lower limit, it varies with intensity, but only slowly, as the sensitivity curve here is particularly steep. This limit, unlike the other, is the terminal point of sensitivity; beyond it nothing at all is heard.

It is apparent that the upper limit of pitch is much more simply accounted for than the lower limit. It results from the concurrent failure of the various receptive processes, both mechanical and neural. In contrast, as we have seen, the lower limit of pitch lies in the midst of prominent distortion processes.

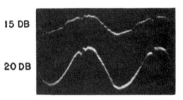

15 DB

20 DB

PITCH DISCRIMINATION

Our ability of pitch discrimination is measured as the least difference in frequency between two tones that is barely appreciable. This is in practice a statistical quantity, and its value depends somewhat upon particular psychophysical procedures and treatments of the data. Also it depends upon the frequency region of the tones, their intensity, and the individual capacities of the observer.

FIG. 103. Nerve responses to low tones. The curve shows a cochlear potential wave on which nerve spikes are superimposed. Those at the peaks are obvious, but those at the troughs are barely discernible as a thickening of the trace. (They were easily perceived visually but were too small to photograph well.) The stimulus tone was 60 ~, at an intensity of 10 dynes per sq cm. From Wever, Bray, and Willey.

Of most interest here are the variations with frequency region and intensity. Figure 104 presents results obtained by Shower and Biddulph over a range from 31 to 11,700 ~, at two different levels of intensity, 15 and 40 db above threshold. It is evident that over a considerable range, from 125 to 2000 ~, the value of the just noticeable difference (Δf) is remarkably constant; it lies in the region of 3 ~ for the stronger and 4 ~ for the fainter intensity. At higher frequencies the value of the just noticeable difference mounts rapidly; for the stronger intensity it has risen about 4-fold at 5000 ~ and about 11-fold an octave higher. As mentioned, Shower and Biddulph's observations ended at 11,700 ~. Some additional measurements (Wever and Wedell) made at 15,000 ~ have yielded the relatively enormous value for Δf of 187 $\sim$, which is about 62 times that for low tones of the same loudness level. Evidently in terms of an absolute change of frequency our discrimination of high tones is very poor.

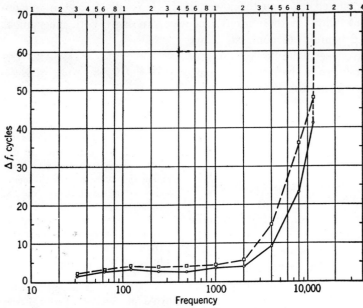

FIG. 104. Pitch discrimination. Shown are the changes in cycles (Δf) that are barely discernible, when the tones are warbled at a rate of 2 per second. The solid curve shows results for tones 40 db above threshold, and the dashed curve shows those for tones 15 db above threshold. These data are from Shower and Biddulph. The nearly vertical broken line at the upper end is leading toward a point at 187 $\sim$ obtained for a tone of 15,000 $\sim$ by Wever and Wedell.

Below 125 $\sim$ the curves show a moderate fall. Shower and Biddulph were inclined to attribute this variation to the introduction of harmonic frequencies. More particularly, it would seem that the presence of a noise pattern that changes rather rapidly with frequency lends assistance to discrimination in this region. It is likely that without this adventitious aid the function would continue to be uniform.

This manner of variation of pitch discrimination is easily understandable on the basis of the volley theory. Over the low-frequency range and partway into the intermediate range, where the nerve impulses afford a precise representation of the stimulus frequency, it is reasonable to find a differentiation that is constant or nearly so in terms of cyclic change. It would seem that the central auditory mechanism is able to appreciate a frequency difference of 3 or 4 $\sim$, under the conditions indicated.

Immediately above 2000 $\sim$ the discrimination begins to grow poorer. This is the region where according to the theory a volley frequency is still maintained, yet the neural pattern is becoming more complicated owing to the increasing number of fibers required to carry the frequency. Still farther along, as 4000 $\sim$ is approached, the discrimination falls off more rapidly, and here it is that inaccuracies of firing of the fibers cause the impulses to become dispersed and partially asynchronous. At higher frequencies still, where the discharge is wholly asynchronous, the only cue available for pitch is the place of action along the basilar membrane, and it is evident that this cue, measured in terms of the change in tonal frequency that is just perceptible, is a rather poor one.

It is of interest that in the middle range, where according to the theory there is both spatial and frequency representation of pitch, the discrimination is no better than in the low range where frequency serves alone. It appears that the frequency cue is so much the more accurate that the presence of the other is of no appreciable benefit to this function.

There is an alternative mode of expression of discrimination data that is often used. It is the relative difference limen, the ratio between the just discriminable cyclic change and the frequency at which it is taken. In Fig. 105 this relative difference limen ($\Delta f/f$) is plotted against the frequency (f).

This function stands in contrast to the one for Δf itself, for now the curve shows the greatest values at the low-frequency end and smaller values elsewhere. The minimum is around 2000 $\sim$, and as the frequency rises there is first a slow and then a rather rapid ascent. Below 2000 $\sim$ the curve rises rapidly, and this occurs naturally because the uniform value of Δf is being divided by smaller and smaller values of f.

The relative difference limen gains meaning as a measure of pitch discrimination if we make certain theoretical assumptions. We recall that on a place theory a change of pitch implies a shift in the locus of stimulation along the basilar membrane. A simple assumption in this relation is that a just discriminable change always involves a shift of some constant distance, regard-

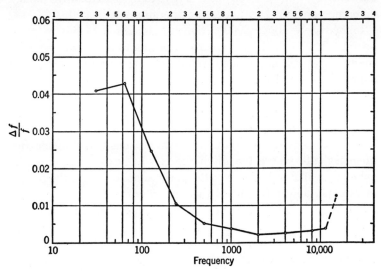

Fig. 105.   Pitch discrimination, expressed as the relative difference limen, $\Delta f/f$. Data as in the preceding figure.

less of the cochlear region concerned.   If now it is further assumed that the pattern of distribution of tones over the basilar membrane is logarithmic, the relative difference limen will be a constant (for on a logarithmic scale a constant step represents a certain relative change).

These assumptions are involved in the frequent assertion that Weber's law holds 'roughly' for pitch in the high-tone region. Yet as we examine the evidence of Fig. 105 we find slender support for this position.   The curve is nowhere horizontal.   It is true, it varies less in the high-tone region than in the low; but it will already be clear that this form of representation is not very meaningful for the low tones, and hence this part of the curve ought not to be used as a basis for comparison.   When we examine the upper portion of the curve in detail we see that it rises by 50 per cent from 2000 to 8000 ~, and then very steeply thereafter. If we accept the first assumption just mentioned, that just discriminable steps occupy constant intervals of length, then we must modify the second and say that in the high-tone region the tones are more closely packed than a logarithmic pattern would call for, and increasingly so as the upper limit is approached.

Indeed, the almost perpendicular ascent of the function at the highest frequencies lends support to a suggestion already made, that in the uppermost octave true resonance ceases and the tones operate only by forcing. It would appear, as Fig. 21 has indicated, that only the 'tail' of a resonance curve is present. Frequency discrimination in this region will depend upon the movements of this 'tail.' Because as frequency rises the sensitivity falls (partly for reasons other than spatial distribution itself), the stimuli must be raised in intensity. This change compensates in part for the frequency rise by spreading out the resonance curve. The result is that the 'tail' moves but slowly for a given change of frequency, and discrimination is correspondingly crude.

We can pursue further the implications of this first assumption, and work out a specific scaling of the basilar membrane. If a just discriminable step represents a constant shift along the basilar membrane, we can begin at one end of the auditory range and lay out the (changing) values of Δf until we reach the other end, and now we can relate this jnd scale to the linear dimension of the basilar membrane. The number of steps on this jnd scale from one end to any chosen frequency in relation to the total number of steps represents a fractional distance along the membrane, and hence locates that frequency's position.

Wegel and Lane were the first to map out the basilar membrane in this manner, by use of Knudsen's discrimination data. Stevens, Davis, and Lurie repeated the calculations with the more extensive data of Shower and Biddulph. Steinberg made the most careful determinations and studied the effects of different assumptions as to loudness level and the end points of tonal representation. Also, he abandoned the notion of a constant distance for each discriminable step and took instead the more reasonable assumption that such a step represents a shift over some constant number of neural elements. This assumption differs from the other if the distribution of the neural elements is not uniform, which the observations of Guild and others had shown to be the case.

According to the theory developed here the low tones do not have any very precise localization, and their discrimination is not a spatial function. For them therefore this kind of scaling operation has no real significance. However, this limitation need not prevent our use of the method for the high tones, and in any case it is of interest to try the method to see what it will yield. Accordingly, calculations were made on the basis of Shower and Biddulph's discrimination data and the detailed results already referred to on the pattern of cochlear innervation. Following Steinberg, the basic assumption here is that discrimination involves some constant shift in the pattern of neural excitation.

The calculations, which are rather complicated, took the following steps:

a. Shower and Biddulph's discrimination data, with the obvious irregularities smoothed out, were used to obtain an integrated curve of just noticeable differences. The integration was from the upper limit of hearing to the lower. This curve is shown in Fig. 106.

b. Different assumptions were made as to the lowest frequency possessing a definite maximum position on the basilar membrane. In one trial, for example, following Steinberg, this lowest localized frequency was taken as 125 $\sim$. The total number of ganglion cells (which averages 30,500 in the 23 ears of the innervation study) was then assumed to be distributed evenly over the number of just noticeable differences from the upper limit to this lowest localized frequency. The number of just noticeable differences is 1378 for the range of 125 to 24,000 $\sim$, and so the density factor, the number of ganglion cells per jnd, is 22.1.

c. For each of several frequencies selected to cover the auditory range the number of jnd's from the upper limit was read off from Fig. 106, and these numbers were multiplied by the density factor to give the number of ganglion cells measured from the upper limit.

d. Reference was then made to the integrated curve of inner-vation, Fig. 91, which shows the total number of ganglion cells as measured from the basal end of the cochlea. This curve was referred to for each of the selected tones for which the total

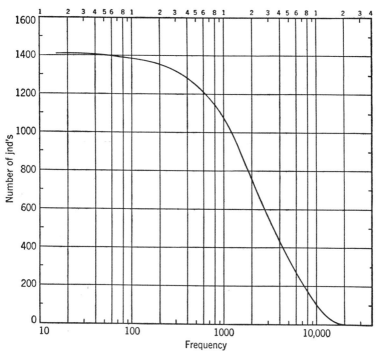

Fig. 106. Integration of jnd's for pitch. The curve shows the number of jnd's measured from the upper limit of hearing to any given point along the frequency scale. Based on Shower and Biddulph's data.

number of ganglion cells had been calculated, and the distance from the basal end (in per cent) was thereby obtained.

Curves *a, b, c* of Fig. 107 show the results of these calcula-tions with three different choices as to the lowest localized fre-quency. It is evident that this choice can be given considerable latitude without making any appreciable difference in the indi-cated positions for the high frequencies.

A comparison of the curves of Fig. 107 with other available data on tone localization, as summarized earlier in Fig. 67, shows no very satisfying agreement. The differences are particularly noticeable for the low frequencies. It is plain that something is wrong in this application of the discrimination data. I think the basic error lies in the assumption that every discriminable difference comes from a movement of the response along the basilar membrane, for low tones and high tones alike. Accord-

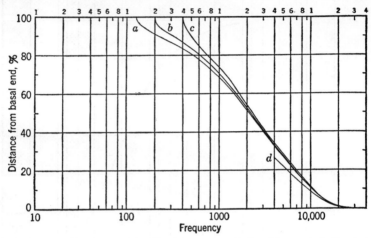

FIG. 107. Patterns of cochlear localization as calculated from pitch discrimination data. Different assumptions were made as to the lowest localized frequency; for curve *a* it was taken as 125 ∼, for curve *b* as 200 ∼, and for curve *c* as 400 ∼. Curve *d* is concerned only with the highest tones.

ing to the theory developed here, the discrimination of low tones has a different basis. The calculation of tonal positions for them in terms of the discrimination data therefore is improper. This is not to say that these low tones do not occupy space on the basilar membrane, but that their broad spatial locations are not primarily serviceable in discrimination.

It is still possible to make the calculations for the high tones, those above about 4000 ∼ where place begins to have significance for pitch discrimination. To do so, however, it is necessary to decide what part of the basilar membrane and hence what share of the total number of neural elements may be assigned to this high-tone range. Fortunately, the data presented in Fig. 67 are in good agreement in locating the tone 4096 ∼. It lies in a region 26 per cent of the distance from the basal end. By extrapolating a little we locate 4000 ⁓ at the 26.5 per cent point, and between here and the basal end we have available, according to Fig. 91, a total of 7440 ganglion cells, or 17 cells per jnd. For this limited range the calculations were carried out just as described above, with results shown as curve d of Fig. 107. This curve agrees reasonably well with other indications on the localization of high tones.

From the above considerations it will now be clear that the absolute difference limen, Δf, is the fairer measure of pitch discrimination for the low tones, and the relative difference limen, $\Delta f/f$, is the fairer one for the high tones. Here again is reflected the dual character of pitch representation.

Another application of the integrated function of just noticeable differences is as a scale of pitch, apart from considerations of localization as such. Stevens, Volkmann, and Newman showed that estimations of the sizes of large distances along the pitch range, when relations to the common musical intervals do not enter, are rather closely related to the number of just noticeable differences contained in these distances. In other words, the pitch continuum can be taken as a scale with the just noticeable difference as the unit. The argument was offered that this evident subjective equality of just noticeable differences really represents a kind of spatial equivalence: every jnd represents a shift of the area of excitation a certain distance along the basilar membrane. However, as the foregoing treatment has shown, this conception becomes more meaningful when the jnd is thought of as the passing over of a number of neural units rather than a simple distance. Moreover, from considerations already indicated, this claim can reasonably be admitted only in part: for the high tones. For the low tones the subjective equality of just noticeable differences can equally well be explained as the direct appreciation of frequency differences. This means simply that in this region two intervals of pitch that seem equal will embrace the same number of cycles.

The variation of the difference limen with intensity has already been indicated in a limited way in Fig. 104. Shower and Biddulph worked with a wide intensity range, at times up to 90 db above threshold. When the data are expressed in terms of Δf

the variations with intensity are large for the high tones and small for the low tones. When on the other hand they are expressed in terms of $\Delta f/f$ this relation is reversed. Actually, the forms of the curves are similar for all frequencies, and if all are plotted relatively, in terms of the degree of change as a function of intensity, they correspond closely. Therefore it is proper to average the results for the different tones used, as has been done for Fig. 108. This figure shows a systematic variation of dis-

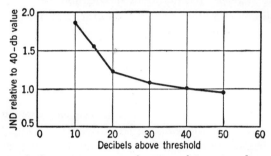

FIG. 108. Pitch discrimination as a function of intensity above threshold. Results for various frequencies are combined after equating them at the 40 db level.

crimination as intensity is changed. As the intensity is raised from the threshold upward the discrimination grows keener, changing at first rapidly and then more slowly, and finally leveling off. The poor performance at the fainter levels evidently reflects the perceptual inadequacies of a vague and ill-defined pattern of neural activity. Once a comfortable loudness is provided the discrimination becomes nearly maximal: the further improvements as the intensity is carried above about 50 db are only slight.

THE INTENSITY-PITCH RELATIONSHIP

It has often been remarked that the pitch of a tone is not determined wholly by the frequency, but under some circumstances and to a limited extent it varies also with intensity. This phenomenon was noticed as early as 1828 by Wilhelm Weber while listening to the sound of a tuning fork as it died away in strength.

What Weber observed was that the tone seemed lower in pitch when it was strong. Many in later years confirmed him, but only recently has the problem been worked out in detail. Zurmühl used tones from 128 to 3072 ~ and found the effect to be marked for the lower tones, but only slight for the higher ones in this range. Stevens repeated the experiment, mostly with a single observer, and after confirming the above result with low tones used still higher tones and found for them a reversal of the relationship. For tones above about 4000 ~ he found the pitch to rise as the intensity increased. For the extreme frequencies the effects seem striking and become as large as 12 per cent (two semitones on a musical scale). The largest changes appear for low tones, around 140 ~ (Snow).

This effect of intensity upon pitch has figured prominently in some of the discussions of auditory theory. Ewald considered it a point of difficulty in the Helmholtz theory. Zurmühl on the contrary found it a point of advantage. He considered it an inevitable feature of the action of vibrating strings. Such strings, he thought, are made to pull more strongly than usual against their end supports when they are vigorously excited, and so effectively they are made more tense. Hence their natural frequencies are raised. The incoming tone then must excite a string that lies lower in the series than it would at a fainter intensity. Therefore a lower pitch is heard.

This theory does not explain why the middle tones show little or no pitch change with intensity. It is even weaker in the face of Stevens' observation of a reversed effect in the high-frequency range. Fletcher bolstered it a bit by suggesting that in the high range the resonators are not like strings but are like tuning forks, whose natural frequencies fall as the intensity is raised. What species of resonators those of the middle range may be has not been made clear. They must be neither strings nor forks, but something else.

Stevens likewise tried to relate the phenomenon to the resonant characteristics of the ear, but without reference to particular types of resonators. He pointed out that the region of frequency where pitch remains stable is that of the ear's greatest sensitivity. Hence, he said, these middle tones lie at the center of the basilar membrane and do not shift their positions with intensity. Other tones, located toward the two ends of the membrane, shift farther outward when the intensity is raised. But why these shifts of position should occur was not made clear.

Later Stevens and Davis offered two other explanations. One was that the changes result from the contractions of the muscles of the middle ear, which occur at high intensities. They assumed that these contractions alter the resonance characteristics of the ear as a whole, including the basilar membrane. Again the details of the action remain obscure.

Their second hypothesis goes farther. It begins with the fact that the cochlear response is linear at low intensity levels and non-linear at high levels. This response ought to reflect the combined action of various segments of the basilar membrane. A given segment, when overloaded, must yield a smaller and smaller response in relation to the applied energy. The point of diminishing returns will be reached soonest in the middle-frequency region where the sensitivity is greatest, and later on the two sides. Hence as the intensity is raised there is a shift in the weight of response away from the middle region. This means for the high tones a shift toward the basal end and a raising of the pitch, and for the low tones a shift toward the apical end and a lowering of the pitch.

This is an ingenious hypothesis. It implies an extensiveness of spread of action in the cochlea not often admitted in a place theory. However, it must face this particular difficulty: the point of overloading of the ear is reached only at a rather high intensity, far beyond the level at which the pitch changes are said to appear. According to Stevens' data these changes are already present at a level of 0.1 dynes per sq cm, whereas in the ears of the experimental animals like the cat and guinea pig, as Fig. 29 will bear out, linearity continues well beyond, up to 1 dyne per sq cm and more. And it is unlikely that the human ear is inferior to other mammalian ears in this respect.

Certain additional evidence regarding the intensity-pitch effect leads us away from explanations like these that depend upon assumed alterations of response patterns among the cochlear resonators. In the first place, the effect has none of the regularity that ought to appear if it were dependent upon some simple peripheral process. Snow's results are especially convincing here.

Some of his subjects showed the changes, others did not. Those that did varied greatly among themselves in the amounts of change, and even a single subject varied from day to day.

In the second place, the changes either do not appear at all, or at least are minimized, when complex tones are used. Fletcher (3) observed only small effects when he used a tone containing 4 or more overtones. Lewis and Cowan had skilled musicians play intervals on the violin or cello first softly and then as loudly as possible and recorded the frequencies produced. There were no significant changes. Evidently the musician does not experience a pitch shift as the intensity rises from pianissimo to fortissimo, or else he fails to heed it in his estimations. Further musical experience is consistent with these results. When a player tunes his instrument he sounds it at any convenient intensity and does not find his adjustment in error as the intensity is altered. Different instruments upon which the same note is played at different intensities do not seem in discord.

Finally, Thurlow (1) showed that the pitch change is not simply a function of the raising of the intensity in the ear in question; it appears also for binaural stimulation. Let the intensity of the tone in the one ear remain unchanged, and add a tone of the same frequency and intensity in the other ear; the pitch then shifts as before.

This binaural phenomenon has all the characteristics heretofore mentioned: the pitch shifts downward for the low tones, upward for the high tones, and remains unchanged for tones in the middle range, as the sound is introduced into the other ear. It is even more significant that the stimulation of the opposite ear need not be with the same frequency as that of the ear where the pitch changes are observed. Any frequency will serve. Not only this, but general stimulation other than auditory is effective in some degree. The changes appear on clenching the fists, tensing the neck muscles, or evidently doing anything that contributes a massive flow of sensory impulses.

This qualitative change that a change of intensity brings about deserves a closer scrutiny. It stands in contrast to the one that frequency causes. It is less certain, more variable. It does not seem the result of any simple, compelling process. Rather, it has the earmarks of a perceptual illusion, an experience based upon equivocal conditions of stimulation. It is not even certain that it is strictly a change of pitch. Anyone who has listened carefully to it will agree that it has a qualitative character, but he cannot have much confidence in its identity with pitch in the more familiar sense. What the experiments show is that some subjects (perhaps the more suggestible ones) experience a change as a result of a variation of intensity that they can match by a change in frequency. Hence in theorizing it is not necessary to find a process dependent upon intensity that is identical with the one by which frequency gives our cue to pitch; it is only necessary to find some process that depends in a peculiar way on both intensity and frequency. Hereafter what has been termed 'pitch' changes as a function of intensity will be regarded in this light, as qualitative variations of some undefined sort. We shall look for the explanation of these variations in some side effects of the frequency and intensity dimensions of stimuli, effects which lead to confusion in the cues afforded us.

Possible conditions for a confusion of cues—or rather, as will appear, two sorts of such confusions—were disclosed in the development of the volley theory. It will be recalled that in this theory the stimulus variables of frequency and intensity in their actions in the cochlea both involve the dimensions of time and space, though in different ways. That these ways are not kept strictly apart, but merge in minor respects, provides a possible basis for the intensity-pitch illusion.

As stimulus intensity is raised there is an increase in the rate of impulses in the nerve fibers in operation, and also in the effective spread of action. As stimulus frequency is raised there is an increase in the rate of nerve impulses and a diminution in the spread of action. The first type of variation with frequency is in the same sense as the variation with intensity (a rise of either increases the rate); the second type is in a contrary sense. May we not expect in the differential workings of these two relations in different parts of the frequency scale an explanation of the peculiar behavior of the illusion? It is only necessary that one relation prevail at one end of the scale, that the other prevail at the opposite end, and that they fade out or neutralize one another in between.

Take first the low end of the scale. The stimulus frequency accurately determines the periodicity of the volleys and provides the cue to pitch. At the same time the frequency determines in a measure the extensiveness of spread of the response: the pattern of action grows broader (for any one intensity) the lower the frequency. An increase of intensity also increases the spread (and at a rapid pace at high levels owing to the generation of overtones). Here we have a linkage of cues. The extension of spread commonly enters into the determination of loudness, but under some conditions we may take it as a fall of 'pitch.' As the frequency rises beyond the low-tone range this kind of confusion diminishes, possibly because the rate of change of spread grows less.

Consider now the high end of the frequency scale. We have seen that as synchronism fails the cue to pitch becomes the locus of action along the basilar membrane; this is the primary role of the stimulus frequency here. We are more interested now in its secondary role. All along this part of the scale the frequency determines the number of excitatory pulses, while the intensity determines (in part) how many of these shall be effective. Thus frequency plays with intensity a quantitative role, already seen clearly in the sensitivity function. This action continues at the upper end of the scale, even after synchronism has ceased.

As the frequency is raised there are increased demands upon the nerve fibers: they are called upon to operate earlier and earlier in their relative refractory periods. One effect of this overdriving is to bring out and emphasize irregularities in timing and thereby to increase the asynchronism. As the intensity is raised much the same thing happens: instability appears in certain fibers owing to overdriving. Accordingly, if one of a pair of matched tones is raised in frequency, the match can in some sense be restored by raising the other tone in intensity. Because the change that is here attributed to the general diffuseness cf the nerve discharge can occur with frequency variations it may be called 'pitch.'

In the middle of the frequency scale these two forms of confusion may be absent, or, a little more likely, they are both present in small degree and confuse one another. The latter supposition is borne out by the general irregularities in the results, and especially the observations of Stevens that tones in this region as they are raised in intensity are not often constant in pitch but show first a slight rise and then a slight fall.

These speculations about the intensity-pitch illusion are sufficiently general to embrace the effects of binaural stimulation, and even the extra-auditory effects. Also they are consistent with the facts about complex tones and with the failure of the effects to obtrude in musical experiences.

THE EFFECTS OF DURATION ON PITCH PERCEPTION

Our discussion of pitch perception so far has assumed that the tonal stimuli have lasted for an appreciable period of time—a quarter of a second or more. When the duration is shorter some complications appear. The tone becomes more or less noisy.

The briefest stimuli, those lasting less than a hundredth of a second, are heard as clicks. As the stimulus is made longer the sound gradually takes on a tonal quality and finally turns into a smooth, pure tone. Bürck, Kotowski, and Lichte (2) distinguished these three—noise, tone-colored noise, and tone—as the main stages in the experience, but actually there is a continuous gradation from noise to tone.

A question often raised is how many cycles are necessary for a tone to develop pitch. The question has been answered variously because different observers adopt different standards in their designation of pitch. If all that is required is that one sound seem different from another, then extremely brief durations are sufficient. Several have reported that a very small number of cycles—Kucharski (1) said less than a single cycle— may give some qualitative character to a sound.* Usually the criterion is somewhat more restricted than this, and it is demanded that the pitch be 'recognizable,' though recognizability is only subjectively defined. The most extensive results obtained under this criterion are those of Bürck, Kotowski, and Lichte

---

* In the study of many, and indeed most, of these experiments it is not possible to determine precisely what the stimulus was. In Kucharski's experiment, for example, we may be sure that his part-cycle stimulus was prolonged into a train of waves through a persistence of activity in the sound-producing apparatus and may have been modified further in its transmission to the ear.

(2), who used tones from 50 to 10,000 ∼, as shown in Fig. 109. A further, and more objective, requirement is that the pitch be adequate for a judgment of discrimination to some tolerable degree of accuracy. Both Békésy (3) and Turnbull showed how pitch discrimination depends upon duration. Turnbull's results

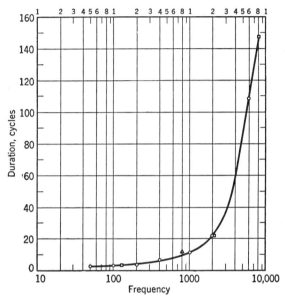

Fig. 109. Pitch in relation to tonal duration. The duration is measured as the number of cycles in the pulse of tone that is just long enough for the pitch to be recognizable (circles, Bürck, Kotowski, and Lichte) or that permits pitch discrimination (triangles, Békésy; and squares, Turnbull).

for the tones 128, 1024, and 8192 ∼, averaged at the lowest level at which all his subjects were able to make reliable discriminations, and Békésy's observations on a single tone of 800 ∼ are given on the same graph as the results of Bürck, Kotowski, and Lichte. As may be seen, these results are closely comparable. Evidently a pitch that is recognizable to the extent that Bürck, Kotowski, and Lichte required is also serviceable in discrimination.

These results show that at the lowest frequencies only a small number of cycles is necessary to determine the pitch sufficiently to satisfy either of these criteria. As the frequency rises the necessary number of cycles grows greater, very gradually at first and then with increasing rapidity. Between 50 and 400 ~ the number rises from 3 to 7 cycles, at 1000 ~ it is 12 cycles, and at 10,000 ~ it has reached the enormous value of 250 cycles.

The results are quite in line with the volley theory. At the lowest frequencies where the nerve fibers are able immediately to take up the full rate of the excitations only a small number of cycles is required. When the frequency exceeds what a single fiber can deliver, and the rotational action described in the volley principle must enter, a larger number of cycles becomes necessary. Several cycles must pass before a suitable volley is achieved. And as the frequency mounts this number rises rapidly. Beyond 4000 or 5000 ~, as asynchronism enters, the number continues to rise both because of the bluntness of the spatial cue in the representation of pitch, and because even in an asynchronous volley it takes time for the discharge to reach its full and settled magnitude.

There is an interesting relation to pitch discrimination, as a comparison with Fig. 104 will show. In the low-tone range the number of cycles required for pitch recognition is of the same order of magnitude as the change in cycles needed to tell one pitch from another. At higher frequencies the number needed for pitch recognition considerably exceeds the size of the pitch discrimination limen. This difference no doubt arises from the feeble and unsettled character of the initial stage of the nerve response to the high tones.

THE PRINCIPLE OF MAXIMUM STIMULATION

As was shown in Chapter 5, the principle of maximum stimulation became a central feature of the modern resonance theory after Gray's formulation of it in 1900. It was regarded as overcoming the difficulty presented by the fact of spread: by the fact that the activity aroused by a simple tone is not confined to a single place on the basilar membrane, but extends widely. By means of this principle, it was thought, the specificity that was given up for the peripheral response could be regained later on in the central processes. According to this principle, the only part of the peripheral activity that has to do with the determination of pitch is the part at the maximum of the response curve; the remaining activity is somehow suppressed.

In view of the crucial importance of the principle of maximum stimulation for the resonance theory it is curious that little attention has been given to its experimental study. Only recently Thurlow carried out two critical investigations.

One of these, on the effect of binaural stimulation upon pitch perception, has already been described. Thurlow found that the changes in pitch that result from raising the intensity of a tone can be obtained as well by introducing another tone in the opposite ear. Now, it is difficult to see how the position of maximum stimulation in the one ear can be altered by adding a stimulus in the other ear. Thurlow therefore argued against the idea that pitch is perceived in terms of the position of maximum stimulation. However, his point is weakened by the consideration that the pitch-intensity illusion may not represent a change of pitch in a true sense.

Thurlow's second experiment was a more direct test of the principle. He showed that the distribution of activity in the cochlea is different for an overtone and for a fundamental tone of the same frequency. His method made use of the fact, already observed in the experiments of Hallpike and Rawdon-Smith and of Culler and others, that a pattern of electrical potentials may be recorded from the cochlear capsule. With fine wire electrodes at several positions on the cochlear wall of the guinea pig ear, Thurlow stimulated, for example, with $1000 \sim$ and recorded the first overtone, which is $2000 \sim$. In this recording he used a wave analyzer, which made it possible to measure one component of the response and to ignore all others. From the several electrode positions he obtained a pattern of $2000 \sim$ potentials, apparently reflecting the distribution of activity representing this component within the cochlea. He then compared this pattern with the one obtained from the same electrode positions on stimulation with $2000 \sim$ itself. The two patterns did not agree. For this and all the other pairs of tones that he used the overtone response became smaller in relation to the fundamental response as the electrode position was displaced apically. Now, a fundamental tone of $2000 \sim$ and a $2000 \sim$ overtone are perceived as of the same pitch, and yet the peripheral pattern is not the same. A reference of pitch to the position of maximum stimulation is evidently unjustified.

This matter of the principle of maximum stimulation need be taken into account in the volley theory only in so far as the spatial type of representation is accepted as the basis of pitch perception, namely, for the high tones. Yet, quite apart from Thurlow's negative evidence, an analytical consideration discloses no advantage to this theory (or to the resonance theory either) in such a principle. Let us follow out the idea from where we left it in the earlier discussion of the resonance theory.

It is agreed that a simple stimulus arouses an extensive peripheral activity that varies in degree; and—under some circumstances—the response shows a maximum at some point. It is generally admitted at the present day that any restriction of activity—any reduction to the point of the maximum—is not peripheral or at least not completely so. Hence the whole activity pattern, or a large part of it, must be represented in the nerve response. That this is true is evidenced by Galambos and Davis' observations that a given auditory nerve element can be stimulated by tones over a very wide range, up to 3 octaves or more when the intensity is strong. This whole pattern must continue to be represented in the neural response up to those portions of the central system through whose activities the pitch is perceived. What is it to assert, as Gray's principle does, that we refer the pitch to the point of the maximum and ignore all else in the activity? It is to imply that these 'ignored' parts are just as important as the point of maximum, for this maximum is only relative to them. It is maximum only by reference to its neighboring regions, and can be perceived so only if all these regions are suitably represented in the neural activity.

It is better to abandon this principle of the maximum and simply to say that the pitch (of high tones) is determined by the whole pattern of activity. Every part of the peripheral response excites its nervous elements and gets its proportionate representation in the total discharge. The different frequencies have somewhat different areas and forms of response and are identified in these terms. The same tone at different intensities will vary in the area covered, but as the intensity is changed this areal variation is continuous and there is much in common from one stage to another. We appreciate the continuity and identify the tone as single.

If in this development the specificity that figured so largely in Helmholtz's theory has been pushed even more remotely than ever beyond our grasp, it is no matter for regret. It will now be obvious that this specificity was lost in fact and even in principle a long time ago—even by Helmholtz himself as soon as he admitted the smallest degree of cochlear spread.

THE QUESTION OF AUDITORY QUANTA

A quantum theory of sensory activity supposes that a sensation is the result of the stimulation of certain separate elements or processes, and that the sensation is changed only by the addition or substitution of a new element or process. A continuous variation of the stimulus therefore causes discontinuous changes of sensation: the sensation alters only by sudden jumps. This quantum character might apply to either the pitch or the loudness of a tone.

Boring in 1926 pointed out that a theory based upon specific energies of nerves is a theory of pitch quanta. A new pitch arises when the stimulus brings in a different neural element. Also, there will be just as many discriminable pitches as there are individual responsive elements. Helmholtz was dealing with this question of quanta when he compared the number of rods of Corti with the number of discriminable pitches.

With loudness the process is one of the addition of elements rather than a substitution of elements. Fig. 110 will make the matter clear. The bar indicates the magnitude of stimulus (16 units) that is sufficient to stimulate the sensory elements shown as shaded: *a, b, c, d, e,* and *f.* If the magnitude should fall to 15 units element *f* would drop out, and the loudness would diminish by 1 jnd. On the other hand, if the magnitude should rise to 18 units the sensation would remain unchanged. It is evident that according to this theory the size of the difference limen will vary periodically with the value of the stimulus. In the example the distances 15–16 (1 unit) and 15–18 (3 units) both represent one discriminable step, whereas 16–18 (2 units) is not discriminable. In general, if the quantum theory holds, the difference limen will have to vary from an indefinitely small value to nearly the magnitude covered by one sensory element. Boring thought that a choice would have to be made between quanta of pitch or of intensity. A resonance theory, he said, is committed to a quantum theory of pitch, but not to one of loudness, because loudness can depend upon the frequency of nerve impulses which is a continuum. The alternative view, which he preferred, is a frequency theory of quality, where pitch depends upon the frequency of nerve impulses and therefore admits of no quanta. In Boring's formulation this theory relates

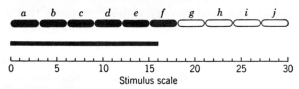

FIG. 110. The theory of auditory quanta. The successive links, identified by letters, represent specific sensory elements, each of which on exposure to stimulation is excited to full activity or not at all. The bar below indicates a certain magnitude of stimulus, which excites the shaded elements, *a* to *f*, and leaves the others unaffected.

loudness to the number of nerve fibers in action, and so makes it quantum-like. He preferred the latter alternative because he thought the extensive work on pitch would long ago have revealed quanta if there were any, whereas the possibilities in loudness had not been so thoroughly explored.

Békésy (4), in studies of loudness discrimination, obtained results that he interpreted as indicating the presence of quanta. The argument, which is based upon the forms of the psychometric functions that he obtained, will not be pursued here. Later, Stevens, Morgan, and Volkmann, by a similar method, obtained results of the same character for both pitch and loudness. However, in their interpretations they regarded these quanta as not peripheral but central: they were said to represent some sort of perceptual units and not single nerve fibers or other simple cochlear processes. These authors reached this conclusion on consideration of the large sizes of the 'quanta,' their variations from time to time, and the fact that they are of different size for binaural and uniaural listening. Their experimental results do not give any firm support even to this species of quanta; and other results seem conclusive in denying their existence. Certainly as the matter stands today peripheral quanta have not been demonstrated. They are not to be expected according to the volley theory. For low and intermediate tones the pitch is a function of volley frequency, which can vary continuously. For high tones, pitch depends upon a spatial pattern, which also can vary without discrete steps. For loudness the nervous correlate is the magnitude of the nerve discharge, which is a continuum because it depends on both the number of fibers and their rates of activity.

CHAPTER 14

AUDITORY ABNORMALITIES

The auditory disturbances that have a particular relevance to theory include tinnitus, diplacusis, and certain of the forms of deafness.

TINNITUS

Very likely everyone on occasion has perceived a ringing or some other kind of sound that is referred to the ear and cannot be traced to any external stimulus; this phenomenon is known as tinnitus. The experience usually is easy to identify as subjective. Nearly always it appears in one ear only and is definitely referred to that ear regardless of the position of the head. Binaural tinnitus is rare, but when it occurs it similarly is referred to the head and seems to move strictly as the head moves.

Tinnitus appears in many forms. It may be tonal or noisy, steady or pulsating, transient or unremitting. The most common type is a tonal tinnitus that comes on suddenly, lasts for a few seconds at full strength, and then gradually dies away. It is usually rather high in pitch, but of a quality not quite pure, hence the appropriateness of the term 'ringing.' Tonal tinnitus of low pitch occurs less often.

Tinnitus has many causes. One type obviously is vascular in origin. The sound is a rushing or throbbing associated with the pulse, and it evidently arises from partial obstruction of a blood vessel in the head, most likely the carotid artery or jugular vein. A second type is muscular, arising from spasms of the neck muscles or perhaps more commonly of the tympanic muscles. Occasionally some of these types of tinnitus can be heard by a second observer, which proves that the sounds are actual. These need no further explanation here.

Other forms of tinnitus arise within the ear itself, either in the cochlea or in the acoustic nervous system, and so are subjective in a narrow sense. A sensory origin is likely for the tinnitus that accompanies Ménière's disease, for this disease evidently is due to an abnormal raising of the endolymphatic pressure or some other condition that causes a general stimulation of endings. A neural origin is likely for the tinnitus that accompanies many neuralgias and neuritic states. For other forms of tinnitus a distinction of sensory and neural cannot easily be made. The tinnitus that often follows exposure to excessively loud sounds is plainly a result of trauma, but whether of sensory cells or nerve fibers, or both, it is not possible to say. The same is true of the many other appearances of tinnitus where no cause is known.

Tinnitus is a prominent symptom in the large majority of ear disorders. Sometimes it amounts to a disease in itself, for it is present unceasingly and in such intensity as to be almost unendurable. In a number of cases where no conservative treatment has been found the patient has submitted to an operation in which the eighth nerve was cut or the whole labyrinth destroyed. The remarkable thing about this treatment is that about half the time the tinnitus persists after elimination of the peripheral system. Such tinnitus obviously is of central origin.

Perhaps the most thoroughgoing study of a case of tinnitus was made by Wegel (1) on his own left ear. His was a faint, continuous, high-frequency tinnitus, like a tone of 3600 or 3700 $\sim$. Tests made by stimulating the ear at low intensities with pure tones of various frequencies revealed certain regions where the resulting perception was one of discord. Beats arose between the tinnitus and the external tone. They appeared in three regions of frequency, around 2400, 3000, and 3600 $\sim$. A beating with a tinnitus has been observed with certainty in at least one other instance, by one of my colleagues, and it was produced by stimulating with a pure tone of nearly the same pitch as the tinnitus itself.

The masking of a tinnitus is a common experience. It appeared in Wegel's tests when he used strong stimuli. Indeed, it is used as a therapeutic measure, to gain temporary relief from an excruciating tinnitus, for evidently a patient will accept a continuing external sound in preference to his subjective one (Jones and Knudsen).

The usual explanation of tinnitus is provided by the place theory, as a local irritation in the cochlea that excites particular hair cells, or an irritation in the nerve that involves particular fibers, in either case giving a quality corresponding to the elements affected.

Wegel in explanation of his experiences employed the frequency principle. He suggested that some toxic or other influence might be at work upon the nerve fibers so as to make them fire at something near their maximum rate. He noted that his three beating regions were 4, 5, and 6 times 600, or approximately that, and thereby inferred that the individual fibers were responding at rates of about 600 per second. If the different fibers were somewhat out of step, so as to make up 4 to 6 groups, they could generate the higher frequencies at which the beating was observed and the apparent pitch around 3600 ~ that the tinnitus itself possessed.

In support of this theory of tinnitus as an adventitious neural discharge it is pertinent to refer to the so-called 'pain' impulses set up in a nerve trunk that has been cut across (Adrian, 5). Sometimes such a discharge is quite irregular, but in other instances it is made up of synchronized impulses of a fairly definite frequency, often as high as 500 to 800 impulses per second. In this latter case the cut end of a fiber seems to excite not only itself but its neighbors also, so that the whole bundle gives a synchronous discharge. Therefore we can easily explain tinnitus, both of tonal and noisy types, as a nerve excitation arising from local injury.

The place and frequency explanations of tinnitus are both reasonable, and probably both hold in particular instances. Tinnitus of high pitch is probably most often due to a local action upon hair cells or nerve fibers, and tinnitus of low pitch is more likely a synchronous neural discharge. Noisy tinnitus may be one or the other.

DIPLACUSIS

A common anomaly of hearing is diplacusis, which literally means 'double hearing.' In the usual form, known as binaural diplacusis, a tone is heard as different in pitch in the two ears.

A rarer form is uniaural diplacusis, in which a tone is heard as double when presented to a single ear.

Diplacusis is often encountered clinically as one of the symptoms of ear disorders. It occurs in fevers, labyrinthitis, Ménière's disease, after acoustic trauma, and especially with infections of the middle ear and upper pharynx. Usually it is transient in character: it appears suddenly when the disease is in an acute stage and then gradually subsides along with the other symptoms. Occasionally it persists for weeks, but even then it will show variations in amount and character from time to time. A subclinical type of diplacusis is found in persons otherwise normal, and is of so slight degree as to go unnoticed unless especially looked for (see Jeffress, for example).

The diplacusis most often reported clinically shows a disparity of pitch between the two ears of the order of 1 or 2 semitones. Larger disparities are sometimes found, up to half an octave or more. Smaller amounts pass unnoticed except by musically trained persons who are annoyed by the disturbance of their pitch perception.

The severe types of diplacusis ordinarily affect only a portion of the auditory range. Tones of certain frequencies are shifted in pitch in the affected ear, while other tones are unaltered. An example is given by Proetz, who measured the effects in himself during a middle ear infection on one side. Tones around 1024 ~ he heard in the infected ear with a pitch about a quarter tone higher than in the other ear. Higher tones showed even more disparity, until at the upper end of his auditory range they were shifted upward by 9 semitones. Tones below 1024 ~ were heard in a normal manner.

In the majority of cases the shift of pitch is upward: a tone seems higher in the affected ear than in the other. Occasionally the shift is downward. Of special interest here are the results obtained in the overstimulation of human ears. Davis, Morgan, and others, after the exposure of subjects to 500, 1000, and 2000 ~ at elevated intensities, observed along with an impairment of sensitivity a marked upward shift of pitch for tones in the region a half octave above the exposure frequency. Rüedi and Furrer obtained similar results for these tones and experimented also with higher tones. They found no pitch displacement after stimulation with 4000 ~ and a reversed effect—a displacement downward—for still higher tones.

A 'recruitment' effect was observed in these tests, and the diplacusis had a systematic relation to it. After the exposure there was a marked impairment of threshold sensitivity, and tones only a little above threshold seemed faint in the exposed ear in comparison with the other. As the stimulus intensity was raised this difference in loudness tended to disappear, until at high levels the loudness in the two ears was nearly the same. Correspondingly, the pitch disparity was marked at the low levels of stimulation and became progressively less as the intensity was raised.

In the large majority of instances the diplacusis is complicated by a qualitative disturbance. The tone in the affected ear is not only changed in pitch but in character as well. It is heard as impure, even noisy. In extreme cases the tonal quality is altogether lost, and only noise remains.

A case unusual in degree and complexity was reported by Minton, who suffered an injury to the right ear as a result of an explosion. He experienced a serious loss of acuity and a diplacusis that varied in amount and quality over the tonal range. In two regions, in the octave from 500 to 1000 ~ and above 4000 ~, the hearing remained normal. In the low-tone region, up to 400 ~, he heard pure-tone stimuli invariably as noises of a complex, nearly random character, and the same was true for tones between 2550 and 4000 ~. Tones in the remaining regions seemed noisy but with recognizable pitch. In the transition zones, between the areas that gave noisy tones and pure noises, a faint stimulus was heard simply as a noise, but as the intensity was raised a tonal component developed. In general, the pitch was displaced upward as compared with the other ear. As time passed the condition changed and perception became normal except for the lowest tones. A curious observation made on occasion was a tonal tinnitus in a region of the scale where objective tones produced only noises.

The rarer uniaural diplacusis is nearly always, and perhaps invariably, of the complex or noisy type. Budde (2) described such a case in himself during an attack of typhus. He heard a single tone as a 'chaos' of tones, yet with pitch of a general sort in the correct region. This condition prevailed over the whole auditory scale and then vanished two or three days later.

Three explanations of diplacusis can be offered. The usual one, based upon the place hypothesis, was formulated by Gray in his development of the principle of maximum stimulation. He pointed out that on this principle anything that altered the position of a tone's maximum on the basilar membrane would change its pitch. A disturbance of the resonance properties of the cochlear elements—a variation in their tension, mass, or the like—ought to change the location and form of the pattern of response. If the maximum point is shifted toward the basal end of the cochlea the pitch will be raised, and if it is shifted toward the apical end the pitch will be lowered. Presumably the mechanical alterations might be general or only regional.

Gray sought to account for the uniaural and noisy types of diplacusis also. If the sensory or neural elements are impaired at the place where the maximum of response falls for some particular stimulating frequency there will seem to be two maxima, one on either side of the impaired region. Then two tones ought to be heard instead of one. Some impairments, he believed, would be so extensive as to give the effect of uniform stimulation over a considerable area and so lead to the perception of a noise.

In the light of the volley theory this explanation needs some modification. We can accept the basic idea of a shift in the pattern of stimulation as a result of a change in the physical condition of the responsive structures, or a shift in the pattern of excitation as a result of the impairment of sensory or neural elements. We ought to think, however, in terms of the whole pattern, and not simply of a point of maximum activity. In so far as pitch depends upon this pattern—as it does for the upper range of tones—it will be altered by these physical or structural changes.

This explanation will not serve so well for the low and intermediate frequencies, for which cochlear localization is not very precise. Only a very grave dislocation of response ought to affect them. Hence this kind of diplacusis ought to be rare in the region of the low tones.

The kind of diplacusis reported by Proetz fits this explanation. The shift of pitch was limited to tones above 1024 ~, where cochlear localization is well defined. It was always in one direction, which would argue for some systematic physical change; Proetz suggested a general relaxation of tension on the basilar membrane. The effect became progressively more pronounced as the frequency was raised; and this we should expect if the physical change was general throughout the cochlea, and if localization becomes more important as a cue to pitch the higher the frequency.

A second explanation of diplacusis arises in the relation of pitch to loudness. Diplacusis typically and perhaps invariably appears in the presence of an impairment of sensitivity of one ear. A tone applied to this ear is less loud than in the other ear, especially when intensities near threshold are used. It follows that in so far as the judgment of pitch depends upon loudness a diplacusis will appear. When the tone is delivered in considerable strength, and through 'recruitment' the loudness in the affected ear approaches that in the other, the diplacusis is reduced. This explanation probably applies best to the milder forms of diplacusis, and to effects observed in the low-tone region where pitch judgments are most affected by loudness.

A third explanation applies particularly to the noisy forms of diplacusis. It is based upon a consideration of the effects of cochlear injury upon volley action. If many of the cochlear nerve fibers are in a pathological condition as a result of injury, toxic conditions in the ear, or the like, they may become hyperresponsive in the presence of a stimulus. The resulting injury currents most likely will be asynchronous and when added to the normal volleys will produce a noisy tone. Indeed, these random discharges may altogether obscure the normal synchronous response and give noise without any tonal character whatever. As the stimulus intensity is raised the nerve fibers will be forced more and more into synchronism, and then the tone will be perceived along with the noise.

The effect of the injury discharge upon pitch is readily seen. In the low- and middle-tone regions where pitch depends upon volley frequency the pitch will be raised. The random impulses add to the over-all frequency and produce a rough tone or a noise whose pitch seems somewhat above that proper to the stimulus tone. This effect will disappear as the high tones are approached, basically because for them frequency no longer serves as a cue to pitch. Its point of disappearance will be somewhat below that at which the frequency cue normally fails, because the usual conditions that limit this cue are now exaggerated. The pathology limits the total number of nerve fibers and even more seriously limits the number available to volley action. Development of the necessary degree of synchronism is now more difficult than normally. It is further likely that a very grave injury will so limit the number of nerve fibers as to prevent the attainment of full synchronism, and so give a noisy sound of a pitch below that proper to the stimulus. Many of the results observed by Davis and his associates and by Rüedi and Furrer after overstimulating the ear fall in with this explanation.

Deafness

There are two general classes of deafness. One is conductive deafness; there is an impairment of the mechanical system for the transmission of vibrations to the inner ear. The other may be called sensory-neural deafness; it includes impairments at any of the three stages of activity following the conductive process: impairments in the cochlea, in the auditory nerve, and in the central auditory pathways and nuclei. The terms nerve deafness and perceptive deafness are often used in a general way for this whole class, but they refer more properly to the difficulties of the second and third stages. They ought to be kept distinct from cochlear deafness.

CONDUCTIVE DEAFNESS

In conductive deafness there is a general loss of acuity to air-conducted sounds which is either fairly uniform over the tonal range or, more typically, is most prominent in the low and middle frequencies. The acuity to bone-conducted sounds is affected relatively little, but may show some variations in the middle range.

A common form of conductive deafness, and perhaps the simplest, is otosclerosis, in which a disease of the bone causes a growth that imbeds the footplate of the stapes and makes it immobile. The acuity falls off in progressive fashion, usually over a period of years, as this process of fixation goes on. The

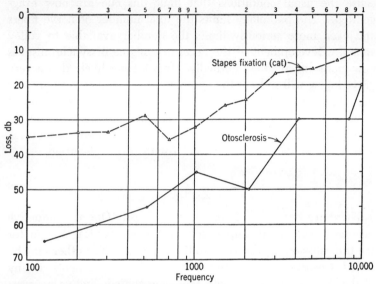

FIG. 111. Conductive deafness. One curve shows a simple case of otosclerosis (in man), and the other shows an artificial impairment of conduction produced in a cat by mechanical fixation of the stapes. Data from Lempert (2) and K. R. Smith (1).

result is shown in Fig. 111, where the solid line represents a typical case of simple otosclerosis (Lempert, 2). The broken line of this figure represents what may be regarded as an artificial case: it shows how the cochlear potentials in a cat were affected after mechanical fixation of the ossicular chain (K. R. Smith, 1). Note that in both cases the severest losses are at the lower end of the frequency scale. The form of these changes is understandable on a consideration of the mechanical resonance of the ear (Fig. 70) and its alteration by the fixation. The fixation adds stiffness and resistance to the mechanical system and therefore reduces the response most seriously in the low frequencies and in the region of mechanical resonance.

SENSORY-NEURAL DEAFNESS

The deafness that results from impairments of cochlear and neural processes is distinguished by the fact that usually, and perhaps always in the early, uncomplicated stages, it is a deafness to high tones. Three forms, two mild and one severe, will take our attention here. The first is the tonal dip, a form in which the loss of sensitivity is confined to a single region of the frequency scale. The second is presbyacusia, or simple old-age deafness, where there is a loss of acuity to the highest tones and therefore a curtailment of the auditory range. The third form is clinical nerve deafness, in which the high-tone loss is severe and disabling.

THE TONAL DIP

An ear that is otherwise normal may show a marked depression of sensitivity in one region of the auditory scale. Such a 'tonal dip' occurs rather frequently in males, but only rarely in females. Almost always it is situated in the medium high frequencies, and particularly in the region from 3000 to 5000 ~. The usual audiometers contain only the tone 4096 in this region and show up the defect in this one place; therefore the defect is commonly referred to as the '4096 dip.' Actually the loss covers at least a third of an octave, and usually more. Dips vary greatly in degree, and in rare instances they reach the profound depth of 75 db below normal.

The cause and basis of the tonal dip are unknown. Of various theories one of the more plausible is the traumatic theory, which ascribes the loss to overstimulation with sounds. Yet a study of the histological condition of the ears of persons with prominent dips has revealed no significant changes of structure such as are typical of animal ears after exposure to damaging sounds (Wever, 7). If the defect lies in the peripheral system it must be of a subtle character, not disclosed in our usual histological procedures.

It is curious and no doubt significant that this impairment almost without exception falls in a certain region of the fre-

quency scale. What special characters does this region possess?
It is for the normal ear the region of the greatest sensitivity.
And it is so, according to the theory developed here, largely on
account of neural factors. This relation brings the thought that
the impairment may lie, in part at least, in these neural processes.
A further relation is possibly significant: this region also is the
one where representation in the auditory nerve in terms of volley
frequency is approaching its limit and will soon give way to

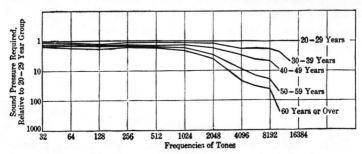

FIG. 112. Age and auditory acuity. Five age groups were tested under
similar conditions, and the results are presented with respect to the young-
est group (20 to 29 years). The curves show for each group the relative
sound pressure required for threshold perception, as a function of frequency.
Data from Bunch and Raiford. From Boring, Langfeld, and Weld [*Introduction to Psychology*, 1939, page 571].

representation by place. It would appear that the neural elements that are responding to these frequencies are operating
near their critical limits, and are easily disturbed or put out of
action. It is conceivable that under these conditions the normal cathodic summation ceases and even gives way to anodic
depression.

PRESBYACUSIA

Zwaardemaker in 1891 formulated what he called his 'law of
presbyacusia,' in which he stated that the upper limit of hearing
grows progressively shortened with age. Others have shown
that all the high tones are depreciated, not just those at the
upper boundary, and that on the average the loss is greater for
each successive decade of life. Figure 112 gives results obtained
by Bunch and Raiford on a population of hospital patients from

which all obvious cases of ear disease had been eliminated. The acuity is normal or practically so for all age groups for frequencies up to 1024 $\sim$ and thereafter falls away systematically in relation to age.

These observations have led some to the view that high-tone loss is the result of tissue changes directly associated with the process of aging. An alternative view, which is perhaps more likely, is that the loss is only indirectly due to age and comes from bouts of infection, acoustic trauma, and other damaging circumstances whose incidence is naturally a function of age. The latter view is favored by the fact that a few fortunate individuals reach an advanced age without any deterioration of hearing. The question might be settled by repeated tests on the same individuals over a long period.

CLINICAL HIGH-TONE DEAFNESS

Some persons, young and old, suffer a serious high-tone loss, well beyond the mild impairments that have come almost to be expected in the aged. The condition is usually progressive: the hearing for the highest tones continues to fade and that for others toward the middle range comes to be impaired.

There are two main types of the disorder, the abrupt and gradual types. In the abrupt type the hearing is good up to some particular frequency, say 1024 or 2048 $\sim$, and then for all following tones it is markedly impaired or altogether absent at practical intensities. In the gradual type the acuity again is within normal limits for the lowest tones but falls away progressively as the frequency is raised (see Fig. 40). The abrupt type of loss is most common in males; the gradual type is found about equally in both sexes. Crowe, Guild, and Polvogt in their study of the pathology of high-tone deafness correlated these disorders with distinctive inner ear lesions. They found the majority of ears with abrupt high-tone loss to have lesions both of the organ of Corti and the nerve fibers of the basal region of the cochlea. Those with the gradual type of loss often showed considerable atrophy of nerve fibers in the basal region but no significant sensory lesions. Other ears of both types contained no atrophies sufficient to account for the hearing loss. It is possible that these losses were due to central nervous lesions, but the experimental situation provided no opportunity to explore this possibility.

The phenomena of high-tone deafness are consistent with the picture of reasonably specific cochlear localization for high tones. When atrophy of sense organ and nerve is present in the base of the cochlea the hearing is severely affected for the uppermost frequencies but not significantly (at threshold levels of stimulation) for the lower tones. In the audiograms the change from normal to defective hearing is abrupt because the high tones have relatively sharp resonance curves on the basilar membrane, and must be raised to high levels to spread enough to bring in appreciably the outlying, normal hair cells. Also, these normal cells may have lost some part of their nerve fibers, especially, we would expect, that which they share with the cells now atrophied. When the organ of Corti is normal but there is a local lesion of nerve fibers in the base of the cochlea the audiogram shows a gradual high-tone loss because the innervation is somewhat diffuse, and fibers are withdrawn from parts of the cochlea over a wide area.

The sensory and nervous lesions found in these ears begin usually at the basal end of the cochlea and extend irregularly upward. Rarely do they run beyond the first 15 mm. Why this is so is unexplained. It would appear that this basal end of the cochlea is particularly fragile or that it is exposed to special hazards.

THE PHENOMENON OF LOUDNESS RECRUITMENT

Ears with partial high-tone deafness usually show a peculiarity of loudness perception. When tones that fall in the impaired region are raised in intensity sufficiently to become audible they come with a rush, as it seems, without passing through an intermediate stage of uncertainty as is usual in the neighborhood of the threshold. A judgment of the presence of these tones is made easily and unhesitatingly.

Then as the intensity is raised above the threshold the loudness grows rapidly, much more rapidly than it would for the same increase in decibels in the normal ear. The sound quickly becomes piercing and disturbing, and arouses a vigorous reaction and complaint. A person with this kind of deafness, when fitted with a hearing aid, cannot tolerate the amplification that might be expected on the basis of the impairment of threshold sensitivity.

Fowler first called special attention to this phenomenon and referred to it as 'recruitment.' He made measurements of the abnormal rise in loudness by using subjects with one normal

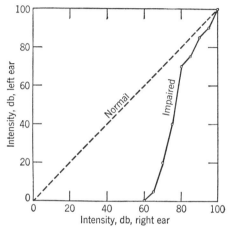

FIG. 113. The recruitment phenomenon. In a person with normal hearing a tone in one ear has to be raised to about the same intensity in the other ear to seem equally loud, and this relation is shown by the broken curve. In a person with one normal ear and one ear impaired by nerve deafness this sort of comparison of loudness gives the solid curve. Data from Fowler, for a patient deafened to 2048 ~ in the right ear. The scales represent decibels above the average normal threshold.

and one deafened ear and having them make binaural loudness balances at various levels. At threshold the sounds must be very different in intensity to balance, but above threshold the difference is smaller, and finally, if the intensity level can be carried high enough, there is no difference at all. Figure 113 shows observations made on a patient whose left ear was normal and whose right ear was impaired for 2048 ~. This tone when presented at threshold intensity for the deafened ear was 60 db above threshold for the normal ear; but when presented at an intensity 40 db higher it seemed equally loud in the two ears.

When this sort of comparison is made by a person with one normal ear and one that has suffered a conductive impairment, as for example that produced by a loss of the auditory ossicles, there is no recruitment of loudness. At all levels of stimulation the loudness in the defective ear is about the same number of decibels below that in the normal ear.

It should be added, however, that recruitment is not invariably associated with high-tone deafness. Dix, Hallpike, and Hood failed to find it in certain ears suffering a high-tone loss due to a diffuse degeneration of the fibers of the auditory nerve. On the other hand, they observed it in some ears suffering from Ménière's disease when the impairment of sensitivity was general. Here are special conditions that will repay further study; but the fact remains that this phenomenon is a common accompaniment of simple high-tone deafness.

The explanation of this phenomenon requires no new assumptions; it follows from the relation already indicated between loudness and nerve discharge, which depends in turn on the way in which stimuli spread over the cochlea and excite nervous action.

As already described, the high tones have rather sharply peaked patterns of cochlear action. For them the stimulus energy is largely concentrated upon a few sensory elements; and when this energy is near threshold there is excitation of only the nerve fibers serving this restricted region. Hence an impairment of either sensory or neural elements in this region is reflected in a disturbance of threshold sensitivity, and it is continued as a reduction of loudness when the intensity is raised further above threshold.

As the intensity is raised to still higher levels, however, the loudness deficiency grows less and less, and ultimately may become inappreciable. This happens because there is a limit to the contribution made by the elements occupying the peak of the response curve (the elements that we have supposed to suffer impairment), and because as the intensity is raised their contribution changes its relation to the whole discharge.

The contribution of any nerve fiber is limited because as intensity rises the rate of its impulses increases rapidly for a time, and then this rate rather sharply approaches a maximum, as

Fig. 87 has shown. Hence the elements serving the peak region of a tone soon reach their combined limits, and further additions to the loudness have to depend upon other elements in adjoining regions. When the level of stimulation is low the contributions of these central elements loom large and their absence is felt; but when the level is high their contributions fade into

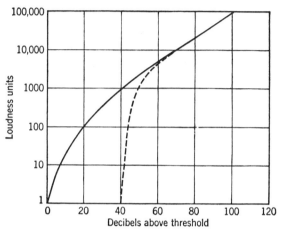

FIG. 114. An explanation of recruitment. The solid line represents the course of the loudness function (Fletcher's curve, Fig. 85) with a logarithmic ordinate, and the broken line is the same function after subtracting 1000 loudness units at every point. After Steinberg and Gardner.

insignificance. Their relation to the whole changes because (according to the theory of loudness presented above) a given increment of loudness is produced at low levels by a very moderate addition to the neural stream, and at higher levels by an increasingly large addition.

This explanation of the recruitment phenomenon combines the hypothesis of Lorente de Nó (4) and Fowler, who spoke of neural elements as readily reaching a point of 'saturation' when strongly stimulated, and the one advanced by Steinberg and Gardner, who pointed out the relation to the loudness function.

Steinberg and Gardner showed that a function like that found in recruitment may be obtained simply by subtracting some constant number of loudness units (corresponding to some constant number of impulses in the nerve discharge, according to the theory) from the number of loudness units represented in the normal loudness function. The curve of Fig. 114 was obtained in this way; and the resemblance to the recruitment function is obvious.

Steinberg and Gardner further pointed out that loudness changes of the kind observed as recruitment in a deafened ear are found in the normal ear in the presence of masking. It is presumed that a masking tone curtails the activity of certain elements, and thereby reduces the discharge representing the other tone to an extent that is serious at low levels but much less so at high levels.

ELECTRICAL STIMULATION OF THE EAR

Of considerable theoretical interest are the phenomena that arise when an electric current is passed through the ear. Sounds are heard that vary in character according to the particular conditions. Direct currents give a dull click when the circuit is closed or opened. Alternating currents give sustained sounds that vary from pure tones to noises, or are a mixture of the two.

Under usual conditions the current is applied through a wire electrode in contact with a quantity of saline solution in the external auditory canal and a second electrode elsewhere on the body. With normal subjects a sinusoidal current gives a tone containing a fundamental (of the frequency of the stimulus) and a rather noticeable overtone. Sometimes this overtone dominates, and the pitch is double what would be heard if the current were first sent through a loudspeaker and converted into aerial vibrations in the ordinary way.

Such effects as these can be explained, as Max F. Meyer (8) pointed out and Stevens and Jones later attested, as an electromechanical action of the peripheral tissues. The skin of the external auditory meatus, the tympanic membrane, or other parts may be set in motion by the varying electric charges, much as the diaphragm of an electrostatic receiver is actuated. After the electrostatic conversion of the alternating currents into sounds, the further processes are the same as when sounds are applied in the usual manner.

Now, the electrostatic receiver and other sound producers of its class have certain distinctive characteristics. When fed by pure alternating current they generate a sound of double frequency. If a direct current is added to the alternating current the fundamental frequency will appear also and will rise in amplitude as a function of the direct-current component.

Stevens and Jones investigated the effects on the ear of various mixtures of direct and alternating currents, as a test of the electrostatic hypothesis. The results followed the pattern to be expected on this hypothesis in that the fundamental rose and fell with the polarizing current, while the harmonic component remained unaltered. However, in one respect there was a departure from expectation: it was not always possible to find a value of the polarizing current that would eliminate the fundamental component altogether. For an electrostatic process such a value should exist; it should be a value that just cancels any internal polarization. This feature of the results remained unexplained except as due to some further process. Despite this difficulty, however, Stevens and Jones accepted the electrostatic explanation. More explicitly, they supposed that the drum membrane and the bony promontory of the cochlea act as the two plates of a condenser, and when this condenser is charged by an alternating current the varying electric tensions cause a vibration of the more mobile of these two plates, the drum membrane, so stimulating the ear.

There seems little doubt that some such electromechanical action can occur. If it were all that occurs our interest in this mode of stimulating the ear would now cease, for once actual sounds appear there are no further distinctive problems. Yet this explanation does not cover all the phenomena. Electric stimuli are still effective in ears in which the drum membrane and ossicles are absent and the electrode is placed on the bony promontory, away from any easily mobile tissue. Under these conditions the subjects report somewhat different experiences. A sinusoidal current often gives a pure fundamental tone, without any noticeable overtone. Sometimes this tone is accompanied by a buzzing noise, and in a few ears nothing but the noise is heard.

Gersuni and his associates, after extensive observations of these phenomena in abnormal ears, became convinced that they were due to some kind of action on the sensory elements of the cochlea (Gersuni and Volokhov; Arapova, Gersuni, and Volokhov). Jones, Stevens, and Lurie accepted this explanation for certain abnormal ears (those that heard pure tones) and tried to make it more explicit. They suggested that the action is the reverse of the one by which sounds elicit the cochlear potentials.

Many physical processes are reversible; a condenser microphone, for example, though designed to convert sound into electric currents, will work the other way, as a sound producer, when currents are applied to it. The argument here is that the hair cells likewise act reversibly when energized by alternating currents.

This hypothesis is in accord with the picture of hair-cell action already presented. If these cells are polarized in the way suggested, they might be forced into changes of length by changes in the electric field about them.

Jones, Stevens, and Lurie developed their views of the action of electric currents within the framework of a simple place theory, and were led into further elaborations. If all the hair cells exposed to the electric field responded by movements and excited their nerve fibers the result would be embarrassing to strict specificity. A vast number of elements throughout the cochlea would be involved for any stimulating frequency. These authors therefore assumed that as the hair cells move they tend to drag the basilar membrane along with them. However, they succeed in doing so only in certain favorable regions: in those regions where the membrane is tuned to the stimulating frequency. The basilar membrane thus imposes its restraints upon the hair cells, and the result is that with electric stimulation only those cells are set in motion that would respond in the ordinary way to sounds. They alone excite their nerve fibers, and specificity holds.

We need to examine further this view that the basilar membrane effectively imposes its resonance properties upon the hair cells. The argument rests upon the assumption of full reciprocity, which means that there is a close mechanical coupling between hair cells and basilar membrane. Movements of the one must be communicated immediately and forcefully to the other. Yet we see in the hair cells (as Fig. 5, page 20, will make clear) only slight mass in relation to the basilar membrane and its pertinent structures, and the connections by way of the Deiters processes seem limited in stiffness. It would appear from anatomical considerations that a hair cell in its expansions and contractions might readily transfer motion to its Deiters process but would encounter resistance at the basilar membrane because of the massiveness of that structure. The forces ought largely to be taken up in lateral bendings of the hair cell and the Deiters process rather than displacements of the membrane. The matter is of course a relative one: if the hair cell really moves as described it must transmit some motion to the membrane.

For such reversed transmission the anatomical conditions seem rather more favorable in the basal region of the basilar membrane than elsewhere. Here the Deiters processes are short and thick, and other parts of the cuticular framework seem correspondingly firm. An appreciable regulation of hair-cell motion by the basilar membrane is perhaps conceivable for this region.

If this much of the hypothesis of Jones, Stevens, and Lurie is admitted, then we can account for the pitch of the tones produced by high-frequency currents along the lines of a place theory, in terms of the resulting spatial patterns on the basilar membrane.

Let us now consider an alternative or at least a supplementary explanation of the electrical phenomena, an explanation based upon the idea that the currents produce a direct excitation of the auditory nerve. This is no new idea; indeed, the early discoverers of the electrical effects took such an action for granted. Of late, however, this simple explanation has largely been neglected. Jones, Stevens, and Lurie accepted it in part, saying that the electric current may have more than one kind of action. In their opinion, the current may produce sounds by electrostatic action, and under appropriate conditions may also excite both sensory cells and nerve fibers.

It would be remarkable if direct auditory nerve excitation did not occur. The stimuli produce widespread effects, evidently by action on various sense organs and nerves about the head. They cause sensations of tickle, itching, pressure, and pain from the near-by cutaneous regions, and nystagmus and even nausea sometimes from labyrinthine stimulation. With so much general stimulation the participation of the auditory nerve can hardly be ruled out.

The acoustic phenomena as described can be accounted for very well as a result of this direct auditory nerve action. If the action is on the more central portions of the fibers, or on their ganglion cells, then alternating currents ought to give a rate of nerve discharge equal to the alternating frequency at levels of current strength near threshold (when the excitation is cathodic only) and double this rate at higher levels (when both cathodic and anodic half-waves become effective). If the action is on the dendritic ends of the fibers in the immediate vicinity of the hair cells, where we have assumed a polarizing potential to be present, this stimulus should give the fundamental rate not only at threshold but at levels well above, up to the point where the amplitude of the alternating potential as made effective on the dendrites exceeds the polarization.

With gross overstimulation, which as we know seriously impairs the excitability and recovery of nerve fibers, an irregular discharge is to be expected. This may be the explanation of the noisy sensations aroused under certain conditions, and observed in general when the currents are strong.

This explanation of the electric effects in terms of a direct action on the nerve has the advantage of avoiding the assumptions that the hair cells move under the influence of the currents and that the basilar membrane exercises specific restraints upon them.

CHAPTER 15

THE PRODUCTS OF TONAL INTERACTION

When two tones are presented simultaneously to the ear they produce one or more interaction phenomena: beats, combination tones, interference, and masking.

BEATS

Beats are of two kinds, classically known as the beats of imperfect unisons and the beats of mistuned consonances. The first-named are the more familiar and arise from two tones whose frequencies differ only a little. The rate of beating is simply equal to the frequency difference. Beats of the second kind appear in the action of two tones whose frequencies depart slightly from some simple interval relationship; for example, the tones 200 and 302, which approximate a musical fifth with a ratio of 2:3, will be heard as beating at a rate of 4 per second. (The rate of beating is found as $mN - nM$, where m/n is the simplest perfect ratio of the interval, and M, N are the actual vibration frequencies of the tones. Thus, in the example, $m = 2$, $n = 3$; $M = 200$, $N = 302$; hence $2 \times 302 - 3 \times 200 = 604 - 600 = 4$ beats per second.)

The character of beats varies according to their rate. Slow beats are heard as surgings in which the periodic rise and fall in the loudness of the sound is the prominent feature. Some, like Helmholtz, have reported a periodic pitch variation as well. With a faster rate this cyclic character disappears, and we hear merely a succession of distinct and seemingly momentary pulses. Finally, with still faster beats, the individual pulses are no longer evident and we hear only a rough whirring of sound. These three stages of surging, intermittence, and roughness appear for all beating regardless of the particular primary tones or the frequency regions from which they come.

How fast the beats may be and still be perceived depends upon a number of conditions. For tones of the middle range, around 1024 ~, surging changes to intermittence at a rate of about 6 per second, and then intermittence goes over into roughness around 166 per second. Roughness extends to 350 per second or so. How much effect frequency region has is still in some doubt, but the available evidence indicates higher limits for the upper frequencies.

These experiences bear a remarkable resemblance to those obtained from single pure tones at the lower end of the frequency scale. The low tones pass through the same three stages of surging, intermittence, and roughness as the frequency is raised, and the critical regions, where one stage gives way to another, have about the same relative locations along the periodicity range.

The theory that up to now has had the most consideration in the explanation of beats is the resonance theory. This theory supposes that two beating tones occupy partially overlapping regions of the basilar membrane, and the movements of the common portion of the membrane represent a resultant of the two vibrations. When the primaries are in phase the vibrations summate to give a maximum displacement, and when a little later they get out of phase the vibrations oppose one another to give a minimum displacement. These changes of amplitude from maximum to minimum have a periodic rate equal to the frequency difference of the primaries, and our perception of them gives the experience of beats.

Incidentally we may note that this explanation of beats runs in the face of Ohm's law and the principle of specificity on which the Helmholtz theory was grounded. A system of independent resonators would resolve the presented stimuli and give a perception of two steady tones without any beats. Within the range of perceptibility of beats the theory is forced to modify its rules of specificity and analysis. This complication only adds to the general difficulty in which the theory finds itself in respect to the problems of spread and specificity, and needs no further attention here.

It is important to note that the above explanation applies only to the simplest beats. The resonance theory cannot handle the beats of mistuned consonances as such but must first find a way of deriving them as a kind of simple beats. The theory does this by means of a subsidiary hypothesis, by supposing that the beats of mistuned consonances are the result of an interaction not of the primaries directly but of overtones either present in the stimuli themselves or produced through distortion in the course of transmission through the middle ear.

It is easy to dispute this explanation of the beats of mistuned consonances. As Koenig stoutly maintained in opposition to Helmholtz, and as modern experiments prove beyond question,

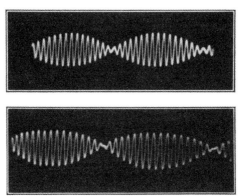

Fig. 115. Beats. The upper curve represents the aerial wave resulting from a combination of two tones of 1000 and 1001 $\sim$. The lower curve shows the form of the cochlear potentials produced in the guinea pig by this sound.

these beats arise in the use of tones in which physical overtones are absent or negligible. They arise also when the level of stimulation is so low that no additional tones are generated within the ear. Here then is exposed a serious weakness of the resonance theory.

The resonance theory suffers further from its failure to account for the similarity of beats produced by primaries chosen from different tonal regions, or for the resemblance between beats and low tones.

The volley theory offers a different and a simpler explanation of beats; simpler because it frees itself more than the resonance theory is able to do from the constraints of specificity and accounts for all beats in the same way, as due in the main to a perception of rhythmic variations in the nerve discharge.

Consider first the simple beats. The motions of the two beating tones are summated in a physical sense in the aerial waves and have precisely the form of the uppermost curve of Fig. 115. Any acoustical system that does not analyze this wave but accepts it as it stands will naturally reflect the amplitude variations shown (the oscillograph used to obtain this picture obviously did so). This pattern is followed by the cochlear response (as the lower curve of this same figure proves) and in turn is translated into nerve activity. This activity consists of a series of bursts of nerve impulses, with the bursts varying in size throughout the beating cycle from a maximum during phase agreement to a minimum during phase opposition.

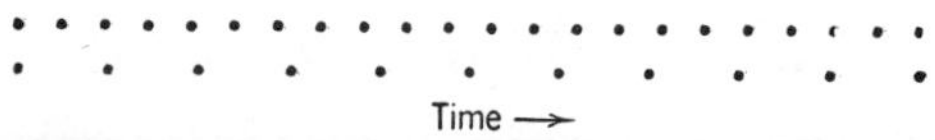

Time →

FIG. 116. A conception of the nerve discharge pattern for the mistuned octave. The upper row of dots represents the pattern of discharge for the higher tone, and the lower row represents the pattern for the lower tone.

The beats of mistuned consonances are best explained if we suppose at first that the primaries act independently and work out the pattern of nerve discharge for each, and then finally put the two patterns together. These two patterns will be found to have coincident volleys at one point in the beat cycle and then progressively less exact coincidences until a complete separation is reached, after which this order of changes reverses itself and coincidence appears once more as the beat cycle ends.

Consider as the simplest example the mistuned octave. Figure 116 is a conceptualization of the discharge pattern. The upper row of dots represents the series of volleys caused by the higher tone, and the lower row represents the series caused by the lower tone. Let us examine these two series in their time relations. Beginning on the left, we have two coincident volleys, then a single volley representing the higher tone only, then two volleys not quite coincident, another single volley, and so on until at the middle of the beat cycle the low-tone volley appears halfway between two high-tone volleys; and thereafter the order reverses until we have coincidence at the end. It should be noted that here we have simply a temporal pattern that recurs at a rate determined by the mistuning; so far no spatial interaction is called for. It may well be that the rhythmic variations perceived in beats are largely determined by these purely temporal conditions. However, it is probable that always, even under the least favorable circumstances, the temporal pattern is reinforced by a spatial interaction. The tones overlap on the basilar mem-

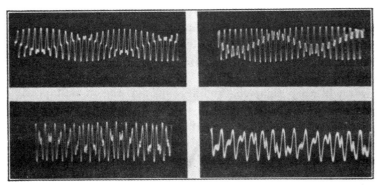

Fig. 117. Forms of complex waves. Upper left, stimulus wave made up of two tones, 1000 and 2001 ∿, forming a mistuned octave; upper right, the cochlear response produced by this sound (in the guinea pig). Lower left, a mistuned fifth (1000 and 1501 ∿), and lower right, a mistuned fourth (900 and 1201 ∿), both as seen in the cochlear responses.

brane and combine their stimulating effects in the sensory elements.

For an idea of the nature of this overlapping we consider the compound wave. Figure 117 shows the form of this wave for the mistuned octave and also for some other more complex intervals. In these pictures we have a visual indication of the periodicities that we perceive as beats. There is not the over-all variation in amplitude that we find in the simple beats. Rather, we see a pattern of disturbances running through the waves. What we hear, when the two beating tones are first equated in loudness, is one tone, the higher, that seems always present, and another that waxes and wanes. The more complex the ratio the more prominent is the steady part of the complex and the less noticeable the beating.

The limits of perceptibility of beats do not represent the limits of overlapping on the basilar membrane; the problem is not so simple as that. Each of the three stages of the experience has its own limit, and each separately needs explanation. The first stage of surging is found at the slow rates where we are still able to observe loudness changes in the course of the beat cycle. Its limit therefore represents the point where we begin to integrate loudness over the cycle and perceive it in 'lumped' form. The limit of 6 per second found for the 1024~ region agrees remarkably well with the data already given on the time interval over which loudness is summated. As we have seen, Békésy in working with 800~ obtained full integration at 0.17 sec, which would indicate a rate of 1/0.17 or 5.88 per second. These figures will vary somewhat with frequency region and possibly with intensity.

Through the stage of intermittence we evidently are integrating the loudness over each beat cycle, for each cycle appears as a definite pulse. In the early part of this stage the pulses are quite distinct, and for the simple beats of equally strong primaries they are separated by appreciable moments of silence. Then as the rates grow faster the separation becomes less until it falls to zero and the limit of intermittence is reached.

Here, where the discreteness of the beating is no longer evident, begins the stage of roughness. The roughness seems to be continuous and colors the whole experience. As the beating rate is further raised this roughness slowly grows less prominent until it is no longer noticeable. No doubt this end point is reached when the irregularities of discharge that the roughness represents are of the same order of magnitude as other irregularities inherent in the nerve discharge and so are swamped by them.

COMBINATION TONES

When two pure tones stimulate the ear at high intensity we hear not only the tones themselves but also other tones whose frequencies are the sums and differences of the primary frequencies and their simple multiples. These are the combination tones. Under ordinary conditions only a few can be observed directly, like the difference tone of the first order whose frequency is the difference between the primary stimuli, and sometimes the summation tone whose frequency is their sum. For example, with stimuli of 2800 and 1000 $\sim$ we may hear the difference and summation tones of $(2800 - 1000) = 1800 \sim$ and $(2800 + 1000) = 3800 \sim$. Careful observation, and the introduction of a third stimulus (exploring tone) of a frequency that will beat with an expected component, will reveal still higher orders of combination tones. An analysis of the electrical response of the cochlea reveals them in great numbers (Wever, Bray, and Lawrence, 3; Wever, 6). All may be expressed as the absolute values of the quantity $(mh \pm nl)$, where h and l are the frequencies of the two primaries, and m and n are any integers. The order of a component is defined as $m + n - 1$. At the same time that the combination tones make their appearance there arise overtones as well, a series for each primary. They are simple multiples of the primary frequency and are expressed also by the formula $mh \pm nl$ if we let m or n become zero.

This appearance of new components not in the physical stimulus constitutes aural distortion. It is explained by the transformation principle, which states that at high levels of intensity the ear's response is no longer directly proportional to the acoustic forces acting upon it but is proportional in some degree to higher powers of those forces. The mathematical expression is

$$X = a_0 + a_1 P + a_2 P^2 + a_3 P^3 + \cdots + a_n P^n$$

where X is the ear's response, P is the force acting, and a_0, a_1, a_2, etc., are constants. Now when P represents the sum of two sinusoidal forces a trigonometric development of the equation yields a long series of terms including the primaries, their overtones, and all their combination tones.

The evidence is in firm support of the transformation principle. A great many of the components predicted by it have been identified. For example, with the tones 100 and 10,000 $\sim$ as many as 35 combination tones have been found in the cochlear responses of the guinea pig. It is equally significant that despite an intensive search no component has ever been found that does not belong to the regular series as indicated by the formula. The theory has the merit of deriving the overtones and the combination tones in the same process and of putting the difference tones and summation tones on the same footing. The magnitudes of the components and their variations as a function of intensity are consistent with theoretical expectations.

The next question to be faced is the locus of the transformation process. Helmholtz placed it in the middle ear and more specifically in the movements of the tympanic membrane and ossicles. It is crucial to a resonance theory thus to locate the process in the periphery. If the new components arise in the periphery they then can be conducted like any other tones to the inner ear for analysis. On the other hand, if only the primaries enter the inner ear they at once are separated spatially in the analytic process and cannot thereafter interact. An incomplete separation such as was admitted by this theory to account for simple beats cannot be carried so far as to account for the combination tones. The range of interaction is too great; it covers the entire scale as the above observation of interaction between 100 and 10,000 ∼ has shown. To accept so extensive a spread over the basilar membrane is to relinquish too much of the specificity on which the simple resonance theory depends.

Unhappily for this theory of Helmholtz's the experimental facts, which have already been referred to, point to the inner ear and not the middle ear as the principal source of the distortion. The clearest evidence comes from the animal studies that employ the cochlear potentials. After the drum and two outer ossicles have been removed and the ear is stimulated by placing a mechanical vibrator in contact with the stapes both the overtone and combination tone patterns appear in essentially their usual forms. There is some contribution to the combination tone pattern by the middle ear when the stimuli are exceedingly strong, but even then by far the major part of the distortion appears beyond the stapes (Wever, Bray, and Lawrence, 1, 2).

Further evidence comes from experiments in which various drastic changes were made in the middle ear apparatus without significantly altering the distortion pattern. Denervating the tensor tympani muscle, cutting its tendon, eliciting its reflex contractions, and applying artificial tension to its tendon are all measures that must seriously modify the operation of the middle ear mechanism. The last two reduce the transmission, yet if the stimulus intensity is raised to compensate for this reduction the distortion becomes the same as before. Raising the air pressure in the middle ear cavity likewise has no appreciable effect. The only measure so far found that very noticeably alters the distortion is the application of tension to the stapedius tendon. It is evident that under normal conditions, and even in the presence of undue stresses, the middle ear apparatus carries out its duties of sound transmission with great faithfulness (Wever and Bray, 7).

If we accept the view that every tone spreads widely over the cochlea the rise of combination tones in the cochlea becomes a simple matter. When two stimuli are very strong they involve portions of the sensory apparatus in common, and they do so with great vigor. Their combined motions exceed the magnitudes to which the system responds in a linear fashion, and they give an effect that is represented by a power series, as the transformation principle states.

The particular locus of distortion in the inner ear has already been suggested. It is, according to the best indications, the basilar membrane and its sensory apparatus. Indeed, two specific processes in the actions of this structure have been put forward as probable sources of the distortion. One of them is the mechanical action by which the hair cells are displaced, and the other is the electromechanical action in the hair cells themselves. The evidence for this locus and for the existence of two separate processes comes from studies of the phenomenon of interference, to which we now turn.

INTERFERENCE

A further phenomenon in the simultaneous action of two tones upon the ear is interference (Covell and Black; Wever, Bray, and Lawrence, 4). This is of recent discovery and so far is known only in the electrical activity of the cochlea. It appears as a reduction in the magnitude of response to one tone on the presentation of another.

To observe the phenomenon one tone is led to the ear and its response measured with a wave analyzer (a highly selective voltmeter) set to its frequency. If now a second or interfering tone is introduced and raised to a sufficient intensity the response to the first tone suffers a reduction in magnitude. The effect is absent at the lower intensities of the interfering tone and then sets in rather suddenly as a critical intensity is reached. Thereafter as the intensity of the interfering tone is raised further the

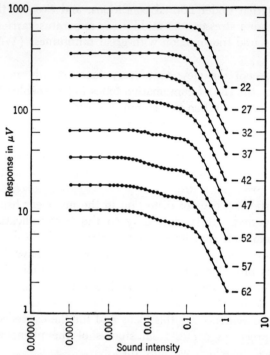

FIG. 118. The interference phenomenon. The curves show the cochlear responses obtained to a 1015∼ tone as measured in the presence of a 3000∼ tone. For each curve the intensity of the 1015∼ tone was constant (shown in decibels relative to 1 dyne per sq cm by the number near its end), and the intensity of the 3000∼ tone (in dynes per sq cm) varied as shown on the abscissa. Guinea pig ear. From Wever, Bray, and Lawrence (4) [*Journal of the Acoustical Society of America*].

effect becomes rapidly more pronounced until at the highest intensities it shows a tendency to level off. Reductions up to 30 db are easily observed, but the maximum effects cannot be ascertained on account of risk of damage to the ear. The responses under extreme interference become unstable, because the ear is being subjected to stresses near its limits of tolerance.

Interference occurs between any pair of tones, whatever their frequencies. It appears for tones only a few cycles apart and for others taken from the very ends of the frequency scale. This does not mean, however, that frequency is irrelevant; it has a significant relation to the degree of interference. Generally

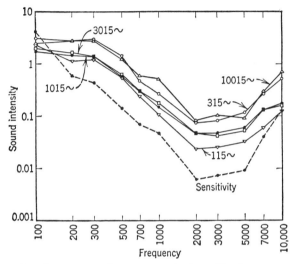

FIG. 119. Interference in relation to sensitivity. The lowermost curve is the cochlear sensitivity curve for a rabbit ear and represents the sound intensity (in dynes per sq cm) required to produce a standard response of 10 microvolts. The other curves are interference curves measured for each of 5 tones in the presence of interfering tones of various frequencies as shown on the abscissa. For each of these curves the stimulus intensity of the tone acted upon was constant, and the various interfering tones were adjusted in intensity so as to produce a standard amount of interference (a loss of 1 db). From Wever, Bray, and Lawrence (4) [*Journal of the Acoustical Society of America*].

speaking, interference is greater for the tones to which the ear is the more sensitive. Evidently, as we would expect, it depends upon the intensity that prevails at the site where it occurs, and so it reflects the sensitivity as shown by the cochlear potentials. However, it does not reflect that sensitivity perfectly; a divergence is found at the two ends of the frequency scale. There the interference is greater than would be expected from the form of the sensitivity curve. Hence it follows that some special condition enters for the extreme tones, a condition that intervenes between interference and the process by which the cochlear potentials are generated. This condition is such as to discriminate against the high and low tones.

Interference bears a close relation to the transformation process. The reduction that is observed in the presence of an interfering tone is in large part due to the diversion of energy into combination tones. When measurements are made of a great many of the components present—the primaries, their overtones, and the combination tones—the total response comes very near to accounting for all the stimulus energy, provided that the tones are not too strong. With very intense tones the total response is always too small for the stimulus energy present, which means that under this condition the ear's efficiency has fallen off. This impairment of efficiency is one of the aspects of overloading.

The locus of the transformation process is now indicated in relation to the other cochlear processes of interference and overloading. Further experiments give this location more anatomic reality. It is easy to prove that interference is independent of the more peripheral parts of the conductive apparatus. Its effect is observed on stimulation by bone conduction, and after the drum membrane and two outer ossicles have been removed and the stimuli are applied to the stapes. More specific information comes from an analysis that makes use of the injury resulting from overstimulation of the ear.

When the ear is overstimulated an injury results that is immediately shown in an impairment of cochlear potentials and whose site is revealed later by histological study. This site is the organ of Corti. We observe a disruption of this organ and a loss of hair cells over a broad area of the basilar membrane. The study of interference functions before and after injury proves that the interference takes place at the site of this injury (Wever and Lawrence, 1). The proof resides in the fact that after injury the forms of the interference functions are significantly changed. If interference occurred in advance of the injury process it would then have to be viewed through the injury supervening, but its functional relations to the stimulus would remain unaltered. Correspondingly, if interference occurred after the injury process it should be unaltered if the injury is compensated for by raising the stimulus intensity until the former level of response is restored. No such stability is found in this situation, and it is evident by a process of elimination that interference must have the same site as the injury: it takes place in the organ of Corti.

Once more we find the facts consistent with the view that all tones spread widely over the basilar membrane. Since interference occurs between any two tones it follows that all tones work on parts of the membrane in common.

MASKING

When two tones applied to the ear are somewhat similar in frequency but one is much stronger than the other the stronger will reduce the other's loudness or even prevent its perception altogether. This effect is called masking. It is primarily a uniaural phenomenon: the effects depend upon the presentation of the tones to the same ear. Binaural masking, from the presentation of the two tones to opposite ears, probably exists as a separate phenomenon, though some have suggested that it appears only by conduction of the stronger tone through the head and therefore is only a form of uniaural masking. In any event it is negligible in amount in comparison with the uniaural form and will not be considered further here.

Masking is quite distinct from interference. As just brought out, interference occurs between any tones whatsoever; but masking demands that the tones be in the same general region of frequency. Also—and even more significant—masking can be shown to be a nervous and not a sensory phenomenon. It is not found in the cochlear potentials but makes its appearance in the nerve action that follows.

The amount of masking depends upon the frequency and intensity of the tones. Wegel and Lane first worked out these relations systematically; and some of their results are given in Fig. 120. Here the amount of masking is defined as the depression of threshold sensitivity for the one tone caused by the introduction of the other.

The figure shows the masking effects of a tone of 1200 ∼ at three different levels of intensity. It is evident that the sensitivity is affected for a broad range of tones in the vicinity of the masking tone. At a level of 60 db above threshold, for example, this tone masks other tones from 600 to 3000 ~, a range of about 2½ octaves. The effect is greatest for tones that are near the primary frequency yet not so near as to give strong beats. At more remote frequencies the masking falls off rapidly at first and then progressively more slowly. When the masking

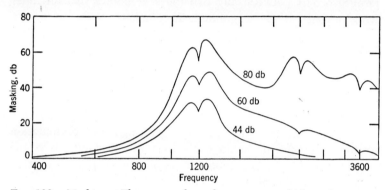

FIG. 120.   Masking.   The curves show the extent to which various tones must be elevated above their normal thresholds when listened to in the presence of a masking tone of 1200 ~. This masking tone was presented at each of 3 levels, as shown in decibels above threshold by the numbers on the curves.   After Wegel and Lane [*Physical Review*].

tone is made stronger the effect extends more widely, and this extension is mainly of the upper end of the frequency band. Secondary elevations appear in the masking curve at frequencies that are multiples of the masking tone.

The range over which masking appears is a function of the frequency of the masking tone. The low tones give broader masking curves than the high tones do, when the results are plotted on a logarithmic scale as in Fig. 120.

The changes in the amount of masking with the intensity of the masking tone are better exhibited by plotting the results for individual frequencies as in Fig. 121. Here it is evident that the form of the masking function varies according to the frequency relation of the two tones. For tones near the masking tone the curves take a rather regular course, with sometimes a slight bending at the highest levels. For tones well above the masking frequency the curves rise only slowly at first, and then flex upward sharply and rise at a rapid rate, until sometimes at high levels they bend over.

The sharp upward rise shown in the functions for tones above the masking frequency is the same feature that appears in Fig. 120 as the introduction of secondary elevations. What is happening, according to Wegel and Lane's interpretations, is that overtones generated in the ear are adding their masking effects.

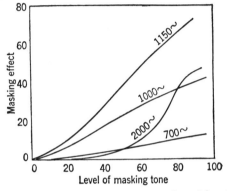

FIG. 121. Masking curves for various tones as affected by 1200 ∼. From Wegel and Lane [*Physical Review*].

The appearance of relatively steep slopes in the curves after their flexures is in agreement with the transformation principle, which states that the increase in the magnitude of an overtone with intensity is more rapid the higher the order of the overtone.

There is good reason to believe that masking arises in the process of excitation of the cochlear nerve fibers. The evidence seems to exclude other possibilities. As already mentioned, masking does not show itself in the cochlear potentials. And, judging by the binaural tests, it is only feeble, if present at all, in the central nervous processes.

According to Wegel and Lane's hypothesis, masking is a product of a spatial interaction. A tone is masked when its maximum amplitude of action on the basilar membrane is exceeded by the action at the same place of another, stronger tone. This idea is indicated in Fig. 122. The largest curve represents the action on the basilar membrane of the primary or masking tone, and the smaller curves represent three different intensities at which the secondary tone might be presented. When the secondary tone at its primary locus has an amplitude below that of the other tone, as at *a* in this figure, the secondary tone *is* masked; when the two tones have the same amplitude at this locus, as at *b*, the secondary tone is at its threshold of percepti-

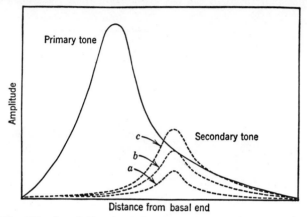

FIG. 122. Wegel and Lane's explanation of masking. A primary tone masks another when its action on the basilar membrane exceeds the action of the other at all points. Tone *a* is masked, *c* is not, and *b* is at the threshold of perceptibility. After Wegel and Lane.

bility; and when the maximum amplitude of the secondary tone rises well above the amplitude of the other at this place, as at *c*, both tones become easily audible.

According to this hypothesis the masking functions, like those of Fig. 120, reflect in a simple way the patterns of response on the basilar membrane. It then becomes possible to extend the exploring tone method, already referred to in the study of combination tones, to a detailed measurement of these patterns.

Wegel and Lane's hypothesis, when considered in its neural aspects, makes masking a matter of the pre-empting of nerve fibers. The stronger tone is supposed to engage a fiber fully and to prevent any action upon it by the weaker tone. Let us consider these neural implications further in the light of the available evidence.

Inhibitory effects of one tone on another are observed in the cochlear nerve potentials. Derbyshire and Davis noted a reduction in the impulses aroused by a tone when a clicking noise was introduced. Galambos and Davis (2) studied this phenomenon more intensively. They found with the microelectrode technique that the response of a particular neural element to one tone is affected by various other tones, over a wide range. Some tones reduce the responses or eliminate them altogether, whereas other tones enhance them. A given tone may inhibit at one intensity and enhance at another. Noises usually inhibit responses to tones, but tones have little or no effect upon the responses to noises. The relationships to frequency and intensity are complex and even rather mystifying; and here further study is necessary.

Lowy proved that central nervous connections are not necessary for the inhibitory effects. He recorded nerve impulses from the round window membrane in response to brief noises (the ticking of a watch was the stimulus), and found them to be masked by certain tones even after the central trunk of the eighth nerve had been narcotized or severed. Central reflex mechanisms are thereby excluded, and masking is indicated as peripheral in origin.

Galambos and Davis, at the time that they regarded their results as representative of the action of nerve fibers, rejected the common explanation of masking as a pre-empting of fibers by the stronger tone. This explanation, they argued, would require that the fiber be in action in response to either one tone or the other, and their findings seemed contrary to this supposition inasmuch as the second tone often renders the fiber altogether inactive.

They offered suggestions as to other forms of neural interaction that might account for masking effects, with a preference for a specific inhibitory mechanism in the cochlea. Later they abandoned this hypothesis in view of the conclusion that their experimental results were representative of secondary neurones. It is plain that for an account of inhibitory effects at this level we have at our disposal all the complex interactions that synapses make possible.

It should be added that inhibition of the sort referred to here is not limited to the ear. It is found in stimulation of the retina by light and of the labyrinth by rotation. Hence in the explanation of masking we ought not to presume any unique character either in the nerve connections or the sensory excitation.

Let us consider another approach to this masking problem. The basic assumption of the foregoing theory, that one or the other of two tones acting at a given place in the cochlea must take exclusive possession of the neural elements there, does not seem a very probable one either from a consideration of the neurophysiological data just referred to or from a consideration of other results on the interaction of tones. It seems more likely that the two tones simply summate their effects; that they combine both in their actions on the membrane and in their excitatory effects. It seems more reasonable, also, to consider the whole pattern of action produced by the tones and not merely the points of maximum stimulation. The problem now is whether or not one tone when added to another produces an appreciable change in the pattern of neural activity.

We have already learned, in our study of loudness and pitch, that the neural patterns aroused by tones may change in two principal ways, either spatially or temporally. We have learned also, in our study of the discrimination of loudness and pitch, that these patterns to be appreciable as changing must vary by amounts that differ according to the conditions, and generally speaking must vary more and more as the level of neural activity rises. We can suppose much the same to be true when these spatial and temporal variables enter into the determination of perception in more complicated ways. We can suppose in this situation, therefore, that the added tone will be perceived if it brings about a substantial alteration in the magnitude of the nerve discharge or in the identity of the elements entering into this discharge. Usually the change will be in both these respects. On the other hand, if these changes are below a certain limiting level the tone will go unnoticed; it then will be masked by the stimulus prevailing.

Masking by Thermal Noise. Fletcher and Munson investigated the masking effects of thermal noise, with results that illuminate further the relation between loudness and masking and the problems of cochlear spread and localization. This kind of noise is wholly random in character, with its energy distributed continuously and uniformly throughout the frequency spectrum. It is produced by applying to the input of a high-gain amplifier the changes in resistance present in any conductor (due to the thermal motions of its molecules), and leading the random currents so obtained into a telephone receiver or loudspeaker. By means of electric filters in the circuit the noise may be split up into bands of frequencies or otherwise modified as desired.

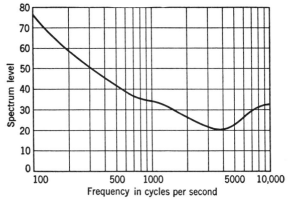

FIG. 123.   The thermal noise spectrogram producing uniform masking. The intensity varied for the different frequency components of the noise as shown by the ordinate. Here 'spectrum level' refers to the intensity level per cycle of the noise (decibels above the reference level of a 1-cycle band). From Fletcher (4) [*Journal of the Acoustical Society of America*].

Fletcher and Munson (2) presented a wide band of this noise, containing frequencies over nearly the whole audible range, and adjusted the intensity of different regions of the band so as to make the masking effect on pure tones of various frequencies as uniform as possible. They found that the regional intensity level of the noise had to be varied in a way shown in Fig. 123 to produce this effect. It is evident that generally speaking this noise had to be stronger at the lower frequencies. They then found that this noise satisfactorily maintained its masking pattern regardless of the general intensity used: once the proper composition was determined the whole could be raised and lowered in intensity, and the masking went up and down accordingly, with the uniformity of its frequency effects maintained, provided that the intensity level was kept within moderate bounds (45 to 100 db).

It is of interest to relate this noise spectrogram to the level of intensity of the tone that it masks. The difference in decibels between the spectrum level of the noise (its intensity level per

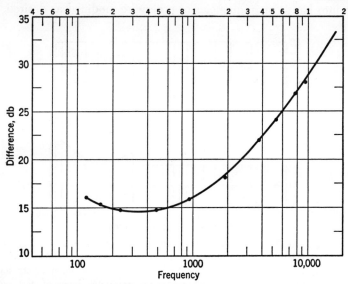

FIG. 124. Thermal-noise masking and the ear's selectivity characteristics. The curve shows the difference in decibels between the spectrum level of the noise (its intensity per cycle) and the intensity level of the tone that it just masks. The differences shown are interpreted as reflecting the increased selectivity of the ear at high frequencies. After Fletcher (4).

cycle) and the intensity level of the tone in the same frequency region that is just masked is shown as a function of frequency in Fig. 124. By this procedure we see the relative effectiveness for masking of the noise energy when operating in different regions of the frequency scale. Plainly the noise has a relatively greater masking effect at the higher frequencies.

This curve is interpreted (Fletcher, 5) as representing the selectivity characteristics of the ear. The argument is that the masking is greater for the high tones because for their region of the basilar membrane the energy contained in any given band of the noise is concentrated upon a few endings, whereas for the low tones the same energy is more widely distributed. In the high-tone region the endings that are called upon to represent the tone are at the same time stimulated strongly by the adjacent bands of noise; but in the low-tone region the overlapping is less.

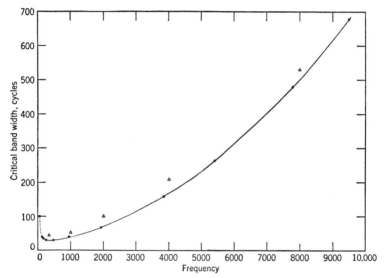

Fig. 125. Critical band widths for thermal noise. As a wide band is narrowed its masking effect remains unchanged until a certain 'critical' width is reached; then any further narrowing of the band reduces the masking. These critical widths vary with frequency. Data from Fletcher (5).

This conception of the varying forms of interaction of tones and noise becomes clearer in a somewhat different approach, in which we deal with 'critical bands' of noise (Fletcher, 6). It was found that the masking effect of a band of noise (of the composition described here) on a tone located in the middle of its range is unchanged as the band width is reduced, so long as the reduction is not carried too far. Beyond a critical point any further narrowing of the band reduces the masking effect. This critical band width varies with frequency in a manner shown by the triangular points in Fig. 125. However, the observations on which these points were based were very difficult to make, and their indications are only rough. Better indications are obtained indirectly from the data already referred to on the effects of broad bands of noise, by taking into consideration the average intensity per cycle of the noise over the general region of the tone being masked. The ratio of the intensity of the tone to the

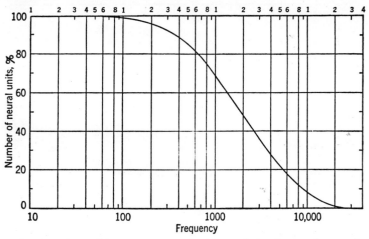

FIG. 126. The cochlear patterns as based on thermal-noise data. This curve is based upon the assumption that a critical band width always represents some constant number of neural units. It represents the relative number of units passed over in going from the upper limit of hearing to any specified frequency. Data from preceding figure.

average intensity per cycle of the noise is taken as the critical band width in cycles. This relation follows from the assumption that when a tone is just masked its response area is fully overlapped by that of the noise, and their common endings are equally stimulated. Then we have equality between the energy of the tone and the effective energy of the noise (and by effective energy is meant the energy spread over the critical area and not the total energy). Therefore if we divide the energy of the tone by the energy per cycle of the noise we come out with the number of cycles over which the noise is effectively operating, which is the critical band width. The results obtained by this method are shown by the circular points of Fig. 125.

Fletcher in using these data to determine a localization function supposed that the critical band widths represent the excitation of some constant number of neural elements regardless of

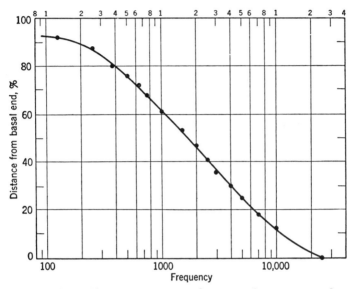

FIG. 127. The cochlear pattern in spatial terms. This curve was derived from the preceding graph by use of the innervation data of Fig. 91.

the region of frequency. This supposition is like the one made when working with the pitch discrimination data, when a jnd was taken as always representing a shift over some constant number of neural elements; and indeed it turns out that a critical band width corresponds to about 20 jnd's. By working simply in terms of relative numbers of neural elements Fletcher avoided at this stage any assumption about the manner of distribution of the elements over the cochlea.

The result of the calculations is a curve like Fig. 126. In deriving this curve, the integration began at the upper end of the frequency scale and proceeded to the lower. (Fletcher integrated in the reverse direction, from the lower end of the frequency scale to the upper.) Any point along this curve represents the percentage of the total number of neural units passed over in reaching that point.

The localization that is indicated only relatively here can be transformed into actual distances if we know the spatial distribution of the neural elements in the cochlea. The innervation data of Fig. 91 have been used for this purpose, with the results shown in Fig. 127. These results agree closely enough with other indications of localization for the very high frequencies, but they fail to do so well for the intermediate and especially the low frequencies. Fletcher suggested that the assumptions on which the procedure is based may not be warranted for the low frequencies.

CHAPTER 16

TEMPORAL PHENOMENA OF AUDITORY PERCEPTION

There are almost unlimited ways in which time can enter into the pattern of action of a sound. Some ways are simple and inescapable, as the manner in which the sound is turned on and off, and how long it lasts. Others are more complicated, such as whether the sound is single or repetitive, rhythmic or irregular. The variations just referred to are of amplitude; and then besides we have an equal number of variations of the other two primary dimensions of sounds: frequency and phase. We can suddenly raise or lower the intensity of a tone, or raise or lower its frequency, or shift its phase. We can make these same changes gradually; and we can also make them repetitively, at various rates.

When we study the behavior of a vibratory mechanism in the presence of these temporal variations we discover certain things about the mechanism itself. When we make a change in the forces acting upon it the mechanism never follows the changes exactly: its own properties intrude themselves and modify the pattern of response. Accordingly, we introduce the changes deliberately and learn about these properties. This procedure we have already come across in our examination of the early development of the resonance theory. It is what Helmholtz used in his famous experiment on 'musical shakes' in which he sought to measure the damping characteristics of the ear in terms of the persistence of its vibrations. We now take up the problem more generally.

To get the physical picture in mind, let us begin with a simple example. Suppose we have a tuning fork that is rigged up so that we can set it in vibration by sending oscillating currents into an electromagnet placed near its prongs. If we turn the current on suddenly the fork does not immediately take up the motion, but lags somewhat, and only gradually attains its final level of action. Then if we cut off the current the fork continues to speak for a while and only slowly dies down to inaudibility. These are the transients of onset and cessation. If the fork is not tuned exactly to the applied current the transients show further complexities. At the beginning we find two frequencies present simultaneously, one the forcing frequency and another the natural frequency of the fork. Quickly the fork frequency subsides and the forcing frequency gains ascendancy until at the close of the onset period it alone is present. When the current is stopped the forcing frequency vanishes and the natural frequency takes its place, and thereafter it gradually decays. The rate of these transitions is a function of the inertia of the mechanism and its damping; if the inertia is small and the damping is great the changes are rapid, and if the inertia is great and the damping is small they take a long while. The character of the transitory response reveals also the natural frequency and the accuracy of the tuning.

Numerous attempts have been made to apply these principles in the investigation of the ear. We take up the results under two headings, dealing first with the effects of single transients and then with the more complex phenomena that appear when the stimulation is repetitive.

AUDITORY TRANSIENTS

TRANSIENTS OF INTENSITY

If a sinusoidal stimulus is presented to the ear for a very short time, say for three or four cycles only, it has no tonal character and is heard as a click. Initial and terminal transients here are fused. They may be separated by prolonging the sound; then we hear one click when the tone comes on and another when it goes off. We can reduce and finally eliminate these transients by fading the tone in and out gradually; and as we do so progressively the click grows softer and more tone-like until at last it loses its noisy quality and we have a simple tone. We can also work with one transient in the absence of the other by making one of the switchings slow and the other abrupt.

Békésy (5) studied the transients of onset by reducing the rate of application of the stimulus to the point where a further reduction made no difference. While doing so he kept the fading-out process sufficiently gradual as to be inappreciable. He argued that once the rate of loading reaches the slowest rate at which the physiological system can operate any further reduc-

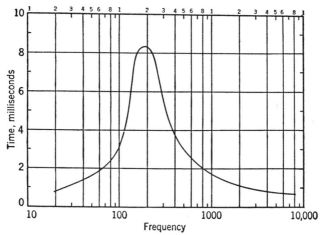

FIG. 128. Transients of onset. The rate of loading of the ear was studied in terms of the time taken to make a change of 60 db in the intensity of a tone when the form of the change was exponential. The times shown here were indistinguishable from still shorter times and are taken as representing the physiological loading time. After Bürck, Kotowski, and Lichte (1) [*Zeitschrift für technische Physik*].

tion can not be perceived. He expressed this critical rate as the time required for a 60 db rise when the form of the rise was exponential. With an 800 ~ tone he found the critical rate to be 60 db in 0.07 sec, irrespective of the intensity. Bürck, Kotowski, and Lichte used the same method with various tones over the frequency range and obtained rates varying with frequency but always much faster than Békésy's, as Fig. 128 shows. Their rates were slowest around 180 ~ (60 db rise in 0.008 sec) and progressively faster for higher and lower tones (60 db rise in 0.001 sec or less). These results become somewhat more meaningful if we translate the times needed to effect a 60 db rise into the number of cycles that the tone has passed through. Figure

129 gives the data in this form. We note that the very low tones require only a fraction of a cycle, and the higher tones a rapidly increasing number.

Békésy used a similar method to arrive at the rate of physiological decay, which he took as the fastest rate of decay of the stimulus that gave an effect indistinguishable from a rate still

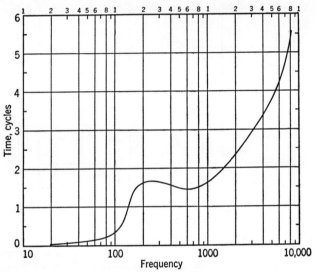

Fig. 129. Loading time of the ear expressed in cycles. Data from the preceding figure.

faster. He worked only with 800 ~ and considered the critical rate to vary with the intensity. The higher the initial intensity the higher the rate of decay, with the result, as interpreted by Stevens and Davis, that if this rate continues the tone ought to grow inaudible after about the same period of time (around 0.14 sec) regardless of its starting point. Other studies of the decay time of the ear have yielded rather disparate results, depending on the particular procedures used. It is clear, however, that the decay processes are much longer drawn out than the processes of onset.

The use of data such as these to calculate the damping and other acoustic constants of the ear encounters a serious difficulty.

We are dealing with no simple system, but rather with two systems, one mechanical and the other electrophysiological, joined end to end. Their effects are inseparable in the experiential phenomena. Hence the above results only indicate limits of the several processes involved and do not allow us to draw final conclusions about the processes themselves. Because the neural processes—and indeed several successive stages of these—are included in the measurements we can be sure that the mechanical operations are a good deal briefer than the over-all results indicate. The mechanical damping in the ear, therefore, must be of a very high order of magnitude.

Our remedy for this experimental difficulty is at hand. It lies in the application of the electrical techniques, by means of which we can deal separately with the cochlear and nervous activities and so achieve at least a partial analysis of the phenomena. This work has only just begun. It has been shown that auditory nerve impulses are more readily aroused by sudden stimuli like clicks than by smooth, continuous tones. This observation is of course in accordance with Du Bois Reymond's principle of neural excitation, according to which the excitatory effect of a stimulus increases with the rate of its application. Clicks contain sharply rising wave fronts. Accordingly, they excite a more extensive array of nervous elements than at least the high tones do.

The above experimental results can be fitted into our present picture of the mechanical and neural activities of the auditory system. When a tone is suddenly applied to the ear it produces a surge of neural activity, both because it contains transients (either of external origin or of origin in the ear itself) and because like a click it excites an extensive series of neural elements. Thereafter the effects vary markedly, depending upon the frequency. If the frequency is low we can expect the surge to be followed by a prompt establishment of a reasonably stable pattern of activity, for there are no restrictions of refractory phase and any fiber can carry the frequency comfortably. So we find that below 1000 ~ only a cycle or two is needed for stability to be reached. On the other hand, if the frequency is high the stabilization process is longer drawn out. Because a rotational activity has to be set up in several groups of fibers a number of cycles must ensue. And the higher the frequency the greater the number of cycles necessary. This explanation follows the outlines of the volley hypothesis.

TRANSIENTS OF FREQUENCY

If a tone is presented to the ear and after it has sounded for a while its frequency is abruptly altered, we hear a click interposed between the old pitch and the new. The click disappears if we make the frequency change gradual, in which case we hear the transition as a glide. Little has been done in a quantitative way in the study of this phenomenon.

SUDDEN SHIFTS OF PHASE

The perception of a sudden shift in the phase of a tone has received particular attention because this problem gave promise of providing a crucial test of the resonance theory. The physical situation is as follows. If a resonator, such as a tuning fork for example, is responding sympathetically to a sustained sound wave of its tuned frequency and the wave is suddenly altered in phase there will be a characteristic change in the action of the resonator. The most marked effect appears when the phase change is half a wave length, which is 180° or π radians of phase. The resonator motion falls away to zero and then builds up again to its former amplitude. It falls away because the action of the stimulus in its new phase relation is in opposition to the motion still going on in the resonator, and the opposition continues until the energy stored in the resonator on account of its inertia is wholly used up. At this moment the motion has ceased. Thereupon the wave restores the motion in accordance with the new phase condition. The process is illustrated in Fig. 130.

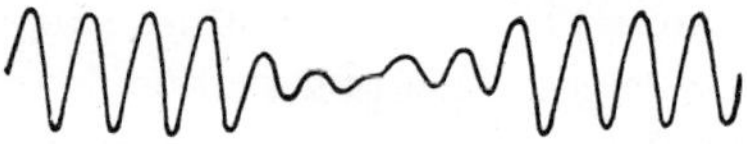

Now the argument that has been advanced is that if the ear contains resonators it will respond to a phase reversal in a tone in precisely the manner just described for the tuning fork; and we shall hear a momentary dip in the loudness.

A number of methods have been tried for the production of phase changes. Perhaps the earliest along this line was the rota-

Fig. 130. The effect upon a resonator of a sudden phase reversal in its actuating tone.

tion of a vibrating tuning fork or metal plate. These like most other sounding bodies send out waves that differ in phase at different spatial positions, and on rotation give a changing phase sequence. Unfortunately, in this situation, there is a summation of waves in the air, and for this reason a phase difference amounts to an intensity difference as well, and the results are now set aside on that ground.

Perhaps the most extensive and critical among the early studies was that of Exner and Pollak. They tried three methods of changing phase and had the most confidence in one that made use of an acoustic switch. They located two tubes near a tuning fork so as to pick up its tone in different phases, one tube with its opening opposite the broad surface of a prong and the other to the side equidistant between the two prongs. A mechanical valve then made it possible to connect a listening tube alternately to one or the other of these pickup tubes. The investigators reported that when the valve was operated the observer heard intensity changes, which at rapid rates of switching sounded exactly like beats. They concluded that the resonance theory had been substantiated.

Hartridge (1) repeated this experiment by a different method. He modified a siren so that while it was operating he could suddenly rotate the position of the wind chest and nozzle with respect to the disc by an amount equal to half the distance between the holes in the disc. This change made the new series of puffs come just out of step with those preceding, and so represented a phase shift of 180°. He reported the auditory effect to be a fall of intensity to zero and a rapid recovery, and sometimes even an overshooting of the former level. Like Exner and Pollak, he found the phenomenon to be similar to beats. In a later study, with the aid of Hallpike and Rawdon-Smith, he repeated the observations with an improved apparatus, the photoelectric siren, and obtained the same results (Hallpike, Hartridge, and Rawdon-Smith, 2).

Békésy (1) performed the experiment with an electronic method of changing the phase, with negative results. His observers were unable to detect any alteration of loudness when the phase shift was made. Hartshorn also used an electronic circuit, with results that were inconclusive. He obtained a loud click at the time of the phase change but was unable to determine whether it arose in the ear or in the apparatus. He suspected the apparatus, and indeed suggested that it is impossible to produce a phase shift in any electrical or acoustical system without producing transient waves. The disturbance of the system causes it to form a broad band of noise that is heard as a click.

A variation of this experiment was carried out by Kellaway. He made use of the fact already discussed above that an electric

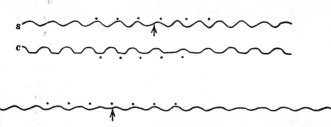

FIG. 131. The effects of a phase reversal upon the cochlear and nerve potentials. Curve *c* is the cochlear response wave and curve *n* is the nerve potential wave, each in response to a stimulus wave (marked *s*) which underwent a phase reversal at the instant indicated by the arrow. From Hallpike, Hartridge, and Rawdon-Smith (1) [*Proceedings of the Royal Society of London*].

current introduced into the ear can be perceived as a sound; and while such a current was being applied he suddenly reversed its phase. He found, just as for acoustic stimuli, that the phase change was attended by a sudden cessation of the sound and then a returning surge of loudness.

Further evidence on this question has been looked for in the electrical potentials of the ear. Hallpike, Hartridge, and Rawdon-Smith (1) introduced a sudden phase change in the sound stimulating a cat's ear while they recorded the electrical responses of the cochlea and also those of the auditory nerve. They reported that as the phase shift occurred the cochlear potentials followed the changes with great fidelity, but the nerve impulses, on the contrary, fell away and then resumed their activity. Figure 131 reproduces some of their records. They inferred from these results not only that a resonating mechanism is present in the ear but that its location is somewhere between the place of origin of the cochlear potentials and the neural elements. They suggested Reissner's membrane as the place of origin of the cochlear potentials and the basilar membrane with its sensory structures as the resonating mechanism. In their view it was this intermediate resonating mechanism that was undergoing a temporary dip in activity that was reflected in the neural response.

The first difficulty in evaluating the above results comes from an uncertainty as to the actual nature of the physical stimulation. Hartshorn's contention that a transient disturbance in the apparatus is inevitable is formally quite correct, but how serious this disturbance is in a practical sense depends upon the conditions of damping. With a sufficiently high degree of damping in the apparatus it is possible to reduce these unwanted transient effects, but whether they can be made altogether negligible is a question in each particular situation and has to be checked experimentally. Most assuredly the effects are not negligible in siren and loudspeaker sounds that are dispersed into the air and allowed to reverberate in enclosed spaces.

What happens in Kellaway's experiment we cannot ascertain; if, as some believe is always true and as assuredly happens under certain conditions, the electric currents applied to the head are transformed into sounds before they reach the cochlea, the problem in this case is no different from the usual one.

A second difficulty in this phase-shift experiment lies in its basic assumption regarding the behavior of a resonator. The picture presented holds for a simple, undamped resonator like a tuning fork, but it does not hold for a resonator that is operating under damping. As damping is introduced the transients diminish in amount and duration, and ultimately the resonator comes to follow the phase changes faithfully.

The observation of Hallpike, Hartridge, and Rawdon-Smith that the cochlear potentials reproduce the phase shifts can be interpreted simply as signifying that the motions by which these potentials arise are subject to heavy damping. We can continue to hold, as our other evidence shows, that these potentials have their origin in the organ of Corti. In this interpretation the results of this experiment are opposed to the more simple type of resonance theory; they do not prove it as these authors claim.

We have still to account for the behavior of the neural elements. If transients are present in the stimulus as often is true, or arise as well within the ear itself, the observed pattern of nerve activity is simply explained. Nerve fibers are very sensitive to changes of stimulation and respond to them oftentimes in a complex manner. Not only are there on-effects and off-effects in response to simple stimuli, but there are also inhibitions and reinforcements when the stimuli are complex.

REPETITIVE STIMULATION

Further questions arise when the changes in the sounds are repetitive. In the language of modern communications engineering we speak of this process as modulation, and we have three kinds: amplitude modulation, frequency modulation, and phase modulation.

AMPLITUDE MODULATION

In considering the changes of intensity that constitute amplitude modulation we begin with two classical problems, auditory flicker and the interruption tones.

The Auditory Flicker Experiments. If we stimulate the eye with brief flashes of light separated by darkness the impression is of flicker when the rate of alternation is low, but eventually, as the rate reaches something of the order of 20 flashes per second, there is a fusion into a perfectly continuous sensation. This phenomenon in vision naturally stimulated a search for a corresponding one in audition. Mayer in 1874 set up the experiment. He placed a disc with a number of holes in it between a tuning fork and its resonance box and rotated the disc so that at the moment when one of the holes was opposite the mouth of the resonator the tone would pass through. A tube then led from the resonator to the ear. The result during rotation of the disc was a series of bursts of sound that could be varied in rate as desired. Mayer found that these bursts blended into a smooth sensation at a certain critical rate.

The critical rate varied with the frequency of the tone being interrupted, from 16 per second for a tone of 64 $\sim$ to 135 per second for a tone of 1024 $\sim$. The reciprocals of these figures are the durations of the individual bursts and are 0.0625 sec for the 64 ~ tone and 0.0074 sec for the 1024 ~ tone. Later by a somewhat improved method and with musically trained subjects Mayer obtained somewhat faster rates, from 23 to 170 per second over the same range. Weinberg and Allen repeated these observations with similar results, as also did Belikoff and Pasternak.

Others, however, failed to get fusion. Kucharski (3) used a tone of 200 ~ and by an electronic method interrupted it 100 times per second; the subject perceived a discontinuous tone with emptiness between the pulses. A tone of 1000 ~ interrupted 500 times per second was not so clearly discontinuous but still was rough in quality. In both instances the tone maintained its proper pitch.

The work of Bishop and Wingfield explained this inconsistency, at least in part. Bishop with the rotating-disc method obtained results like Mayer's when he reproduced the same conditions, but he found fault with those conditions because they failed to give complete interruptions of the tone. Sound leakage through the disc and out into the room in general gave a degree of continuity of the stimulation that was only partially broken by the rotation of the disc. He then took precautions to eliminate the leakage. He stationed the observer beyond a wall through which the sound tube was run and cut down the intensity of the sound to a point where it was inaudible when the disc blocked the conduction tube. Then when the disc was rotated there was no fusion: the bursts of sound were separate as long as any tone remained. At the fastest speeds the tone became masked by a noise that evidently arose from the rotation of the disc itself.

Wingfield improved on this apparatus further by using a heavy disc whose surface, including the holes, was covered with a thin rubberized cloth. The purpose of the covering was to let sound pass through but to prevent disturbance of the air by the holes during rotation, which was responsible for much of the interfering noise in the previous experiments. Under these conditions, with tones from 250 to 2500 ~ and interruption rates from 3 to 40 per second, there was never any fusion of the sounds but a continuing perception of flutter. Under other conditions, when the apparatus was adjusted to give only a partial interruption of the sound, or when the intensity was reduced to a point near the threshold, the pulses faded out and a continuous sensation resulted. These changes evidently reduced the fluctuations below the level of discrimination.

Wingfield, as Bishop had done, concluded that the ear, unlike the eye, does not fill up gaps in its stimulation by a persistence of activity. This conclusion of course ought to be limited to the range of interruption rates used in the experiments, which in no case exceeded 40 per second.

If these phenomena are analogous to the ones encountered with beating tones, as we have every reason to suppose, then a further increase in the interruption rate should lead finally to a disappearance of the primary intermittence. With beats, according to the rather meager evidence, the critical rate at which this disappearance occurs is a function of the frequency, and for tones over 1000 ~ it is in the region of 150 to 250 per second. Kucharski evidently had passed the critical rate with a 1000 ~ tone when interrupted 500 times per second. Again, as is true of beats, we shall expect roughness to remain long after the disappearance of intermittence; and Kucharski in this instance described his tone as noticeably rough in quality. Moreover, as the interruption rate is raised the roughness will vary periodically according to the ratio between the frequency of the tone and its rate of interruption, as Bishop pointed out.

The Interruption Tone Experiments. When Helmholtz held a certain tuning fork opposite the opening of his siren, with one of the disc holes exposed, he observed a strong resonance of the fork tone, and on setting the siren in rotation the resonance occurred periodically. Then he could hear, in addition to the fork tone, two other tones, one higher and one lower in pitch. These additional tones he accounted for as a kind of combination tone, of the composition $n + m$ and $n - m$, where n is the fork frequency and m the number of times per second that a hole is exposed. Similarly, Mayer in one of his flicker experiments noticed what he called secondary sounds, one above and one below the fork tone and differing from it by an amount depending upon the speed of rotation of the disc. These tones were later named variation tones.

Koenig (1) first clearly observed in this kind of situation a tone of the frequency of the interruption itself. He obtained it by varying the size of the holes in a siren disc. In one of his arrangements, for example, he varied the sizes of the holes periodically around the disc from a maximum of 6 mm to a minimum of 1 mm. On rotating the disc rapidly he heard a tone whose pitch corresponded to the total number of puffs both large and small, which in one trial was 768; and he heard also a tone equal to the rate of the periodic changes of intensity, which in the same trial was 128.

Dennert repeated these observations and also varied the arrangement. He used a siren disc in which he varied the positions of the holes in a regular pattern. For example, one disc had 4 holes and then 4 blank spaces, 4 holes and 4 blank spaces, and so on around the circle; and when it was rotated he heard two tones, one the same in pitch as if there

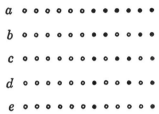

FIG. 132. Patterns used in the siren experiments of Schaefer and Abraham. These patterns of siren holes gave sounds containing the same fundamental and interruption tones.

had been holes in every space in perfectly regular order, and the other of a pitch 2 octaves lower. The latter tone is called an interruption tone, or sometimes an intermittence tone. Its frequency is always equal to the rate of appearance of a periodic group in the stimulation.

Schaefer and Abraham tested this generalization more thoroughly. They found various kinds of periodic alterations in the stimulation to be effective. Thus the following patterns, repeated at any one convenient rate, gave the same pair of fundamental and interruption tones: 4 large and 4 small holes, 7 large and 1 small, and 1 large and 7 small. Here the interruption tone always had a frequency one-eighth that of the fundamental. Even more striking is the equivalence of patterns in which the second half of a recurring group of holes is disturbed in a variety of ways, as Fig. 132 illustrates. These produced the same fundamental and interruption tones, and always the interruption tone was one-twelfth the frequency of the fundamental. It is evident from this study that the periodic group operates as a unit, whatever its specific nature, and it gives an interruption tone of a pitch equal to the rate of appearance of the group.

Modern Experiments on Amplitude Modulation. We now have in electronic circuits very convenient and precise means of producing periodic changes of amplitude. Nevertheless, modern experiments on these problems are strangely few. One such experiment is that of Stowell and Deming. They produced a sinusoidal modulation of a number of tones of the middle range at the single rate of 60 per second. Their observers were usually able to hear the 60 ~ modulating tone (or interruption tone in the older terminology). The frequency of the tone being modulated was an important condition, and the region about 1000 ~ gave the best results. Tones below about 350 ~ and above 3200 ~ when modulated failed to give the 60 ~ tone. These authors implied but did not specifically state that the variation tones (which for 1000 ~ would be 940 and 1060) were regularly heard along with the fundamental.

How are these phenomena to be explained? The oldest theory was developed in the study of beats and combination tones. Its originator was Robert Smith. In 1749, in a treatment of the mathematical theory of recurrent patterns, he suggested that two simultaneous tones that constitute a mistuned consonance (that is, whose frequencies depart a little from a simple ratio) produce resultant displacements that are heard as beats. Thomas Young, and more specifically Koenig, developed this idea as the beat-tone theory of combination tones. They supposed that the changes of amplitude that when slow are heard as beats will turn into a combination tone when sufficiently rapid. By a broadening of this theory they accounted for the resultant tones and interruption tones. Any periodic change in the stimulation they regarded as a basis for the perception of a tone.

This explanation met vigorous opposition on the part of Helmholtz and his followers because it is inconsistent with the assumptions made in connection with the resonance theory. If a complex wave is analyzed by a process wherein each component goes to its specific place in the cochlea, there can be no interaction and accordingly no perception of resultant displacements.

It is true, these writers found it necessary to yield a point in regard to the simple beats, and to say that for tones of adjacent frequencies there is a degree of overlapping on the basilar membrane and thus far a failure of analysis; but they were not willing to carry this concession to the point of including the combination tones, resultant tones, and interruption tones. As they saw it, to have done so would have lost the virtue of specificity.

Their alternative, as we have seen, was to explain the combination tones as products of distortion and to handle the other tones as special cases. Schaefer and Abraham were able in some instances to get reinforcement of the resultant tones with physical resonators and therefore argued that these tones were present in the aerial waves. No aural explanation then was needed for them. They thereupon derived the interruption tone as a difference tone between one of the variation tones and the fundamental. Thus, for example, if 1000 ~ is interrupted 60 times per second and the tones 940 and 1060 are thereby introduced as physical tones, the interactions 1000 − 940 and 1060 − 1000 both generate a 60 ~ tone. This explanation encountered two difficulties that Schaefer and Abraham could not circumvent: under some conditions they were unable to resonate the variation tones, and often—indeed more often than not—these tones either were not discernible at all to the ear or were much fainter than the interruption tone that they were presumed to generate. Stowell and Deming similarly assumed that the 60 ~ tone observed in their experiment was a product of distortion. They first observed it when the tone being modulated attained a pressure in the neighborhood of 1 dyne per sq cm, which is just possibly sufficient to overload the ear. It is unfortunate that their modulation rate was so low as to throw the interruption tone into a region of frequency where the ear's sensitivity is at its poorest. It is likely, in view of the older evidence, that a higher rate would have given an interruption tone at a stimulation level well below the overloading point.

A somewhat different explanation, accepted by many of the modern representatives of the Helmholtzian school, derives from the mathematical treatment of modulation. Mathematically an amplitude-modulated wave is the equivalent of three simple waves, which in the language of the above discussion are the fundamental and the variation tones and which in communications theory are referred to as the carrier wave and its two side tones (or side bands). The side tones differ from the fundamental by the modulation frequency and have amplitudes that depend upon the degree of modulation—the greater the degree of modulation the larger they become. The phases of these three waves must be chosen in a certain way in order for the mathematical equivalence to hold. Another way of expressing this equivalence is to say that we shall have the same stimulus, and hear the same thing, regardless of whether we present a single tone modulated in amplitude or present three tones simultaneously with certain frequencies, amplitudes, and phase relations.

At this point a rather general misapprehension has arisen. From the above equivalence the conclusion is drawn that the ear must perceive an amplitude-modulated tone as three simple tones. This conclusion of course follows tradition in the view that the ear is an analyzer and ought to reduce the complex wave to its elementary constituents. Yet the fact of equivalence does not imply so much. It does not specify just what the ear —or any other acoustic device for that matter—will do under the circumstances. It requires only that the two procedures yield the same results.

Already in the older studies we have had an indication of what the procedures yield for the ear. The modern observations are less disturbed by impure stimuli and therefore cleaner cut.

At slow rates of modulation we perceive only one tone, whose pitch corresponds to the fundamental frequency or something near it and which undergoes periodic variations of loudness. As the modulation rate is speeded up, the loudness variations lose detail and turn into more and more discrete pulses. At this stage we have a very rough and unpleasant jangle of sound in which the original simple pitch has been beclouded. Later, as the modulation rate is made more rapid still, the complex takes on a somewhat more agreeable character, and out of it we may analyze—if we have the skill—the three tonal components already referred to. Hence the ear takes cognizance of each aspect of our mathematical expression of equivalence and portrays it under the proper conditions; and it gives as well a whole series of transition phenomena that our mathematics provides no reckoning of.

Closely analogous to this series of experiences is the one obtained with beating tones when the rate of the beating is progressively increased.

For an amplitude modulation the stimulus has the form shown in Fig. 133, and this same form appears in the movements of the middle ear and in the cochlea also as revealed in its potentials. We need more information before we can say what is the

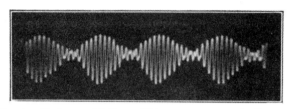

FIG. 133. Amplitude modulation. This curve represents the cochlear response wave obtained by stimulating with three tones whose frequencies, amplitudes, and phase relations were suitably adjusted as indicated in the text. Cf. Fig. 135.

pattern of activity along the basilar membrane, but it seems likely that the nature of our changing experiences as the modulation rate varies is determined largely by the neural portion of the receptive system.

Somewhere in this system is a process by which the intensity is roughly integrated over a short period of time. Probably this process is based upon a temporal dispersion of the nerve impulses arising from any momentary excitation. Indeed, it may be little more than this dispersion and our failure to discriminate in terms of loudness the variations in the magnitude of the neural stream when these variations fall below some minimum value. If this is so we can explain the changes in our experiences as a function of modulation rate.

When the rate is slow, and the modulation period is long with respect to the interval over which an integration of intensity occurs in the ear, we shall have continuous indications of the intensity, and we perceive the sound as undergoing regular undulations. When the modulation period approaches but still slightly exceeds the integration interval we shall have one indication of intensity per period, and we perceive the sound in discrete pulses. The pulsating or intermittent quality vanishes when the modulation period grows smaller than the period of integration. Thereafter we hear roughness, because the integration is incomplete: the modulation period contains no empty space, yet there are irregularities in the discharge that are still discernible. If the modulation rate is carried high enough we can expect this roughness too to disappear, as the irregularities become negligible in the total nerve discharge. This aspect of the phenomenon has had little study as yet. In the observation of beats a disappearance of roughness has been observed when the beating rate reaches about 350 per second, for a 1024 ∼ tone. For modulation itself we have only Kucharski's observation that at 500 interruptions per second, in a 1000 ∼ tone, he had passed the limit for intermittence but had not reached the limit for roughness.

FREQUENCY MODULATION

Variation in the frequency of a wave constitutes frequency modulation. The important variables are the range of modulation, which is the amount of the change of frequency above and below the central frequency, the rate of the modulation, which is the number of cyclic changes per second, and also the form of the changes, which can be abrupt or graduated in various ways.

A special form of frequency modulation that has long excited theoretical interest is the changing note of the siren as the rate of rotation is raised or lowered. The auditory effect is a wailing or gliding of pitch. Scripture once contended that the existence of such a glide cannot be explained on a resonance theory. As he put it, any frequency occurs only once; and he might have added that it lasts but an infinitesimal time. Hence, he argued, a frequency is not sustained long enough to activate any single specific resonator in the ear. The answer is of course that the responsive elements are not very sharply tuned, and each differential part of the wave excites many elements; each element then summates the effects of many such differentials. Scripture was right, in that this phenomenon is inexplicable on an assumption of simple, isolated resonators; but no discerning advocate of the resonance theory when pressed has carried specificity so far.

A familiar sort of frequency modulation is the vibrato, often used in musical performance. The violinist produces it by trembling the finger with which he stops a string. The singer achieves the same result with the vocal apparatus. By listening alone it is puzzling to decide whether the changes are of frequency or intensity or both, but analysis of the waves has proved that they are mainly of frequency. For the most pleasing effects in singing the modulation rate is around 6 or 7 per second, and the range of modulation (from one extreme to the other) is of the order of a semitone.

The simplest kind of frequency modulation is that in which we make equal changes above and below the base frequency, make them at a constant rate, and give each change a sinusoidal form. Then when the range of modulation is fixed at some arbitrary value and the modulation rate is varied the experience changes in a way that corresponds in some respects to that described for amplitude modulation. At slow rates the pitch glides slowly up and down. As the rate is increased the pitch changes more rapidly, until a point is reached where the changes are no longer of pitch but of loudness. Then we hear a tone of a single pitch that is pulsating in loudness. A still higher rate gives a pulsating complex in which other tones appear. The rate at which the gliding pitch changes into a pulsing complex was determined by Ramsdell as around 7 per second (for a few specific base tones and modulation ranges).

The mathematical treatment of frequency modulation shows that it, like amplitude modulation, can be expressed as a combination of simple tones of certain fixed frequencies, amplitudes, and phases. In this instance, however, the number of components is theoretically unlimited. The pattern is made up of a series of tones arranged symmetrically on either side of the fundamental frequency and separated from one another by frequency steps that are equal to the modulation rate. The relative amplitudes of the components depend upon the modulation rate and its amount, or, more specifically, upon the ratio of these two factors, called the modulation index. When the frequency variation is sinusoidal in form, and the modulation index is small (the frequency variation is small with respect to the modulation rate), there is one large component (the fundamental) with a smaller one on either side, while other components are negligible. As the modulation index grows larger additional components become important, and the central component loses its dominating position, as will be seen from the samples presented in Fig. 134.

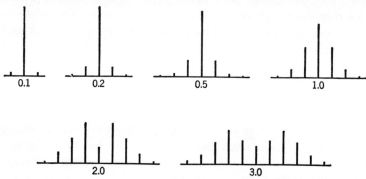

Fig. 134. Frequency modulation; the effects of the modulation index. The vertical lines show the relative magnitudes of the components produced in frequency modulation when the modulation index is given various values as indicated. The components are separated in frequency by amounts equal to the modulation rate, which here is represented as constant.

Of special interest is the first case mentioned, where the modulation index is small and only three components are appreciable, for these three components are identical in frequency with the ones that result from an amplitude modulation of the same modulation rate. There is a difference only in phase relations; the fundamental component in one differs by 90° of phase from what it is in the other. We shall discover the importance of this case presently.

THE PERCEPTION OF PHASE

Helmholtz raised the question whether the phase of a sound has anything to do with its perception and approached it experimentally in his study of artificial vowels. He found that he could imitate the vowel sounds by setting in vibration an array of tuning forks of the proper frequencies and intensities. He then set out to discover whether changes in the phase relations of these fork tones would affect the quality of the sound.

His method was ingenious, though rather difficult in execution. Each fork was placed near the mouth opening of its resonator chamber, and a little vane was mounted between in such a manner that it could be drawn partway across the mouth opening. This blocking of the opening alters the tuning of the resonator and changes the phase of the tone emitted. It changes the intensity as well, but Helmholtz found that he could compensate for this change by adjusting the distance between fork and resonator. Such manipulations gave random variations in the phase relations of the components entering into the vowel sounds.

The variations caused no perceptible changes in the musical quality of the sounds. Helmholtz's conclusion, which came into wide acceptance as a basic principle of sound perception, was that "the quality of the musical portion of a compound tone depends solely on the number and relative strength of its partial simple tones, and in no respect on their differences of phase" (2).

We must be careful to observe Helmholtz's exact language here: he confined his conclusion to the 'musical' portion of the sound; and this is a distinction (almost one might call it a subtlety) that was destined to confuse the issue for a long time to come. We can surmise that Helmholtz really observed changes of quality when he altered the phase relations—but he set them aside as belonging to the 'non-musical' aspects of his sounds and so of no relevance to the problem. What he probably heard were changes of roughness, for at the end of his discussion he suggested that the noises and the dissonances resulting from the interaction of upper partials very likely are dependent upon phase relations. He described also what he referred to as an 'apparent exception' to his rule, which was a change of quality when two notes slightly mistuned produced a faint beating. This change, however, he attributed to intensity variations, and not to the phase variations as such.

It is probable that in making the above distinction of musical and non-musical effects of phase Helmholtz was guided by his conception of two sorts of receptive mechanisms, one in the cochlea for tones and another in the ampullary and vestibular organs for noises. In line with this hypothesis the noisy quality that appeared as a result of his manipulations of phase would be ascribed to the second species of receptors, and be considered as separate from the action of the cochlear resonators.

Koenig (2) a little later repeated the above experiments with his wave siren, an instrument that permitted a more immediate comparison of the sounds. This siren makes use of a narrow slit through which air is blown and a rotating metal band whose edge is cut out so as to control the width of exposure of the slit. By giving the band the proper form any kind of complex sound is produced. Koenig prepared several sets of bands to give sounds containing the same components but in different phase relations.

On listening to these sounds Koenig observed clear differences of quality. The qualitative changes bore a systematic relation to the phase structure, or more specifically to the shapes of the waves. Waves with prominent peaks seemed loud and brilliant; those with broad, smooth contours were weak and dull in quality. Koenig's conclusion from these results was that we really perceive phase relations.

Many have repeated these experiments with a variety of methods. For the most part they have verified Koenig in the observation of qualitative changes as a result of the phase shifts. In their interpretations, however, they have divided, apparently along lines of theoretical predisposition. Most have agreed with Helmholtz's dictum, yet (as so often happens in the perpetuation of the ideas of a great authority) they have failed to note the restriction that he placed upon it. In missing this restriction and in trying to reconcile their observations with what they took the principle to be, they have promulgated an explanation that is remarkable for its obliquity. Over and over in the literature on this subject we find it said that the qualitative changes that appear as a result of phase shifts are really due to the beating of components of adjacent frequencies. Overtones of higher orders are usually blamed as the offending components.

This explanation evidently arose in a misunderstanding of Helmholtz's 'apparent exception' and a use of it that he did not contemplate. We have here a confusion of two sorts of phase change, the dynamic sort that gives beats and the static sort that is really under consideration in these experiments. As we well know, two waves that differ slightly in frequency can be looked upon as undergoing continuous variations of phase relation; they are sometimes in coincidence and sometimes in opposition, and we hear the cycles of change as beats. If we stop the tones and then start them again in a new phase relation we may find ourselves at a different point in the beat cycle from what we would be if no interruption had occurred, but from there the cyclic changes go on as before. There will be no change in the character of the beating. The evidence of a long list of investigators —Hermann (2), Lindig, Lloyd and Agnew, Schulze, and perhaps others—which they themselves explained away as due to the presence of beating components may therefore be regarded in some seriousness as demonstrating the effectiveness of phase.

There is, however, the possibility of a second kind of tonal interaction that can cause changes of quality that only indirectly are to be attributed to phase. When the components are so strong as to undergo non-linear distortion in the ear they produce combination tones; and it is reasonable to suppose that the distortion will be greater, and the combination tones correspondingly stronger, for those particular phase relations that give waves with the higher peaks. Trimmer and Firestone emphasized the importance of this condition, and then Chapin and Firestone and also Schouten described changes of loudness and quality that they attributed to this effect of phase relation.

Certain recent experiments in which consideration was given to the intensity of the stimuli and possible overloading of the ear show plainly that distortion is not the only way in which phase can make itself known. Beasley worked at 25 to 30 db above threshold, a level that will not overload the ear, and obtained clear evidence of the perception of qualitative changes due to phase differences.

The latest and most definitive results are those of Mathes and Miller. They used modulator circuits to obtain three tones of equally spaced frequencies and any desired amplitudes and varied the phase of one of them. Such a stimulus arrangement for one phase and amplitude relation is the equivalent of a 100 per cent amplitude modulation of the central frequency, and the resulting wave has already been shown in Fig. 133. When the phase of the central frequency is changed 90° the combination of these tones becomes approximately the same as a frequency-modulated wave whose modulation index is unity; this wave is illustrated in Fig. 135. Therefore by changing the phase back and forth all gradations of wave form between those shown in Figs. 133 and 135 are the result. When the sound is listened to, these changes produce a remarkable qualitative effect. The features vary somewhat according to the modulation rate. At

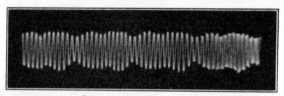

Fig. 135. Frequency modulation, as shown in the cochlear potentials. The stimulating conditions were the same as for Fig. 133 except that one of the three tones was altered in phase. Note that the separation of the waves varies periodically in time. This is only an approximate frequency modulation; if it were perfect the wave amplitude would be constant.

very slow rates the wave with the widely undulating envelope (Fig. 133; amplitude-modulated wave) gives a definite surging of loudness, while the wave with the more uniform envelope (Fig. 135, frequency-modulated, approximately) exhibits a fluctuation of pitch. (The envelope would become perfectly uniform for true frequency modulation, which would require additional components.) As the modulation rate reaches 7 to 10 per second the amplitude-modulated form grows discontinuous and rough, and the frequency-modulated form becomes a warble. The most noticeable differences are exhibited when the modulated frequency is 1000 ~ and the modulation rate is around 50 ~, which gives the equivalent of three frequencies of 950, 1000, and 1050 ~. Then the amplitude-modulated form is fluttering and raucous, while the other is continuous and smooth, disturbed only by the addition of a tone of 100 ~. This tonal component that is added to the other three in the frequency-modulated case corresponds to the undulations shown in the envelope of Fig. 135.

The frequency range over which these phenomena occur will need further exploration, but in the region from 500 to 2000 ~, which was studied in this experiment, the upper limit at which modulation gave the effects described was about 40 per cent of the frequency of the modulated tone (hence 800 per second for a 2000 ~ tone).

The above observations were made usually at a level of 60 db above threshold. The effects were still present, however, at intensity levels as low as 20 db above threshold and were prominent at 35 db above threshold. For these levels of stimulation subjective tones were looked for by the exploring-tone method and were not found in appreciable magnitudes. Hence we cannot consider overloading of the ear as a contributing condition.

We conclude from these results that the ear does not act as a perfect analyzer, for if it did so it would resolve both the forms of wave exhibited here into the same pattern and would not distinguish them. Instead it gives to the neural centers, in momentary detail, a portrayal of the composite wave. We are brought back to the old resultant displacements theory, according to which the instantaneous amplitude is perceived, and when it varies rapidly enough is appreciated as a tone.

This explanation is of course inconsistent with a pure place theory and requires a representation of frequency in the nerve discharge. We must suppose that within the range covered in these observations the true composite wave form, or a close approximation to it, is preserved in the neural excitatory processes. Then bursts of impulses will occur at each of the wave peaks represented in Figs. 133 and 135, in the one case periodically varying in numbers from few to many and in the other case varying only slightly in numbers but more prominently in temporal distribution. And it must be emphasized that even a slight variation in numbers when the variation is periodic will come to be perceived as a tone of the appropriate frequency.

CHAPTER 17

BINAURAL PHENOMENA

Already we have seen that the two ears working together give keener perceptions of loudness and pitch than one ear does alone. When the ears are stimulated identically the effects evidently are brought together in the central nervous processes and effectually fused. Now we have to consider the situation where the binaural stimulation is somewhat disparate; then the fusion is incomplete and other phenomena arise, among them the phenomena of sound localization.

THE LOCALIZATION OF SOUNDS IN SPACE

When a source of sound is directly ahead of an observer and there are no near-by objects to disturb the paths of the sound waves, the two ears are stimulated equally. If the observer's ears are functioning alike, or he can compensate for their differences, he will localize the sound correctly in the median plane. If now the source is displaced to the right or left the waves reaching the ears will differ in some respects, and (within certain limits) he will localize the sound to one side. Our problem is, what are the binaural disparities that the situation presents, and how are they represented in the actions of the acoustic mechanism?

There are three principal ways in which the waves reaching the two ears may differ when the source is displaced to one side. They are the intensity, the time of arrival, and the phase. Sometimes also there is a fourth, the wave composition.

To be concrete, let us suppose that the source lies well to the right of the median plane. The right ear will be stimulated the more strongly, both because it is nearer to the source and because the other ear lies somewhat in a 'shadow' cast by the head. Likewise because it is nearer to the source the right ear will receive the sound somewhat earlier. Then, as the sound is maintained, its wave changes will always take place sooner

424

for the right ear, or in other words the waves in this ear will constantly lead in phase. Finally, if the stimulus gives a complex wave, the wave form may differ at the two ears. The head casts a more effective shadow for high tones than for low tones, and therefore the sound reaching the averted ear will have its high components relatively weakened.

All these forms of disparity are possible, but how effective they are in the actual location of sounds is a further matter. In the natural situation they operate concurrently, but they may be isolated experimentally and separately studied.

Binaural Intensity. An intensity difference, when fairly large, causes a displacement of localization toward the more favored ear. There is still doubt of the effectiveness of this factor in the natural situation, however. If the sound comes from afar, the path difference to the ears gives only a negligible intensity ratio. Also, for low tones, whose wave lengths are large, the head is but a small obstacle, and its shadowing effect is slight. Only for the high tones is the intensity difference of much significance.

Time of Incidence. If the ears are stimulated with very brief clicks, one delivered a little ahead of the other, a single click is heard on the side where the stimulation is prior. As little as a few microseconds of time difference is effective—something like 30 microseconds, according to Hornbostel and Wertheimer. The lateral displacement of the sound grows greater as the time difference increases, until as 630 microseconds is approached the sound is directly opposite the favored ear; and finally if the difference is made still greater two separate sounds are heard, one on one side and then one on the other.

For a sustained sound, a time difference may obtain not only on its onset but also on its cessation, and at any noticeable change of character during its course. Very likely the greater ease with which we localize noises in comparison with simple tones comes from the fact that their fitful patterns afford a multiplicity of temporal cues.

Phase. If the stimulation reaching the two ears is initially the same in all respects, and then it is advanced a little in phase in one ear, the sound will seem to move out of the median plane toward this ear. As the phase difference is increased the sound moves farther to the side, until it comes to be directly opposite the favored ear. Then, for a still larger phase difference, it suddenly appears on the opposite side.

This description holds for simple tones of frequencies up to 600 or 1000 ~. Higher tones give more complex perceptions. According to usual descriptions, they do not produce so extensive displacements, and those in the extreme range around 2000 to 4000 ~ give only a slight wavering from the neutral position. At the same time, under some conditions, there are multiple images: the sound seems to be coming from two or three places at once.

These complications in the perceptual behavior of the high tones have an objective basis, as Rayleigh pointed out in 1907 and Hartley then showed in detail. They arise in the natural situation from the relation between the wave length of the sound and the difference in the two pathways to the ears. Suppose we keep the source in a constant position and raise the frequency, which means reducing the wave length. When we reach a frequency where half the wave length is equal to the difference in distance between the two paths we have exact phase opposition, a phase difference of 180°. Now bearing in mind that we are dealing with a continuous series of waves we see that neither ear has any phase advantage: the stimulation is equivocal. (A simple analogy that gives a clear picture of the situation is a pair of runners on a circular track; if the swifter of them gains just half a lap on the other a casual observer—one who has no knowledge of preceding events—will be at a loss to say which of the two is ahead.) Now when the frequency is raised a trifle more the phase relation formerly obtaining becomes reversed: the side where the phase has been leading now is the one of lagging phase. (Consider our runners again: if the fleeter gains more than half a lap he seems—from the instantaneous view—to be the one behind.) As the frequency is raised further the phase difference is narrowed until complete phase agreement is reached (a 360° phase difference is the same as zero phase); and then this cycle of changes begins anew. We get these same shifting phase relations with a high tone of constant frequency when its source is moved in an arc from the median position toward the side; the relation between wave length and the difference in pathways is varying as before. Thus it is no wonder that our localization of high tones in terms of phase is confused. Moreover, this cue is often in conflict with the other auditory cues, as well as with visual evidence of the true location. Such a fallible cue we learn to suppress; and so perhaps we account for the confusingly varied results often obtained in experiments on phase perception.

At many times in the past the perception of phase differences has been denied altogether. The effects observed when phase is varied have been attributed to some other condition, allegedly uncontrolled; and in some of the experiments this supposition bears weight. Parenthetically I may add that a further influential consideration here, and by no means a negligible one, has been the fact that the conventional resonance theory is embarrassed by this matter of phase and can find no way of its representation in the ear's response.

The first unassailable evidence of the operation of a binaural phase difference came in observations of a phenomenon arising in the rather confused area of the binaural beats. When the two ears are stimulated separately with two tones a little different in frequency—tones that in the same ear would give uniaural beats of a very slow rate, say one per minute or so—there is a perception of a tone that seems to swing back and forth from one side of the head to the other. This binaural shift phenomenon, as it is properly called, is a dynamic form of the more usual phase localization. We have in the stimulus situation a cyclic variation in phase relations at the two ears; the phase leads now on one side and now on the other, and the apparent location of the tone varies accordingly.

The stimulus situation is simple enough here that there is no doubt that the effects are due to the phase relations. The only question—and for theory an important one as we shall see—is the upper limit of frequency to which the effects obtain. Rayleigh got shifts for tones up to 640 $\sim$, and probably to 768 $\sim$. Lane found limits of 800 to 1000 $\sim$. With very slight frequency differences, which make the shiftings slow, I have obtained effects up to 3000 $\sim$.

For further data on the upper limit of frequency at which a phase difference is effective we return to the more usual static situation. The judgment is easier when the sound image seems stationary; and in the more recent experiments where electronic and electromagnetic devices are used to produce the phase changes there is good reason to believe that the old objection of uncontrolled variables has been avoided. Stewart (2) obtained effects up to 1280 ~ for three subjects; Banister (1) got them up to 1705 ~ for his best two subjects in a group of five; Trimble got to 2000 ~ for three subjects and to 4000 ~ for a fourth; and

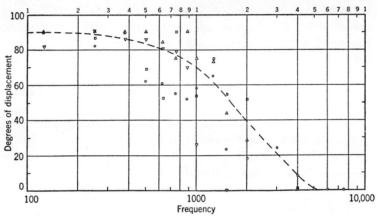

Fig. 136. Apparent displacement of tones from the median plane as a result of binaural phase difference. Results for four subjects are shown by the different kinds of points. Data from Trimble.

finally Hughes got to 2000 ~ for two subjects and perhaps to 4000 ~ for a third. Figure 136 reproduces Trimble's results and shows clearly how the amount of the observed displacement from the median plane grows smaller as the frequency is raised. It seems clear that phase permits easy judgments of sound direction for all tones up to about 1000 ~, rather less certain ones in the next octave up to 2000 ~, and gives only difficult indications in the octave beyond. The upper limit of effectiveness of the phase cue thus seems to lie around 4000 ~.

It is proper to say that these results are crucial to auditory theory. They cannot be accounted for on a simple place theory. They require, over the range indicated, that the periodicity of the sound somehow be preserved in the auditory nerve action. Many have appreciated this fact—Rayleigh in 1907, and Banister

(2) and Fletcher (1) more recently—and have sought to modify the place theory accordingly. They proposed to add to the place hypothesis the condition that in the low frequencies where binaural phase differences are effective the auditory nerve carries the stimulus frequency.

This modification of the place theory will seem merely a minor one if it concerns just the lower portion of the auditory range, up to a few hundred cycles, as was usually suggested. If, however, it has to extend as far as 4000 ～—covering 8 out of the total of 10½ octaves—it is hardly an incidental matter. Rather, it is a matter to be given as serious consideration as any other basic aspect of hearing. Especially to be considered is the way in which the phase is represented in the nerve discharge.

The volley theory shows how this representation is possible. It is possible because, over the range indicated, the actual frequency of the sound is reflected in the nerve discharge.

The indicated limit of 4000 ～ for effective phase action agrees well with the limit of frequency representation in the nerve discharge as already indicated. The considerable difficulties in the use of the phase cue through the upper part of this range, from 1000 ～ to 4000 ～, need further comment. These difficulties are better ascribed to the perceptual complexities than to any limitations in the fidelity of auditory nerve representation. No doubt they arise, as already suggested, because for the high tones the phase cue becomes inconsistent with itself and with the other cues present and gives an unreliable or false indication. It therefore is largely suppressed. The suppression evidently varies somewhat among different subjects. Some carry it far and fail altogether to use the cue for the upper middle tones; others use it here for the smaller displacements from the median plane where it still works satisfactorily. It is likely that a course of special training would lead all subjects to make more use of this cue than ordinarily they do.

Some recent results of Loesch and Kapell support the above suppositions. They gave their subjects intensive practice in observing both the binaural shift and binaural beats and found a rapid and progressive improvement in the maximum frequencies at which the phenomena appeared. The limits attained after only a few sessions, when the experiment had to be discontinued, are higher than usually reported, as Table VIII will show. The practice curves for one of the subjects, typical of the group, are shown in Fig. 137. From the trend of these curves it seems certain that further practice would have raised the upper limits higher still.

TABLE VIII

Subjects	Upper Limit for Binaural Shift	Upper Limit for Binaural Beats	Total Practice Time (Hours)
A	2000	2400	8
B	2300	2500	10
C	1300	1500	5
D	2300	2500	14
E	900	1100	6

According to the volley hypothesis, an auditory nerve fiber in responding to a tonal excitation fires at some fairly regular phase position; the sinusoidal excitation is translated into a discrete series of nervous pulses, and the phase is represented by the periodic time. Binaural stimulation in which the phase is different at the two ears will produce two series of pulses in which the moments of firing are different. Each nerve impulse in the ear where the phase is leading will precede the corresponding impulse in the opposite ear by some fraction of a period. Phase localization therefore becomes a special case of time localization.

There is further evidence that phase is translated into time. If to the two ears we present one tone with a certain binaural phase difference, and then another tone of different frequency with the same binaural phase difference, the two tones in general will not be localized at the same angular position. On the other hand, if for these two tones we choose binaural phase relations that are different in terms of phase but which represent the same time differences, their localizations will then correspond. We see this same relationship in the following situation. A sound coming from a certain position displaced from the medial plane is localized there (within the limits of error) regardless of the frequency, provided of course that the frequency is not too high. The binaural phase difference for such a position varies with the frequency: the higher the frequency the larger the phase difference. When converted into time, however, the differences are the same.

Our explanation of phase localization requires not only that the tonal periodicity get into the cochlear nerve discharge, but also that it be maintained in the central nervous channels up to some point where the discharges from the two ears come together and interact. There is evidence that at least a part of this interaction occurs at a low level of the nervous system. As

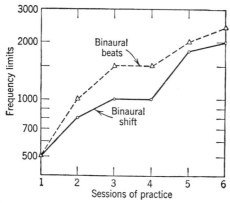

Fig. 137. Effects of practice on the upper limits of perception of binaural beats and the binaural shift. The results are those of subject A in Table VIII.

already mentioned, Bard and Rioch found that a decorticate cat was able to follow a person about, seemingly by the sound of his footsteps.

This behavior of the decorticate cat can be accounted for if we assume that the auditory centers of the brain stem produce a reciprocal innervation of the postural and locomotor muscles. We suppose that the impulses from one ear are relayed chiefly to the muscles on one side of the body, and so dispose as to turn the head and body in the direction of that ear. In addition these impulses are carried across to the opposite side and either reinforce or block the impulses in those corresponding pathways, depending on the time relations. When there is phase coincidence, both right and left paths conduct and the animal continues to face the sound, and perhaps to approach it. When there is near coincidence there is partial reinforcement and a slight reorientation toward the sound. Finally, when the phase difference is great enough, the impulses from one side get through but those from the other are wholly blocked, and a maximum turning movement follows.

Our conscious perception of the direction of a sound may be something similar to this reflex action at a higher, cerebral level; or it may be simply our appreciation of slight movements of orientation. If it is the first we must preserve the phase relations in good form in the course of transmission through the acoustic nervous channels, probably all the way to the temporal cortex. If it is the second there is no necessity for complete fidelity in this transmission. It is further possible that in the higher centers both the direct and indirect cues are made use of in the perception of sound direction.

BINAURAL BEATS

In 1877, Thompson reported well-controlled experiments in which he led tones of slightly different frequencies to the two ears and obtained a beating somewhat similar to the well-known uniaural beats. He used precautions to prevent any leaking of the sound on one side to the opposite ear, and concluded that the results were due to a central, neural integration. Ewald (1) a little later repeated the experiments with still more exacting tests against sound leakage and agreed with Thompson that the beats were truly binaural.

In the decades following many others observed the phenomenon, but after extended discussion it came generally to be believed that these beats were uniaural and the result of cross conduction either by way of the air or through the head. First Rostosky and then Wilson and Myers were emphatic in this contention. The phenomenon therefore came to be regarded as an artifact, and attention turned to the other aspect of the situation, the localization effect, already treated in the preceding section.

Stewart (1) made one of the more extensive studies of the problem. He paid particular attention to the nature of the cyclic changes of loudness and reported two secondary maxima as well as a primary maximum in each cycle of phase changes. His explanation was an elaborate one involving cross conduction through the head, and also the assumption of two distinct sound receptors in each ear. He regarded the effects as unilateral if not strictly uniaural.

Lane without much question obtained the beats under conditions that excluded cross conduction. He used telephone receivers fitted with rubber cushions that reduced both aerial leakage and the communication of vibrations to the head. Previously he and Wegel in tests made on persons totally deaf in one ear had found that this arrangement gives effective isolation of the ears until the stimulation rises to about 60 db above threshold. Yet with intensities safely below this level all his observers heard the binaural beats.

It is interesting to remark, however, that Lane explained away these experiences as not true beats but a kind of perceptual illusion. The observer, he thought, was not experiencing a fluctuation of loudness in the strict sense but was making a judgment that reflected his degree of definiteness of localization. When the sound was referred to the median plane or to one of the ears it was easier for him to attend to, and accordingly it seemed louder; whereas in other, less definite locations he could not so readily take it in his grasp, and it seemed fainter. Hence the fluctuations of loudness, he affirmed, were really due to rapid variations in the apparent position of the sound.

I have recently taken up this matter of binaural beats, and am assured that they are binaural and are loudness fluctuations in the strict sense. My own observations are confirmed by those of several other subjects, under conditions that exclude cross conduction of any kind.

What is experienced as a result of the binaural stimulation depends very much on the frequency difference of the two tones. With a slight frequency difference, where the phase cycle occupies several seconds, it is difficult if not impossible to perceive any systematic intensity fluctuations. This is however the best condition for the observation of the movement of the sound from side to side, described above as the binaural shift phenomenon. Now when the frequency difference is made greater, and the phase cycles occur 3 or more times a second, the sound seems no longer to wander from place to place, but to undergo loudness variations. The beats have something of the character of uniaural beats, but they vary in several respects. They lack the crisp, staccato quality of these other beats at the favorable rates of 3 to 6 per second and are instead rather fuzzy and at times even slightly irregular. The adjustment of the intensity at the two ears is highly critical for their appearance.

These binaural beats are most easily heard with low-frequency stimuli, but they still are found, when the conditions are favorable, for all tones up to 3000 ~. I have not been able to hear them at 5000 ~. The upper limits at which they were observed by five other subjects have already been given in Table VIII.

A binaural beat with tones as high as 3000 ~ calls for an accurate representation of frequency in the neural channels for the two ears up to some integrative center, just as phase localization does. Indeed, the evidence points to a common process that yields either shifts of localization or fluctuations of loudness according to the rate of the phasic changes. The rates that give the most prominent loudness variations (3 to 6 per second, representing periods of 0.33 to 0.16 sec) fall in the range of the periods for optimal summation of loudness, which Békésy found to be 0.17 sec and Munson considered to be a little longer, about 0.2 to 0.5 sec. It appears that the impulses from the two ears summate readily if they strike the common center within an interval around 0.1 to 0.5 sec, but less adequately if they are separated by longer and shorter intervals of time.

As already mentioned, these results are crucial to auditory theory. They cannot be explained on a simple place theory in which the neural elements only relay information as to the locus of the peripheral activity and give no account of the temporal conditions. Much more is necessary: the nervous messages must reveal the temporal changes, and they must do so not just in a gross fashion, but in great detail, cycle by cycle. So to account for these binaural phenomena we must employ the frequency principle.

CHAPTER 18

THE VOLLEY THEORY IN REVIEW;
CONCLUDING OBSERVATIONS

In the historical chapters of this book we have traced the appearance and development of two main types of explanation of auditory phenomena, one based upon the place principle and the other upon the frequency principle. We have observed how, over many years, these two were maintained and defended as distinct and exclusive accounts of the actions of the ear; and then we have come to see how they may be adjusted and reconciled to form a single theory.

There seems little room for argument now as to the validity of the two principles. Each rests upon substantial evidence. Yet, as we have found, neither by itself is sufficient: one alone is unable to account for all the phenomena of auditory experience. It is only in their harmonious combination that we come to a full realization of our explanatory purpose; together, assisting and supplementing one another, they produce a complete theory.

There may be a degree of uncertainty still as to the particular spheres of operation of these principles and as to their relative effectiveness in the areas where they overlap. My own suggestions on these problems are sketched in the foregoing chapters; and it will remain for further experimentation and discussion to determine how reasonable they are and to work out the revisions, large and small, that are found to be necessary.

Generally speaking, the explanations offered for the various phenomena have called impartially upon the two principles. Both are deemed indispensable in our accounts of nearly every one of the basic manifestations of hearing: both play their parts in the phenomena of pitch and loudness; in the disturbances of the ear's performance seen in auditory fatigue and more seriously in tinnitus, diplacusis, and various forms of deafness; in the interactions disclosed as beats, combination tones, interference, and masking; and the others. Only as regards the temporal phenomena, for a single ear or both, do we find a notable supremacy of one principle, which is naturally the frequency principle; and even so the operation of the other principle here is by no means negligible. In general, from the character of the spatial and temporal representations, the frequency principle is paramount in respect to the low tones, the place principle takes that position for the high tones, and the two often share the honors in the intermediate region.

In the treatment of the above phenomena, the place and frequency principles have been assigned their respective roles as well as may be on a basis of the evidence now at hand; yet it must be appreciated that there are many uncertainties of detail that can be cleared up only by further experimental work. Especially do we need to know in terms as precise as possible the limits and modes of operation of these two principles.

The Limits of the Frequency Principle. For the auditory nerve itself the upper limit of synchronism of 4000 to 5000 $\sim$ as now observed agrees so well with the indirect indications that any substantial revision on the basis of further study seems rather unlikely.

For the higher acoustic tracts, however, the contrary is true; for them it is almost certain that refinements of technique, and especially a proper handling of the problems of anesthetic depression and the anatomical dispersion of elements will considerably extend the limits now known. When we have more dependable information on the representation in these higher tracts we should be able to conceive with greater definiteness and understanding than is possible now the nature of the central acoustic processes.

The Form of Place Representation. In our dealing with the problem of cochlear localization it is well to bear in mind that here at the periphery are three stages of activity, in each of which we have a spatial representation of tonal stimuli. These stages are, in order, the mechanical action, the sensory response, and the neural discharge. The patterns of representation undergo changes from one of these stages to the next.

The mechanical activity represents the acoustic stimulus as conveyed to the cochlea, and its pattern is determined by regional variations in vibratory characteristics within the structure. The transmission by the middle ear is evidently simple, uncomplicated by serious distortion at any tolerable intensities. In the mechanical action of the cochlea, however, a degree of distortion is likely when the stimulation is strong, and its effect will be to reduce the peak amplitudes of the vibratory movements.

There is good reason to believe that the sensory activity that follows is, region by region, a faithful copy of the mechanical activity, except for the stronger intensities for which further distortion appears, evidently contributed by the sensory cells themselves. The effect of this distortion is to exaggerate the changes caused by the first variety and so further to flatten out the peaks of the response pattern.

The neural activity reproduces the sensory pattern only in a general way. There are three complicating conditions. The first is a limitation of range imposed by the fact that a nerve fiber has a threshold: the fiber responds only when its excitation exceeds some limiting amount. Hence at the lowest level only those elements are involved that lie in the region of peak stimulation; and then as the intensity is raised other elements add themselves to the discharge. A second condition is neural distortion. The rate of impulses in any one fiber bears a linear relation to the stimulus intensity for only a short course, and thereafter its rise decelerates and the rate ultimately reaches a maximum. The effect is to flatten out the higher contours of the response pattern, just as the other kinds of distortion do. Then, finally, there is the diffuse arrangement of the cochlear nerve supply, which tends to iron out any abrupt changes of excitatory effect and so contributes further to the broadening and rounding off of the tonal patterns.

From these conditions it is clear that the pattern of activity as developed in the cochlear nerve and represented to the higher centers for any given tone is not of fixed form, but changes with the intensity. It changes with particular rapidity just above threshold, and again as the highest intensities are passed through. Specificity changes accordingly; it is at its maximum at threshold and diminishes from that point on. It is evident that specificity operates in the face of distinct limitations.

Let us now review the variations of specificity as a function of frequency. All the evidence goes to show that there are characteristic differences in the patterns for low and high tones. For the low tones the patterns are broad, and especially so at high levels of intensity. As can be proved most decisively from the experiments on stimulation deafness and on the maximum potentials of the cochlea, these tones at high levels involve the great mass of hair cells, and perhaps every cell, in vigorous activity. For the high tones, and especially the very high ones, so massive a response does not occur for stimuli within our limits of tolerance, but for them certain cochlear areas are strongly involved and others only moderately. The difference comes from the more selective mechanical action of these tones, which is such as to produce a high concentration of stimulus energy on certain cochlear areas. As the stimulus is raised to high levels it begins to cause serious distortion in these more favored areas before it has greatly involved the other areas. If the intensity were raised sufficiently it would indeed bring up the activity of the peripheral areas, but only at the impracticable cost of destroying the central areas.

SPECIFICITY AND ITS CONSEQUENCES FOR THEORY

We have traveled far from the original conception of specificity in the cochlear activity. No one now can take seriously the notion of a separate element for every discriminable pitch. Indeed, this simple notion, attractive as it seems at first acquaintance, had no firm status even in the beginning when Helmholtz made it the foundation of his resonance theory. For not even Helmholtz was able to remain true to his principle: knowing the physical nature of resonance, having to account for such phenomena as beats and glides of pitch, and forced to reconcile the niceties of discrimination with the indicated paucity of resonators, he found himself compelled to admit a small degree of cochlear spread.

Then, as we have seen, later considerations of the phenomena of hearing, and especially of the cochlear anatomy as it gave evidence of high damping and the interconnection of moving parts, led to further modifications of the picture of specificity. Still further considerations, all leading away from strict specificity and toward a conception of broad cochlear activity in response to simple tones, have brought us to our present understanding of this problem.

What was not often appreciated, and plainly was never apparent to Helmholtz himself, was the seriousness of a departure from strict specificity. If a given tone excites elements that are also excited by other tones, the problem looms as to how any specific pitch can be determined. The reservation that the overlapping may be only moderate, as Helmholtz conceived it— with perhaps about a score of elements operating in common to two tones that are just discriminable—does not mitigate the difficulty. Why, as Hostinsky wondered, do we not perceive a manifold of tones from a single stimulus, and how do we sort out the sensations from two neighboring stimuli? We have already seen how he tried to solve the problem by means of central interactions.

Gray faced the problem too, with a theory no more meritorious than Hostinsky's but one that historically proved more successful. His solution, as we know, was the now famous principle of maximum stimulation. Specificity in the initial action of tones on the basilar membrane he yielded up, and then he sought to regain it farther along in the course of the acoustic activity through this principle of the maximum. He supposed that somehow—the means was never quite clear—only those elements at the maximum of the response pattern had any final consequence for pitch perception. Truly it may be said that this principle of Gray's rescued the resonance theory from the threat of oblivion that hung over it at the close of the past century. It was at a time when the theory's critics were many and its rivals were gathering strength; Gray's pronouncement turned the tide of favor and established the theory in a position in which it has stood seemingly unassailable over the years.

In the light of this development it is a curious fact, and ironical almost, that the benefit to specificity lent by Gray's principle is entirely specious. Strict specificity—specificity in its original sense as a definite representation of quality by an individual sensory or neural element—is not recovered by this principle. Such specificity would have to be recovered in the peripheral processes, and Gray's principle concerned some undefined sort of central processes, not peripheral ones. There seems to have been a poor apprehension of this fact by Gray himself, and by others after him, perhaps because to speak of a maximum point of stimulation gives an appearance of objectivity and independent existence. Gray's hypothesis was accepted and made use of with a tacit assurance, unwarranted by its actual assertions, that this maximum point could function as a physical point and could find a representation in just those nerve fibers serving its limited place on the basilar membrane. Otherwise it must have been appreciated from the outset that the strict kind of specificity is utterly lost and that there remains only a pattern relationship.

A Pattern Theory of Auditory Perception. Assuredly, a pattern theory is what the facts sustain. Every neural element relays two sorts of information, the position along the membrane that it serves and the periodicity of its excitation. This information from all the active elements forms a central pattern on which our perceptions depend. The form of the pattern will bear a resemblance to the peripheral action but will not be a precise copy of it, because, as will now be clear, the representations are inexact in both their positional and intensive aspects. The positional representation is modified by neural diffusion and interconnection, and the intensive representation is limited at one end of the intensity scale by neural thresholds and at the other end by mechanical, sensory, and neural departures from linearity. All these conditions combine in broadening and blurring the represented pattern. Yes, despite these limitations, enough remains of the form of the pattern to join with the factor of frequency representation in serving our perceptual purposes.

It cannot be too much emphasized that we have to deal with this pattern as it stands, in all its fullness. In our concentration upon the problem of pitch we are not to resort to the devices of Hostinsky and Gray, and others after them, by which some central process is presumed to effect a loss of all the pattern except its point of maximum and thereby to convert its complexities into an ultimate singularity. As I have already insisted, a maximum point has a reality only by reference to the lesser points beside it, and indeed only by reference to the whole context in which it appears. Then, too, we must recall that to lose the outlying area of the pattern would jeopardize our handling of other problems of our auditory experience, like the problem of loudness, in which we must make use of every active element. What happens to the peripheral patterns as they are transmitted centrally we do not know in detail. We have some inklings of the variables made use of in the central processes, but about the processes themselves we are deeply ignorant. We know only that the higher centers accept and work upon the response patterns, and out of them we glean our knowledge of pitch and loudness and the other qualities of sounds. Here is a challenging field for investigation.

Still another problem that remains unsolved is the physical basis of cochlear differentiation. There are many theories in the field, as we have found. Among the ones under serious discussion in recent years is the tube-resonance hypothesis of Ranke and Reboul. This hypothesis stands in some favor nowadays, perhaps in a measure just because it is of recent formulation and has come late enough to take account of many of the modern observations, and in Reboul's version to embrace the volley principle. Yet there appears to be a serious drawback in attributing systematic discriminatory powers to an anatomical feature seemingly so wayward as the form and size of the cochlear canals. It becomes difficult in terms of such a variable, even when it is aided by others, to account for the considerable similarities in the hearing of animals whose cochleas differ greatly in dimensions. The possibilities here need to be explored further, but from what we know now it seems better to look elsewhere for the differential conditions. And in this quest, as the evidence now stands, we can do no better than was done in classic theory, and though perchance with a more critical eye with respect to the details of our conception, still to look for the basis of our specific variables in the basilar membrane and its pertinent structures. We can now pursue this problem with more comfort than heretofore because we need not load the whole burden of theory upon the mechanical conditions, but can allow the frequency variable to take its share.

DEFINITIONS AND SYMBOLS

Cycle (~). The simplest pattern of changes in a sound wave that continually recurs. For simple waves (sine waves) we can think of a cycle as a rise from zero to a positive peak, then a fall through zero to a negative peak (or a trough), and finally a return to zero. In older terminology the cycle was a 'complete' or 'double' vibration, in distinction from a 'single' vibration. A 'single' vibration is either a positive or negative half-cycle. Old tuning forks, like those made by Koenig, are often marked in 'single' vibrations, and their frequencies are but half the numbers they bear.

Damping. A force that tends to reduce the amplitude of a vibration. For example, the friction of the air against the prongs of a tuning fork is a damping force, and after the fork is struck it quickly brings the motion to an end.

Decibel (db). A kind of ratio between two quantities, as for example two sound intensities. If one sound contains 25.9 per cent more energy than another, it is stronger by 1 db. In general, we find the difference in decibels between two energies by means of the formula

$$N = 10 \log_{10} R$$

where N is the number of decibels and R is the ratio between the energies. Specifically, we divide one energy by the other, look up the common logarithm of this quotient in a logarithm table, and multiply by 10; the result is the difference in decibels. If we have divided the larger energy by the smaller the result is positive, and if we have done the reverse the result is the same number of decibels but negative. It is easier to use a decibel table, where the last two operations have been combined: with such a table we have only to compute the ratio R and look it up to obtain the answer in decibels. To go from decibels to ratios we reverse the process.

Actual sound measurements usually deal with sound pressures rather than with energies, and then, if we can assume

443

constant conditions of acoustic impedances (as we usually can for sounds in air), we may use the alternative formula for decibels,

$$N = 20 \log_{10} \frac{P_1}{P_0}$$

where P_1, P_0 are the pressures of the two sounds. In this formula the constant is doubled because for a given sound the pressure varies as the square root of the energy, and accordingly for a pair of sounds the pressure ratio varies as the square root of the energy ratio. It follows that the logarithm of the pressure ratio is only half as large as the logarithm of the energy ratio, but then by doubling the constant we come out with the same number of decibels as before. The difference between two sounds in decibels is the same regardless of our use of energy or pressure units, but we must be careful to take account of the kind of units in doing the computation. Particle velocities are treated in the same way as pressures in this reckoning.

Δf (read as *'delta f'*). A change in the frequency of a tone that is just discriminable; called the absolute jnd or difference limen for pitch.

$\Delta f/f$. The just discriminable frequency change divided by the frequency itself; called the relative jnd or relative difference limen for pitch.

ΔI (read as *'delta I'*). A change in the intensity of a tone that is just discriminable; called the absolute jnd or difference limen for loudness. The intensity may be considered in either energy or pressure units, and it is necessary to state which is used.

$\Delta I/I$. The just discriminable intensity change divided by the intensity itself; called the relative jnd or relative difference limen for loudness. It makes a difference whether energy or pressure units are used.

Dynes. A unit of force. One gram under the pull of gravity exerts a force of 980 dynes (at sea level and certain latitudes). A dyne per square centimeter is the unit of sound pressure.

Frequency. The number of cycles per second.

Intensity. The magnitude of a stimulus. Preferably, the intensity of sounds is stated in units of energy flow, as in watts, or, because a watt of sound is a very large amount indeed, we use microwatts (millionths of a watt), or even micro-microwatts. Sounds may also be measured in pressure units (dynes per square centimeter) or in particle velocity units (centimeters per second).

Intensity level. The intensity level of a sound is its number of decibels above a chosen reference intensity.

Just noticeable difference (jnd). A change of stimulus that is just discriminable, under certain prescribed conditions of observation. See Δf, ΔI.

Loudness. The quantitative dimension of an auditory sensation. It is to be distinguished from *intensity*, which is a physical quantity.

Loudness level. For a 1000 $\sim$ tone, the loudness level is the same as its intensity level. For any other sound, it is the intensity level of the 1000 $\sim$ tone that seems equally loud.

Microvolts (μV). Millionths of a volt.

Milliseconds (ms or msec). Thousandths of a second. Sometimes, especially in physiological literature, it is called *sigma (σ).*

Period. The time required for one cycle of a wave; the reciprocal of the frequency.

Phase. Relative position within a cycle, expressed either as a fraction of the period, and measured in seconds, or, more commonly, in angular units, either as degrees or radians. Angular measure is applicable because a simple wave (sine wave) can be derived geometrically as a projection of uniform motion around a circle. Therefore, carrying over this measure, we designate a whole cycle as 360° or 2π radians, half a cycle as 180° or π radians, and so on. Two waves whose phase relation is zero or 360° are in phase: they are executing the same motions in complete synchronism. Two whose phase relation is 180° are in opposite phase: every motion of one is contrary in direction to the motion of the other.

Pressure (sound pressure). A particle in motion exerts a force on any object that it strikes, and if we add up over a unit area all the forces of many particles whose reciprocating motions constitute a sound we have a sound pressure. Its magnitude is expressed in dynes per square centimeter. Actually, the pressure varies continually during a cycle; that at any instant we speak of as the instantaneous pressure. Of more practical use is the peak pressure, which is the maximum attained during the cycle, and the root-mean-square (rms) pressure, which is a kind of average through the cycle. The rms pressure is considered in this way: as the result of taking the values of pressure attained at small intervals throughout the cycle, squaring each one, adding them, dividing by their number, and finally extracting the square root. The rms pressure is the one in most general use and is to be understood unless there is some indication to the contrary. In a sine wave, the rms pressure equals the peak pressure divided by the square root of 2.

Reference intensity. An intensity from which sound levels in decibels are reckoned. The most generally accepted reference intensity is 10^{-16} watts per square centimeter. For sounds in air this is (roughly) equivalent to a sound pressure of 0.0002 dynes per square centimeter.

Spectrum level. Applied to bands of noise; it is the intensity level per cycle of the noise.

Velocity. There are two kinds of velocity pertaining to sounds: propagation velocity and particle velocity. *Propagation velocity* is the rate of transmission of the sound through a medium; in air under ordinary conditions this rate is about 344 meters per second (1129 ft per second). *Particle velocity* is the rate of motion of the molecules of the substance that is in vibration. Because this motion varies from moment to moment within the cycle we must either consider it instantaneously or, what is more practical, take it at its peak value or else take it in a kind of average sense over the cycle, just as described under *Pressure.*

REFERENCES

ADES, H. W., METTLER, F. A., and CULLER, E. A. Effect of lesions in the medial geniculate bodies upon hearing in the cat, *Amer. J. Physiol.*, 1939, 125, 15–23.

ADRIAN, E. D. (1) Wedensky inhibition in relation to the 'all-or-none' principle in nerve, *J. Physiol.*, 1913, 46, 384–412. (2) The all-or-none principle in nerve, *J. Physiol.*, 1914, 47, 460–474. (3) *The basis of sensation*, 1928. (4) Impulses in sympathetic fibres and in slow afferent fibres, *J. Physiol.*, 1930, 70, *Proc. Physiol. Soc.*, xx–xxi. (5) The effects of injury on mammalian nerve fibres, *Proc. Roy. Soc. Lond.*, ser. B, 1930, 106, 596–618. (6) The microphonic action of the cochlea; an interpretation of Wever and Bray's experiments, *J. Physiol.*, 1931, 71, xxviii–xxix.

ADRIAN, E. D., and BRONK, D. W. (1) The discharge of impulses in motor nerve fibres; Part I, Impulses in single fibres of the phrenic nerve, *J. Physiol.*, 1928, 66, 81–101. (2) The discharge of impulses in motor nerve fibres; Part II, The frequency of discharge in reflex and voluntary contractions, *J. Physiol.*, 1929, 67, 119–151.

ADRIAN, E. D., BRONK, D. W., and PHILLIPS, G. The nervous origin of the Wever and Bray effect, *J. Physiol.*, 1931, 73, 2P–3P.

ADRIAN, E. D., CATTELL, McK., and HOAGLAND, H. Sensory discharges in single cutaneous nerve fibres, *J. Physiol.*, 1931, 72, 377–391.

ADRIAN, E. D., CRAIK, K. J. W., and STURDY, R. S. The electrical response of the auditory mechanism in cold-blooded vertebrates, *Proc. Roy. Soc. Lond.*, ser. B, 1938, 125, 435–455.

ADRIAN, E. D., and LUCAS, K. On the summation of propagated disturbances in nerve and muscle, *J. Physiol.*, 1912, 44, 68–124.

ADRIAN, E. D., and ZOTTERMAN, Y. (1) The impulses produced by sensory nerve-endings; Part 2, The response of a single end-organ, *J. Physiol.*, 1926, 61, 151–171. (2) The impulses produced by sensory nerve endings; Part 3, Impulses set up by touch and pressure, *J. Physiol.*, 1926, 61, 465–483.

ALEXANDER, G. (1) Zur vergleichenden, pathologischen Anatomie des Gehörorganes; I, Gehörorgan und Gehirn einer unvollkommen albinotischen, weissen Katze, *Arch. f. Ohrenheilk.*, 1900, 50, 159–181. (2) Zur vergleichenden, pathologischen Anatomie des Gehörorganes, *Zeits. f. Ohrenheilk.*, 1904, 48, 378–381.

ARAPOVA, A. A., GERSUNI, G. V., and VOLOKHOV, A. A. A further analysis of the action of alternating currents on the auditory apparatus, *J. Physiol.*, 1937, 89, 122–131.

ASHCROFT, D. W., HALLPIKE, C. S., and RAWDON-SMITH, A. F. On the changes in histological structure and electrical response of the cochlea of the cat following section of the VIII nerve, *Proc. Roy. Soc. Lond.*, ser. B, 1937, 122, 186–197.

AYERS, H. Vertebrate cephalogenesis; II, A contribution to the morphology of the vertebrate ear, with a reconsideration of its functions, *J. Morphol.*, 1892, 6, 1–360.

BACINSKY, B. (1) Zur Physiologie der Gehörschnecke, *Akad. d. Wiss.*, *Berlin, Sitzungsber.*, 1883, 685–688. (2) Die Function der Gehörschnecke, *Virchows Arch. f. path. Anat. Physiol.*, 1883, 94, 65–85.

BANISTER, H. (1) The effect of binaural phase differences on the localisation of tones at various frequencies, *Brit. J. Psychol.*, 1925, 15, 280–307. (2) A suggestion towards a new hypothesis regarding the localization of sound, *Brit. J. Psychol.*, 1926, 17, 142–153.

BARD, P., and RIOCH, D. M. A study of four cats deprived of neocortex and additional portions of the forebrain, *Bull. Johns Hopkins Hosp.*, 1937, 60, 73–147.

BAST, T. H., and EYSTER, J. A. E. Symposium: Is there localization in the cochlea for low tones? *Ann. of Otol., Rhinol. and Laryngol.*, 1935, 44, 792–803.

BAUHIN, CASPAR (1560–1624). *Theatrum anatomicum*, Francofurti ad Moenum, 1605.

BEASLEY, W. (1) The monaural phase effect with pure binary harmonies; I, Frequency ratio 2:3, *J. Acoust. Soc. Amer.*, 1930, 1, 385–402. (2) Differential responses to cyclic phase variations in compound sounds, *J. General Psychol.*, 1931, 5, 329–351.

BEAUREGARD, H., and DUPUY, E. Sur la variation électrique (courant d'action) déterminée dans le nerf acoustique par le son, *Arch. internat. laryngol., otol., etc.*, 1896, 9, 383–386.

BECK, A. Die Bestimmung der Localisation der Gehirn- und Rückenmarksfunctionen vermittelst der elektrischen Erscheinungen, *Centralbl. f. Physiol.*, 1890, 4, 473–476.

BÉKÉSY, G. VON. (1) Zur Theorie des Hörens; Die Schwingungsform der Basilarmembran, *Phys. Zeits.*, 1928, 29, 793–810. (2) Zur Theorie des Hörens; Über die Bestimmung des einem reinen Tonempfinden entsprechenden Erregungsgebietes der Basilarmembran vermittelst Ermüdungserscheinungen, *Phys. Zeits.*, 1929, 30, 115–125. (3) Zur Theorie des Hörens; Über die eben merkbare Amplituden- und Frequenzänderung eines Tones; Die Theorie der Schwebungen, *Phys. Zeits.*, 1929, 30, 721–745. (4) Über das Fechnersche Gesetz und seine Bedeutung für die Theorie der akustischen Beobachtungsfehler und die Theorie des Hörens, *Ann. d. Phys.*, 1930, 7, 329–359. (5) Über die Hörsamkeit der Ein- und Ausschwingvorgänge mit Berücksichtigung der Raumakustik, *Ann. d. Phys.*, 1933, 16, 844–860. (6) Physikalische Probleme der Hörphysiologie, *Elektr. Nachr. Techn.*, 1935, 12, 71–83. (7) Über die

Herstellung und Messung langsamer sinusförmiger Luftdruckschwankungen, *Ann. d. Phys.*, 1936, 25, 413–432. (8) Über die Hörschwelle und Fühlgrenze langsamer sinusförmiger Luftdruckschwankungen, *Ann. d. Phys.*, 1936, 26, 554–566. (9) Über die Messung der Schwingungsamplitude der Gehörknöchelchen mittels einer kapazitiven Sonde, *Akust. Zeits.*, 1941, 6, 1–16. (10) Über die Elastizität der Schneckentrennwand des Ohres, *Akust. Zeits.*, 1941, 6, 265–278. (11) Über die Schwingungen der Schneckentrennwand beim Präparat und Ohrenmodell, *Akust. Zeits.*, 1942, 7, 173–186. (12) Über die Resonanzkurve und die Abklingzeit der verschiedenen Stellen der Schneckentrennwand, *Akust. Zeits.*, 1943, 8, 66–76. (13) Über die Frequenzauflösung in der menschlichen Schnecke, *Acta oto-laryngol.*, 1944, 32, 60–84. (14) The variation of phase along the basilar membrane with sinusoidal vibrations, *J. Acoust. Soc. Amer.*, 1947, 19, 452–460.

BELIKOFF, P. N. (1) Über die Gültigkeit des Talbotschen Gesetzes für das Gehör, I, *Pflüg. Arch. ges. Physiol.*, 1925, 209, 537–539. (2) Ueber die Verschmelzung der pulsierenden Töne, *J. f. Psychol. Neurol.*, 1929, 38, 292–300.

BELL, CHARLES. Reprint of the "Idea of a new anatomy of the brain, submitted for the observations of his friends," arranged by A. Shaw, *J. of Anat. Physiol.*, 1869, 3, 147–182. [Original privately printed in 1811.]

BERENDES, —. Die Spannung der menschlichen Basilarmembran, *Zeits. f. Hals- Nasen- Ohrenheilk.*, 1934, 36, 338–342.

BERENGARIO DA CARPI, JACOPO. [Work not seen; quoted by Fallopius and Schelhammer.]

BISHOP, H. G. On Mayer's "Residual sonorous sensation," *Amer. J. Psychol.*, 1930, 42, 38–50.

BLAIR, E. A., and ERLANGER, J. A comparison of the characteristics of axons through their individual electrical responses, *Amer. J. Physiol.*, 1933, 106, 524–564.

BOETTCHER, ARTHUR. *Ueber Entwicklung und Bau des Gehörlabyrinths*, Dresden: Blochmann, 1869.

BONNIER, PIERRE (1861–). (1) De la nature des phénomènes auditifs, *Bull. sci. de France et Belg.*, 1895, 25, 367–397. (2) Le limaçon membraneux considéré comme appareil enregistreur, *Compt. r. soc. biol.*, 1895, 47, 127–129. (3) Fonctions de la membrane de Corti, *Compt. r. soc. biol.*, 1895, 47, 130–131. (4) L'audition, 1901.

BORING, E. G. Auditory theory with special reference to intensity, volume, and localization, *Amer. J. Psychol.*, 1926, 37, 157–188.

BORING, E. G., and TITCHENER, E. B. Sir Thomas Wrightson's theory of hearing, *Amer. J. Psychol.*, 1920, 31, 101–113.

BRAMWELL, E. A case of cortical deafness, *Brain*, 1927, 50, 579–580.

BRECHER, G. A. Die untere Hör- und Tongrenze, *Pflüg. Arch. ges. Physiol.*, 1934, 234, 380–393.

BREMER, F., and DOW, R. S. The cerebral acoustic area of the cat, *J. Neurophysiol.*, 1939, 2, 308–318.

BRESCHET, G. Recherches anatomiques et physiologiques sur l'organe de l'ouïe et sur l'audition dans l'homme et animaux vertébrés, *Mém. acad. roy. med.*, Paris, 1836, 5, 229–523.

BROWN, G. L. Reported by Newman, H. W., Doupe, J., and Wilkins, R. W. Some observations on the nature of vibratory sensibility, *Brain*, 1939, 62, 31–40.

BRYANT, W. S. Die Lehre von den schallemfindlichen Haarzellen, *Arch. f. Ohrenheilk.*, 1909, 79, 93–102.

BUCK, A. H. On the mechanism of hearing, *New York Med. J.*, 1874, 19, 561–579.

BUDDE, E. (1) Über die Resonanztheorie des Hörens, *Phys. Zeits.*, 1917, 18, 225–236, 249–260. (2) Mathematische Theorie der Gehörsempfindung, in Emil Abderhalden's *Handbuch der biologischen Arbeitsmethoden*, division 5, part 7, 1–194.

BURCK, W., KOTOWSKI, P., and LICHTE, H. (1) Hörbarkeit von Regelvorgängen in dynamikgeregelten Verstärkern und Film- Reintonsystemen, *Zeits. f. tech. Phys.*, 1935, 16, 522–525. (2) Frequenzspektrum und Tonerkennen, *Ann. d. Phys.*, 1936, 25, 433–449. (3) Logarithmische und lineare Lautstärkenskala, *Ann. d. Phys.*, 1936, 27, 664–668.

BUNCH, C. C. Auditory acuity after removal of the entire right cerebral hemisphere, *J. Amer. Med. Assoc.*, 1928, 90, 2102.

BUNCH, C. C., and RAIFORD, T. S. Race and sex variations in auditory acuity, *Arch. of Otolaryngol.*, 1931, 13, 423–434.

BUYTENDIJK, F. J. J. On the negative variation of the nervus acusticus caused by a sound, *Akad. van Wetensch., Amsterdam, Proc. Sci. Sect.*, 1911, 13, part 2, 649–652.

BUYTENDIJK, F. J. J., and MEESTERS, A. Duration and course of the auditory sensation, *Commentationes Pontif. Acad. Sci., Rome*, 1942, 6, 557–576.

CATON, R. The electric currents of the brain, *Brit. Med. J.*, 1875, 2, 278.

CATTELL, McK., and HOAGLAND, H. Response of tactile receptors to intermittent stimulation, *J. Physiol.*, 1931, 72, 392–404.

CAUSSÉ, R., and CHAVASSE, P. Études sur la fatigue auditive, *Année psychol.*, 1947, 43–44, 265–298.

CHAPIN, E. K., and FIRESTONE, F. A. The influence of phase on tone quality and loudness; the interference of subjective harmonics, *J. Acoust. Soc. Amer.*, 1934, 5, 173–180.

CHLADNI, E. F. F. *Traité d'acoustique*, 1809.

CHURCHER, B. G. A loudness scale for industrial noise measurements, *J. Acoust. Soc. Amer.*, 1935, 6, 216–226.

CIOCCO, A. A statistical approach to the problem of tone localization in the human cochlea, *Hum. Biol.*, 1934, 6, 714–721.

CLAUDIUS, M. Bemerkungen über den Bau der häutigen Spiralleiste der Schnecke, *Zeits. f. wiss. Zool.*, 1856, 7, 154–161.

COITER, VOLCHER. *De auditus instrumento*, in *Externarum et internarum principalium humani corporis*, partium tabulae, Noribergae, 1573, 88–105. [First appeared separately, 1566.]

COPPÉE, G. (1) La pararésonance dans l'excitation par les courants alternatifs sinusoidaux, *Arch. internat. physiol.*, 1934, 40, 1–58. (2) Distribution systématique des neurones, des voies auditives dans le mésencéphale, *Bull. acad. roy. méd. Belg.*, 1939, 216–239.

CORTI, ALPHONSE. Recherches sur l'organe de l'ouïe des mammifères, *Zeits. f. wiss. Zool.*, 1851, 3, 109–169.

COTUGNO, DOMINICO = COTUNNIUS, DOMINICUS. *De aquaeductibus auris humanae internae.* Viennae, 1774. [First ed., Neap. 1760; not seen.]

COVELL, W. P., and BLACK, L. J. The cochlear response as an index to hearing, *Amer. J. Physiol.*, 1936, 116, 524–530.

CRAMER, —. Letters to de Mairan, *Journal des Sçavans*, Amsterdam, 1741, 124, 167–202.

CROWE, S. J. (1) Anatomic changes in the labyrinth secondary to cerebellopontile and brain stem tumors, *Arch. of Surg.*, 1929, 18, 982–991. (2) Ménière's disease, *Medicine*, 1938, 17, 1–36.

CROWE, S. J., GUILD, S. R., and POLVOGT, L. M. Observations on the pathology of high-tone deafness, *Bull. Johns Hopkins Hosp.*, 1934, 54, 315–379.

CULLER, E. A. Symposium: Is there localization in the cochlea for low tones? *Ann. of Otol., Rhinol. and Laryngol.*, 1935, 44, 807–813.

CULLER, E. A., COAKLEY, J. D., LOWY, K., and GROSS, N. A revised frequency-map of the guinea-pig cochlea, *Amer. J. Psychol.*, 1943, 56, 475–500.

DANDY, W. E. (1) Removal of right cerebral hemisphere for certain tumors with hemiplegia, *J. Amer. Med. Assoc.*, 1928, 90, 823–825. (2) Ménière's disease: diagnosis and treatment, *Amer. J. Surg.*, 1933, 20, 693–698. (3) Physiological studies following extirpation of the right cerebral hemisphere in man, *Bull. Johns Hopkins Hosp.*, 1933, 53, 31–51. (4) Treatment of Ménière's disease by section of only the vestibular portion of the acoustic nerve, *Bull. Johns Hopkins Hosp.*, 1933, 53, 52–55. (5) Ménière's disease, *Arch. of Otolaryngol.*, 1934, 20, 1–30. (6) The effect of hemisection of the cochlear branch of the human auditory nerve, *Bull. Johns Hopkins Hosp.*, 1934, 54, 208–210. (7) The treatment of bilateral Ménière's disease and pseudo-Ménière's disease, *Acta neuropath. in hon. L. Puusepp*, 1935, lx, 10–14.

DANILEWSKY, B. Zur Frage ueber die electromotorischen Vorgänge im Gehirn als Ausdruck seines Thätigkeitszustandes, *Centralbl. f. Physiol.*, 1891, 5, 1–4.

DAVIS, H. (1) The physiological phenomena of audition, in C. Murchison's *Handbook of general experimental psychology*, 1934, 962–986. (2) The electrical phenomena of the cochlea and the auditory nerve, *J. Acoust. Soc. Amer.*, 1935, 6, 205–215.

DAVIS, H., DERBYSHIRE, A. J., KEMP, E. H., LURIE, M. H., and UPTON, M. Functional and histological changes in the cochlea of the guinea pig resulting from prolonged stimulation, *J. General Psychol.*, 1935, 12, 251–278.

DAVIS, H., DERBYSHIRE, A. J., LURIE, M. H., and SAUL, L. J. Further analysis of cochlear activity and auditory action currents, *Trans. Amer. Otol. Soc.*, 1933, 23, 106–116.

DAVIS, H., MORGAN, C. T., HAWKINS, J., GALAMBOS, R., and SMITH, F. W. Temporary deafness following exposure to loud tones and noise, *Comm. on Med. Res.*, OSRD, 1943; *Laryngoscope*, 1946, 56, 19–21.

DEITERS, OTTO. *Untersuchungen über die Lamina spiralis membranacea,* Bonn, 1860.

DENNERT, H. Akustisch-physiologische Untersuchungen, *Arch. f. Ohrenheilk.*, 1887, 24, 171–184.

DERBYSHIRE, A. J., and DAVIS, H. The action potentials of the auditory nerve, *Amer. J. Physiol.*, 1935, 113, 476–504.

DIX, M. R., HALLPIKE, C. S., and HOOD, J. D. Observations upon the loudness recruitment phenomenon, *Proc. Roy. Soc. Med.*, 1948, 41, 516–526.

DUVERNEY, JOSEPH GUICHARD. *Traité de l'organe de l'ouie*, Paris, 1683.

EBNER, V. VON. In Albert Kölliker's *Handbuch der Gewebelehre des Menschen*, 6th ed., Leipzig, 1902, vol. 3, 889–960.

ECHLIN, F. A., and FESSARD, A. (1) La sensibilité vibratoire et le récepteur de tension, *Compt. r. soc. biol.*, 1937, 124, 1199–1202. (2) Synchronized impulse discharges from receptors in the deep tissues in response to a vibrating stimulus, *J. Physiol.*, 1938, 93, 312–334.

ERLANGER, JOSEPH, and GASSER, H. S. *Electrical signs of nervous activity,* 1937.

ESTEVE, —. *Traité de l'ouïe*, Avignon, 1751. [Work not seen; quoted by S. von Stein.]

EUSTACHIUS, BARTHOLOMAEUS. *Opuscula anatomica*, Venetiis, 1564, 148–164.

EWALD, J. R. (1855–1921). (1) Die centrale Entstehung von Schwebungen zweier monotisch gehörten Töne, *Pflüg. Arch. ges. Physiol.*, 1894, 57, 80–88. (2) Ueber eine neue Hörtheorie, *Wien. klin. Wochenschr.*, 1898, 11, 721. (3) Zur Physiologie des Labyrinths, VI, Eine neue Hörtheorie, *Pflüg. Arch. ges. Physiol.*, 1899, 76, 147–188. (4) Zur Physiologie des Labyrinths, VII Mitt., Die Erzeugung von Schallbildern in der Camera acustica, *Pflüg. Arch. ges. Physiol.*, 1903, 93, 485–500. (5) Über die neuen Versuche, die Angriffsstellen der von Tönen ausgehenden Schallwellen im Ohr zu localisieren, *Pflüg. Arch. ges. Physiol.*, 1910, 131, 188–198.

EWALD, J. R., and JÄDERHOLM, G. A. Die Herabsetzung der subjektiven Tonhöhe durch Steigerung der objektiven Intensität, *Pflüg. Arch. ges. Physiol.*, 1908, 124, 29–36.

EXNER, S. Zur Lehre von der Gehörsempfindungen, *Pflüg. Arch. ges. Physiol.*, 1876, 13, 228–253.

EXNER, S., and POLLAK, J. Beitrag zur Resonanztheorie der Tonempfindungen, Zeits. f. Psychol., 1903, 32, 305–332.

FALLOPIUS, GABRIEL. Observationes anatomicae, ad Petrum Mannam, Venetiis, 1561.

FIELD, H., JR., and BRÜCKE, E. T. Über die Dauer des Refraktärstadiums des Nerven bei Ermüdung und Erholung, Pflüg. Arch. ges. Physiol., 1926, 214, 103–111.

FISCHER, O. Über ein von Max Wien geäussertes Bedenken gegen die Helmholtzsche Resonanztheorie des Hörens, Ann. d. Phys., 1908, 25, 118–134.

FLANDERS, P. B. A method of measuring acoustic impedance, Bell System Tech. J., 1932, 11, 402–410; and J. Acoust. Soc. Amer., 1932, 4, Suppl., following p. 96.

FLETCHER, HARVEY. (1) Speech and hearing, 1929. (2) A space-time pattern theory of hearing, J. Acoust. Soc. Amer., 1930, 1, 311–343. (3) Newer concepts of the pitch, the loudness and the timbre of musical tones, J. Franklin Inst., 1935, 220, 405–429. (4) Loudness, masking and their relation to the hearing process and the problem of noise measurement, J. Acoust. Soc. Amer., 1938, 9, 275–293. (5) The mechanism of hearing as revealed through experiment on the masking effect of thermal noise, Proc. Nat. Acad. Sci., Washington, 1938, 24, 265–274. (6) Auditory patterns, Revs. Mod. Phys., 1940, 12, 47–65.

FLETCHER, H., and MUNSON, W. A. (1) Loudness, its definition, measurement and calculation, J. Acoust. Soc. Amer., 1933, 5, 82–108. (2) Relation between loudness and masking, J. Acoust. Soc. Amer., 1937, 9, 1–10.

FOÀ, C., and PERONI, A. Primi tentativi di registrazione delle correnti d'azione del nervo acustico, Arch. di fisiol., 1930, 28, 237–241; and Valsalva, 1930, 6, 105–109.

FORBES, A., and GREGG, A. Electrical studies in mammalian reflexes, Amer. J. Physiol., 1915, 39, 172–235.

FORBES, A., MILLER, R. H., and O'CONNOR, J. Electric responses to acoustic stimuli in the decerebrate animal, Amer. J. Physiol., 1927, 80, 363–380.

FOURIER, J. B. J. (1) La théorie analytique de la chaleur, Acad. des sci., Paris, Mém. acad. roy. sci., 1829, 8, 581–622. (2) Le mouvement de la chaleur dans les fluides, Acad. des sci., Paris, Mém. acad. roy. sci., 1833, 12, 507–530. (3) The analytical theory of heat, trans. by A. Freeman, 1878.

FOWLER, E. P. (1) Marked deafened areas in normal ears, Trans. Amer. Otol. Soc., 1928, 18, 262–275; and Arch. of Otolaryngol., 1928, 8, 151–155. (2) Measuring the sensation of loudness, Arch. of Otolaryngol., 1937, 26, 514–521.

FRANK, O. Die Theorie der Pulswellen, Zeits. f. Biol., 1926, 85, 91–130.

FRENCH, R. L. Auditory acuity in monkeys after destruction of the auditory cortex, Psychol. Bull., 1942, 39, 604.

GALAMBOS, R., and DAVIS, H. (1) The response of single auditory-nerve fibers to acoustic stimulation, *J. Neurophysiol.*, 1943, 6, 39–57. (2) Inhibition of activity in single auditory nerve fibers by acoustic stimulation, *J. Neurophysiol.*, 1944, 7, 287–303. (3) Action potentials from single auditory-nerve fibers? *Science*, 1948, 108, 513.

GALEN, CLAUDIUS [*sic*]. *Opera omnia*, medicorum Graecorum opera quae exstant, ed. by D. C. G. Kühn, Lipsiae, 1822, II, 837 *ff.*; III, 644 *ff.* [The name 'Claudius,' often applied to Galen, is considered to be a misinterpretation of the older appellation 'Clarissimus' when abbreviated as 'Cl.']

GALILEI, GALILEO. *Unterredungen und mathematische Demonstrationen über zwei neue Wissenszweige, die Mechanik und die Fallgesetze betreffend*, trans. by A. von Oettingen, Leipzig, 1890; from Galileo's works of 1638.

GARNER, W. R., and MILLER, G. A. Differential sensitivity to intensity as a function of the duration of the comparison tone, *J. Exper. Psychol.*, 1944, 34, 450–463.

GASSER, H. S., and GRUNDFEST, H. Action and excitability in mammalian A fibers, *Amer. J. Physiol.*, 1936, 117, 113–133.

GEFFCKEN, W. Untersuchungen über akustische Schwellenwerte, III, Über die Bestimmung der Reizschwelle der Hörempfindung aus Schwellendruck und Trommelfellimpedanz, *Ann. d. Phys.*, 1934, 19, 829–848.

GELDARD, FRANK A., and WEITZ, J. Status report to the Office of Naval Research, on research under contract to the University of Virginia, September, 1948.

GERARD, R. W., MARSHALL, W. H., and SAUL, L. J. Electrical activity of the cat's brain, *Arch. of Neurol. Psychiat.*, 1936, 36, 675–735.

GERSUNI, G. V., and VOLOKHOV, A. A. On the effect of alternating currents on the cochlea, *J. Physiol.*, 1937, 89, 113–121.

GILDEMEISTER, M. (1) Zur Theorie des elektrischen Reizes, IV, Polarisation durch veränderliche Ströme, *Akad. d. Wiss.*, *Leipzig, Ber. Saechs. Akad. Wiss., math-phys. Kl.*, 1929, 81, 287–302. (2) Probleme und Ergebnisse der neueren Akustik, *Zeits. f. Hals- Nasen- Ohrenheilk.*, 1930, 27, 299–328.

GILMER, B. VON H. The measurement of the sensitivity of the skin to mechanical vibration, *J. General Psychol.*, 1935, 13, 42–61.

GIRDEN, E. (1) The role of the auditory area of the cortex, *Amer. J. Psychol.*, 1940, 53, 371–383. (2) The acoustic mechanism of the cerebral cortex, *Amer. J. Psychol.*, 1942, 55, 518–527.

GOEBEL, O. Über die Tätigkeit des menschlichen Hörorgans, *Arch. f. Ohrenheilk.*, 1911, 87, 42–60; 1912, 87, 89–122; 1912, 89, 39–58, 112–136, 238–255; 1912, 90, 134–153; 1913, 90, 155–171.

GOODFELLOW, L. D. The sensitivity of the finger-tip to vibrations at various frequency levels, *J. Franklin Inst.*, 1933, 216, 387–392.

GOTCH, F. The submaximal electrical response of nerve to a single stimulus, *J. Physiol.*, 1902, 28, 395–416.

GRAY, A. A. (1) On a modification of the Helmholtz theory of hearing, *J. of Anat. Physiol.*, 1900, 34, 324–350. (2) The application of the principle of maximum stimulation to clinical otology, *J. of Laryngol.*, 1929, 44, 817–826.

GRUBER, J. Ein Fall von Ausstossung des oberen zwei Windungen, *Monatsschr. f. Ohrenheilk.*, 1885, 19, 225–229.

GRUENEBERG, H., HALLPIKE, C. S., and LEDOUX, A. Observations on the structure, development and electrical reactions of the internal ear of the shaker-1 mouse (*Mus musculus*), *Proc. Roy. Soc. Lond.*, ser. B, 1940, 129, 154–173.

GUILD, S. R. (1) A graphic reconstruction method for the study of the organ of Corti, *Anat. Rec.*, 1921, 22, 141–157. (2) The width of the basilar membrane, *Science*, 1927, 65, 67–69. (3) The circulation of the endolymph, *Amer. J. Anat.*, 1927, 39, 57–81. (4) Correlations of histologic observations and the acuity of hearing, *Acta oto-laryngol.*, 1932, 17, 207–249. (5) Symposium: Is there localization in the cochlea for low tones? II, Discussion from the point of view of studies on human temporal bones, *Ann. of Otol. Rhinol. and Laryngol.*, 1935, 44, 738–753. (6) Symposium: The neural mechanism of hearing; Comments on the physiology of hearing and the anatomy of the inner ear, *Laryngoscope*, 1937, 47, 365–372.

GUILD, S. R., CROWE, S. J., BUNCH, C. C., and POLVOGT, L. M. Correlations of differences in the density of innervation of the organ of Corti with differences in the acuity of hearing, *Acta oto-laryngol.*, 1931, 15, 269–308.

GUTTMAN, J., and BARRERA, S. E. Persistence of cochlear electrical disturbance on auditory stimulation in the presence of cochlear ganglion degeneration, *Amer. J. Physiol.*, 1934, 109, 704–708.

HALLER, ALBERTUS VON. *Primae lineae physiologiae*, Gottingae, 1751.

HALLPIKE, C. S. Recent advances in the electro-physiology of hearing, *J. of Laryngol. Otol.*, 1935, 50, 672–687.

HALLPIKE, C. S., and CAIRNS, H. Observations on the pathology of Ménière's syndrome, *J. of Laryng. Otol.*, 1938, 53, 625–655.

HALLPIKE, C. S., HARTRIDGE, H., and RAWDON-SMITH, A. F. (1) On the electrical responses of the cochlea and the auditory tract of the cat to a phase reversal produced in a continuous musical tone, *Proc. Roy. Soc. Lond.*, ser. B, 1937, 122, 175–185. (2) The response of the mammalian cochlea to phase-reversal in a continuous musical tone, *Proc. Phys. Soc. Lond.*, 1937, 49, 190–193.

HALLPIKE, C. S., and RAWDON-SMITH, A. F. (1) The Helmholtz resonance theory of hearing, *Nature*, London, 1934, 133, 614. (2) The "Wever and Bray phenomenon," *J. Physiol.*, 1934, 81, 395–408. (3) The origin of the Wever and Bray phenomenon, *J. Physiol.*, 1934, 83, 243–254.

HALLPIKE, C. S., and WRIGHT, A. J. On the histological changes in the temporal bones of a case of Ménière's disease, *Proc. Roy. Soc. Med.*, 1939, 32, 1646–1656.

HARDESTY, IRVING (1866–   ). (1) On the nature of the tectorial membrane and its probable role in the anatomy of hearing, *Amer. J. Anat.*, 1908, 8, 109–179. (2) On the proportions, development and attachment of the tectorial membrane, *Amer. J. Anat.*, 1915, 18, 1–73. (3) A model to illustrate the probable action of the tectorial membrane, *Amer. J. Anat.*, 1915, 18, 471–514.

HARDY, M. (1) Observations on the innervation of the macula sacculi in man, *Anat. Rec.*, 1934, 59, 403–418. (2) The length of the organ of Corti in man, *Amer. J. Anat.*, 1938, 62, 291–311.

HARTLEY, R. V. L. The function of phase difference in the binaural location of pure tones, *Phys. Rev.*, 1919, 13, 373–385.

HARTLINE, H. K., and GRAHAM, C. H. Nerve impulses from single receptors in the eye, *J. Cell. Comp. Physiol.*, 1932, 1, 277–295.

HARTRIDGE, H. (1) A vindication of the resonance hypothesis of audition, *Brit. J. Psychol.*, 1921, 12, 142–146. (2) A criticism of Wrightson's hypothesis of audition, *Brit. J. Psychol.*, 1921, 12, 248–252.

HARTRIDGE, H., and BANISTER, H. Hearing II, in Carl Murchison's *Foundations of experimental psychology*, 1929, 313–349.

HARTSHORN, L. The audible effect of a sudden change of phase in the current supplied to a telephone receiver, *Proc. Phys. Soc. Lond.*, 1937, 49, 194–197.

HASSE, CARL (1841–1922). (1) Die Schnecke der Vögel, *Zeits. f. wiss. Zool.*, 1867, 17, 56–104. (2) Die vergleichende Morphologie und Histologie des häutigen Gehörorganes der Wirbelthiere, *Anat. Stud., Suppl.*, 1873, 1, 1–96.

HELD, H. (1) Die centrale Gehörleitung, *Arch. f. Anat. Physiol., Anat. Abt.*, 1893, 201–248. (2) Zur Kenntniss der peripheren Gehörleitung, *Arch. f. Anat. Physiol., Anat. Abt.*, 1897, 350–360. (3) Untersuchungen über den feineren Bau des Ohrlabyrinthes der Wirbeltiere, I, *Akad. d. Wiss., Leipzig, Abh. k. Saechs. Gesellsch., math-phys. Kl.*, 1904, 28, 1–74. (4) Die Cochlea der Säuger und der Vögel, ihre Entwicklung und ihr Bau, in A. Bethe's *Handbuch der normalen und pathologischen Physiologie*, 11, *Receptionsorgane*, 1926, I, 467–534.

HELD, H., and KLEINKNECHT, F. Die locale Entspannung der Basilarmembran und ihre Hörlücken, *Pflüg. Arch. ges. Physiol.*, 1927, 216, 1–31.

HELMHOLTZ, HERMANN L. F. (1821–1894). (1) Ueber physikalische Ursache der Harmonie und Disharmonie, *Gesellsch. deutsch. Naturf. u. Aerzte. Amtl. Ber.*, 34 Versamml., 1859, 34, 157–159. [Lecture in Carlsruhe in 1858.] (2) *Die Lehre von den Tonempfindungen als physiologische Grundlage für die Theorie der Musik*, 1st ed., 1863; 3rd ed., 1870. Eng. trans. by A. J. Ellis, *On the sensations of tone*, 2nd Eng. ed., 1885. (3) Ueber die physiologischen Ursachen der musikalischen Harmonie, *Populäre wissenschaftliche Vorträge*, 2nd rev. ed., 1876, part 1, 55–91 (1st ed. in 1865). Eng. trans. by E. Atkinson, *Popular lectures on scientific subjects*, 1873, 61–106. [A lecture given in Bonn during the winter of 1857.] (4) Ueber die Schallschwingungen in der Schnecke des Ohres, *Wissenschaftliche Abhandlungen*, 1883, II, 582–588. [Originally appeared in *Verh. natur-hist-med. Verein.*, Heidelberg, 1869, 5, 33–38.]

HENSEN, V. Zur Morphologie der Schnecke des Menschen und der Säugethiere, *Zeits. f. wiss. Zool.*, 1863, 13, 481–512.

HERMANN, L. (1) Zur Theorie der Combinationstöne, *Pflüg. Arch. ges. Physiol.*, 1891, 49, 499–518. (2) Beiträge zur Lehre von der Klangwahrnehmung, *Pflüg. Arch. ges. Physiol.*, 1894, 56, 467–499.

HILL, A. V. Excitation and accommodation in nerve, *Proc. Roy. Soc. Lond.*, ser. B, 1936, 119, 305–355.

HILL, A. V., KATZ, B., and SOLANDT, D. Y. Nerve excitation by alternating current, *Proc. Roy. Soc. Lond.*, ser. B, 1936, 121, 74–133.

HOAGLAND, H. Electrical responses from the lateral-line nerves of fishes. IV, The repetitive discharge, *J. General Physiol.*, 1933, 17, 195–209.

HODGKIN, A. L. (1) A local electric response in crustacean nerve, *J. Physiol.*, 1937, 91, 5P–7P. (2) Evidence for electrical transmission in nerve, Part I, *J. Physiol.*, 1937, 90, 183–210. (3) Evidence for electrical transmission in nerve, Part II, *J. Physiol.*, 1937, 90, 211–232. (4) The subthreshold potentials in a crustacean nerve fibre, *Proc. Roy. Soc. Lond.*, ser. B, 1938, 126, 87–121.

HOESSLI, H. Die durch Schall experimentell erzeugten Veränderungen des Gehörorganes, *Internat. Zentralbl. f. Ohrenheilk.*, 1913, 11, 303–315.

HORNBOSTEL, E. M. VON, and WERTHEIMER, M. Über die Wahrnehmung der Schallrichtung, *Akad. d. Wiss.*, Berlin, *Sitzungsber.*, 1920, 388–396.

HORTON, G. P. (1) The effect of intense and prolonged acoustical stimulation on the auditory sensitivity of guinea pigs, *J. Comp. Psychol.*, 1934, 18, 405–417. (2) An experimental study of stimulation deafness in guinea pigs, *Ann. of Otol. Rhinol. and Laryngol.*, 1935, 44, 252–259.

HOSTINSKY, OTTOKAR. *Die Lehre von den musikalischen Klängen*, Prag, Dominicus, 1879.

HOWE, H. A. The relation of the organ of Corti to audioelectric phenomena in deaf albino cats, *Amer. J. Physiol.*, 1935, 111, 187–191.

HOWE, H. A., and GUILD, S. R. Absence of the organ of Corti and its possible relation to electric auditory nerve responses, *Anat. Rec.*, 1932–33, 55, Suppl., 20–21.

HUGHES, J. W. The upper frequency limit for the binaural localization of a pure tone by phase difference, *Proc. Roy. Soc. Lond.*, ser. B, 1940, 128, 293–305.

HUGHSON, W., CROWE, S. J., and HOWE, H. A. Physiology of the ear, *Acta oto-laryngol.*, 1934, 20, 9–23.

HUGHSON, W., THOMPSON, E., and WITTING, E. G. An experimental study of bone conduction, *Ann. of Otol., Rhinol. and Laryngol.*, 1936, 45, 844–858.

HUGHSON, W., and WITTING, E. G. An objective study of auditory fatigue, *Acta oto-laryngol.*, 1935, 21, 457–486.

HURST, C. H. A new theory of hearing, *Trans. Liverpool Biol. Soc.*, 1895, 9, 321–353. [Meeting of Nov. 9, 1894.]

HUSCHKE, EMIL. (1) Ueber die Gehörzähne, einen eigenthümlichen Apparat in der Schnecke des Vogelohrs, *Arch. f. Anat. Physiol.*, 1835, 335–346. (2) Lehre von den Eingeweiden und Sinnesorganen des menschlichen Körpers, in S. T. von Sömmerring's *Vom Bau des menschlichen Körpers*, 1844, vol. 5.

INGLIS, A. H., GRAY, C., and JENKINS, R. A voice and ear for telephone measurements, *Bell System Tech. J.*, 1932, 11, 293–317.

INGRASSIA, GIOVAN FILIPPO. [Work not seen, quoted by Schelhammer.]

JEFFRESS, L. A. Variations in pitch, *Amer. J. Psychol.*, 1944, 57, 63–76.

JOHNSON, E. P., JR. *Localization of response in the cochlea as determined by electrical recording*, Thesis, Brown Univ., 1940.

JOHNSON, H. M. Audition and habit formation in the dog, *Behav. Monog.*, 1913, 2, No. 8.

JONES, I. H., and KNUDSEN, V. O. Certain aspects of tinnitus, *Laryngoscope*, 1928, 38, 597–611.

JONES, R. C., STEVENS, S. S., and LURIE, M. H. Three mechanisms of hearing by electrical stimulation, *J. Acoust. Soc. Amer.*, 1940, 12, 281–290.

KALISCHER, O. Weitere Mitteilung über die Ergebnisse der Dressur als physiologischer Untersuchungsmethode auf den Gebieten des Gehör-, Geruchs- und Farbensinns, *Arch. f. Anat. Physiol., Physiol. Abt.*, 1909, 303–322.

KATZ, BERNHARD. (1) Experimental evidence for a non-conducted response of nerve to subthreshold stimulation, *Proc. Roy. Soc. Lond.*, ser. B, 1937, 124, 244–276. (2) *Electric excitation of nerve*, 1939. (3) Nerve excitation by high-frequency alternating current, *J. Physiol.*, 1939, 96, 202–224.

KEITH, A. (see WRIGHTSON, THOMAS, and KEITH, A.). *An enquiry into the analytical mechanism of the internal ear*, Appendix, 1918, 156–254.

KELLAWAY, P. The electrophonic response to phase reversal, *J. Neurophysiol.*, 1944, 7, 227–230.

KEMP, E. H. (1) A critical review of experiments on the problem of stimulation deafness, *Psychol Bull.*, 1935, 32, 325–342. (2) An experimental investigation of the problem of stimulation deafness, *J. Exper. Psychol.*, 1936, 19, 159–171.

KEMP, E. H., COPPÉE, G. E., and ROBINSON, E. H. Electric responses of the brain stem to unilateral auditory stimulation, *Amer. J. Physiol.*, 1937, 120, 304–315.

KIRCHER, ATHANASIUS. *Phonurgia nova*, 1673.

KISHI, K. Corti'sche Membran und Tonempfindungstheorie, *Pflüg. Arch. ges. Physiol.*, 1907, 116, 112–123.

KNUDSEN, V. O. (1) The sensibility of the ear to small differences of intensity and frequency, *Phys. Rev.*, 1923, 21, 84–102. (2) "Hearing" with the sense of touch, *J. General Psychol.*, 1928, 1, 320–352.

Koch, H. (1) Die Ewaldsche Hörtheorie, *Zeits. f. Sinnesphysiol.*, 1928, 59, 15–54. (2) Die Schwingungsformen der Basilarmembran, *Ber. ges. Physiol.*, 1931, 61, 362–363.

Kock, W. E. A new interpretation of the results of experiments on the differential pitch sensitivity of the ear. *J. Acoust. Soc. Amer.*, 1937, 9, 129–134.

Koelliker, Albert. (1) *Mikroskopische Anatomie oder Gewebelehre des Menschen*, 1852, II, Part 2, 737–763. (2) Über die letzten Endigungen des Nervus Cochleae und die Function der Schnecke, *Festschrift f. Friedrich Tiedemann*, Wurzburg, 1854. (3) *Handbuch der Gewebelehre des Menschen*, 1896, II.

Koenig, R. (1) Über den Zusammenklang zweier Töne, *Ann. d. Phys.*, 1876, 157, 177–237; and *Phil. Mag.*, 1876, 1, 417–446, 511–525. (2) Bemerkungen über die Klangfarbe, *Ann. d. Phys.*, 1881, 14, 369–393; and *Quelques expériences d'acoustique*, 1882, 218–243.

Kreidl, A., and Yanase, J. Zur Physiologie der Cortischen Membran, *Zentralbl. f. Physiol.*, 1907, 21, 507–510.

Kryter, K. D., and Ades, H. W. Studies on the function of the higher acoustic centers in the cat, *Amer. J. Psychol.*, 1943, 56, 501–536.

Kucharski, P. (1) La sensation tonale exige-t-elle une excitation de l'oreille par plusieurs périodes vibratoires, une seule période ou une fraction de période? *Année psychol.*, 1923, 24, 151–170. (2) Sur le loi d'excitation de l'oreille, *Compt. r. soc. biol.*, 1925, 92, 690–693. (3) Sur la persistance des sensations auditives, *Compt. r. soc. biol.*, 1927, 97, 691–693.

Kuile, Emile ter. (1) Die Uebertragung der Energie von der Grundmembran auf die Haarzellen, *Pflüg. Arch. ges. Physiol.*, 1900, 79, 146–157. (2) Die richtige Bewegungsform der Membrana basilaris, *Pflüg. Arch. ges. Physiol.*, 1900, 79, 484–509.

Kurtz, R. Zur Messung von Absorptions- und Empfindlichkeitskurven des menschlichen Ohres, *Akust. Zeits.*, 1938, 3, 74–79.

Kwiek, M. Über Lautstärke und Lautheit, *Akust. Zeits.*, 1937, 2, 170–178.

Lane, C. E. Binaural beats, *Phys. Rev.*, 1925, 26, 401–412.

Larionow, W. Ueber die musikalischen Centren des Gehirns, *Pflüg. Arch. ges. Physiol.*, 1899, 76, 608–625.

Larsell, O., McCrady, E., Jr., and Larsell, J. F. The development of the organ of Corti in relation to the inception of hearing, *Trans. Amer. Acad. Ophthal. Otolaryngol.*, 1944, 48, 333–357; and *Arch. of Otolaryngol.*, 1944, 40, 233–248.

Larsell, O., McCrady, E., Jr., and Zimmermann, A. A. Morphological and functional development of the membranous labyrinth in the opossum, *J. Comp. Neurol.*, 1935, 63, 95–118.

Lehmann, Alfred. Ueber die Schwingungen der Basilarmembran und die Helmholtzsche Resonanztheorie, *Folia Neurobiol.*, 1910, 4, 116–132.

Leiri, F. Eine neue Hörtheorie, *Acta oto-laryngol.*, 1929, 13, 419–473.

LEMPERT, J.   (1) Improvement of hearing in cases of otosclerosis: a new one-stage surgical technic, *Arch. of Otolaryngol.*, 1938, 28, 42–97.   (2) Fenestra nov-ovalis: a new oval window for the improvement of hearing in cases of otosclerosis, *Arch. of Otolaryngol.*, 1941, 34, 880–912.

LEMPERT, J., WEVER, E. G., and LAWRENCE, M.   The cochleogram and its clinical application, *Arch. of Otolaryngol.*, 1947, 45, 61–67.

LEWIS, D.   Pitch: its definition and physical determinants, *Iowa Stud. Psychol. Music*, 1937, 14, 346–373.

LEWIS, D., and COWAN, M.   The influence of intensity on the pitch of violin and 'cello tones, *J. Acoust. Soc. Amer.*, 1936, 8, 20–22.

LEWY, F. H., and KOBRAK, H.   The neural projection of the cochlear spirals on the primary acoustic centers, *Arch. of Neurol. Psychiat.*, 1936, 35, 839–852.

LICKLIDER, J. C. R.   An electrical study of frequency localization in the auditory cortex of the cat, *Psychol. Bull.*, 1941, 38, 727.

LICKLIDER, J. C. R., and KRYTER, K. D.   Frequency-localization in the auditory cortex of the monkey, *Fed. Proc. Amer. Soc. Exper. Biol.*, 1942, 1, 51.

LIFSHITZ, S.   (1) Two integral laws of sound perception relating loudness and apparent duration of sound impulses, *J. Acoust. Soc. Amer.*, 1933, 5, 31–33.   (2) Apparent duration of sound perception and musical optimum reverberation, *J. Acoust. Soc. Amer.*, 1936, 7, 213–221.

LINDIG, F.   Ueber den Einfluss der Phasen auf die Klangfarbe, *Ann. d. Phys.*, 1903, 10, 242–269.

LIPMAN, ELI A.   (1) Comparative exploration of the auditory cortex in the dog by conditioning and electrical methods, *Psychol. Bull.*, 1940, 37, 497.   (2) *Frequency localization in the auditory cortex of the dog*, Thesis, Univ. of Rochester, 1941.

LLOYD, M. G., and AGNEW, P. G.   Effect of phase of harmonics upon acoustic quality, *Bull. Bureau Stand.*, 1909, 6, 255–263.

LOESCH, JOHN G., and KAPELL, B. L.   *The frequency limit for the perception of binaural beats and for cyclic binaural localization*, Thesis, Princeton Univ., 1948.

LORENTE DE NÓ, R.   (1) Anatomy of the eighth nerve; The central projection of the nerve endings of the internal ear, *Laryngoscope*, 1933, 43, 1–38.   (2) Anatomy of the eighth nerve; III, General plan of structure of the primary cochlear nuclei, *Laryngoscope*, 1933, 43, 327–350.   (3) The sensory endings in the cochlea, *Laryngoscope*, 1937, 47, 373–377.   (4) Discussion of E. P. Fowler's paper on The diagnosis of diseases of the neural mechanism of hearing by the aid of sounds well above threshold, *Trans. Amer. Otol. Soc.*, 1937, 27, 219–220.

LOWY, K.   Some experimental evidence for peripheral auditory masking, *J. Acoust. Soc. Amer.*, 1945, 16, 197–202.

LUCAE, A.   Beiträge zur Lehre von den Schallempfindungen, *Arch. f. Ohrenheilk.*, 1909, 79, 246–290.

LURIE, M. H. Studies of the waltzing guinea pig, *Laryngoscope*, 1939, 49, 558–565.

LURIE, M. H., DAVIS, H., and HAWKINS, J. E., JR. Acoustic trauma of the organ of Corti in the guinea pig, *Laryngoscope*, 1944, 54, 375–386.

LUX, F. (*see* BUDDE, E.).

MAGENDIE, FRANÇOIS. *Précis élémentaire de physiologie*, 1816, I.

MARX, H. Untersuchungen über experimentelle Schädigungen des Gehörorganes, part C, *Zeits. f. Ohrenheilk.*, 1909, 59, 333–343.

MATHES, R. C., and MILLER, R. L. Phase effects in monaural perception, *J. Acoust. Soc. Amer.*, 1947, 19, 780–797.

MATTHEWS, B. H. C. (1) The response of a single end organ, *J. Physiol.*, 1931, 71, 64–110. (2) Nerve endings in mammalian muscle, *J. Physiol.*, 1933, 78, 1–53.

MAYER, A. M. (1) Researches in acoustics, paper No. 6, *Amer. J. Sci.*, 1874, 108, 241–255. (2) A redetermination of the constants of the law connecting the pitch of a sound with the duration of its residual sensation, *Amer. J. Sci.*, 1875, 109, 267–269. (3) Researches in acoustics, No. IX, *Phil. Mag.*, 1894, 37, 259–288.

McCRADY, E., JR., WEVER, E. G., and BRAY, C. W. (1) The development of hearing in the opossum, *J. Exper. Zool.*, 1937, 75, 503–517. (2) A further investigation of the development of hearing in the opossum, *J. Comp. Psychol.*, 1940, 30, 17–21.

METZ, O. The acoustic impedance measured on normal and pathological ears, *Acta oto-laryngol.*, Suppl. 63, 1946.

MEYER, MAX F. (1873–). (1) Über Kombinationstöne und einige hierzu in Beziehung stehende akustische Erscheinungen, *Zeits. f. Psychol.*, 1896, 11, 177–229. (2) Zur Theorie der Differenztöne und der Gehörsempfindungen überhaupt, *Zeits. f. Psychol.*, 1898, 16, 1–34. (3) Zur Theorie des Hörens, *Pflüg. Arch. ges. Physiol.*, 1899, 78, 346–362. (4) E. ter Kuile's Theorie des Hörens, *Pflüg. Arch. ges. Physiol.*, 1900, 81, 61–75. (5) An introduction to the mechanics of the inner ear, *Univ. Missouri Stud.*, Sci. ser., 1907, 2, No. 1. (6) Die Morphologie des Gehörorgans und die Theorie des Hörens, *Pflüg. Arch. ges. Physiol.*, 1913, 153, 369–384. (7) The hydraulic principles governing the function of the cochlea, *J. General Psychol.*, 1928, 1, 239–265. (8) Hearing without cochlea? *Science*, 1931, 73, 236–237.

MILLS, C. K. On the localisation of the auditory centre, *Brain*, 1891, 14, 465–472.

MINTON, J. P. Diplacusis and acuity of hearing, *Arch. of Otolaryngol.*, 1946, 44, 184–190.

MOOS, S., and STEINBRÜGGE, H. Ueber Nervenatrophie in der ersten Schneckenwindung, *Zeits. f. Ohrenheilk.*, 1881, 10, 1–15.

MORGAN, C. T., and GALAMBOS, R. A reinvestigation of the relation between pitch and intensity, *J. Acoust. Soc. Amer.*, 1943, 15, 77.

MORTON, W. B. On Sir Thomas Wrightson's theory of hearing, *Proc. Phys. Soc. Lond.*, 1919, 31, 101–110.

462 REFERENCES

MUELLER, JOHANNES. (1) Zur vergleichenden Physiologie des Gesichtssinnes, 1826, 44–55. (2) Handbuch der Physiologie des Menschen, 1838, II, book 5.

MUNK, H. Ueber die Functionen der Grosshirnrinde, 2nd ed., Berlin, 1890.

MUNSON, W. A. (1) The growth of auditory sensation, J. Acoust. Soc. Amer., 1947, 19, 584–591. (2) Sound and hearing, in O. Glasser's Medical physics, II.

MYGIND, S. H. La théorie de l'audition, Ann. des mal. oreille, 1928, 47, 726–735.

NATANSON, —. Analyse der Funktionen des Nervensystems, Arch. f. physiol. Heilk., 1844, 3, 515–535.

NEFF, W. D. The effects of partial section of the auditory nerve, J. Comp. Physiol. Psychol., 1947, 40, 203–215.

NEWMAN, H. W., DOUPE, J., and WILKINS, R. W. Some observations on the nature of vibratory sensibility, Brain, 1939, 62, 31–40.

NUEL, J. P. Beitrag zur Kenntniss der Säugethierschnecke, Arch. f. mikr. Anat., 1872, 8, 200–215.

ODA, D. Observations on the pathology of impaired hearing for low tones, Laryngoscope, 1938, 48, 765–792.

OHM, G. S. Ueber die Definition des Tones, nebst daran geknüpfter Theorie der Sirene und ähnlicher tonbildener Vorrichtungen, Ann. d. Phys., 1843, 59, 497–565.

OSTERHOUT, W. J. V. Electrical phenomena in large plant cells, Physiol. Revs., 1936, 16, 216–237.

OSTERHOUT, W. J. V., and HILL, S. E. Positive variations in Nitella, J. General Physiol., 1935, 18, 369–375.

PASTERNAK, J. Ein Beitrag zur Lehre von den akustischen Intermittenzerscheinungen, Arch. f. ges. Psychol., 1931, 81, 1–48.

PATTIE, F. A., JR. A further experiment on auditory fatigue, Brit. J. Psychol., 1929, 20, 38–42.

PEARCE, C. H. The pitch specificity of auditory adaptation, J. General Psychol., 1935, 12, 358–371.

PERRAULT, CLAUDE. Du bruit, in C. and P. Perrault, Oeuvres diverses de physique et de mechanique, Aleide, 1721, I. [Du bruit first appeared in 1680.]

PFAFFMANN, C. Afferent impulses from the teeth resulting from a vibratory stimulus, J. Physiol., 1939, 97, 220–232.

PIPER, H. (1) Ueber das Hörvermögen der Fische, Münscher med. Wochenschr., 1906, 53, 1785. (2) Aktionsströme vom Gehörorgan der Fische bei Schallreizung, Zentralbl. f. Physiol., 1906, 20, 293–297. (3) Die akustischen Funktionen des inneren Ohres und seiner Teile, Med. Klin., 1906, No. 41, 2, 1073–1078. (4) Aktionsströme vom Labyrinth der Fische bei Schallreizung, Arch. f. Anat. Physiol., Physiol. Abt., 1910, Suppl. 1–13.

POLIAK, S. The main afferent fiber systems of the cerebral cortex in primates, Univ. Calif. Publ. Anat., 1932, 2, 81–104.

PRATT, F. H. Response of a muscle fiber-group to apparent stimulation of a single motor fiber in the nerve trunk, *Amer. J. Physiol.*, 1925, 72, 179.

PROETZ, A. Diplacusis binauralis dysharmonica, *Ann. of Otol., Rhinol. and Laryngol.*, 1937, 46, 119–123.

PUMPHREY, R. J., and RAWDON-SMITH, A. F. (1) Synchronized action potentials in the cercal nerve of the cockroach (*Periplaneta americana*) in response to auditory stimuli, *J. Physiol.*, 1936, 87, 4P–5P. (2) 1 to 3 and 1 to 4 alternation in the cercal nerve of the cricket, *J. Physiol.*, 1936, 87, 57P–59P. (3) Hearing in insects: the nature of the response of certain receptors to auditory stimuli, *Proc. Roy. Soc. Lond.*, ser. B, 1936, 121, 18–27.

RAAB, D. H., and ADES, H. W. Cortical and midbrain mediation of a conditioned discrimination of acoustic intensities, *Amer. J. Psychol.*, 1946, 59, 59–83.

RAMON Y CAJAL, S. *Beitrag zur Studium der medulla oblongata,* Leipzig: Barth, 1896.

RAMSDELL, D. A. *The psycho-physics of frequency modulation,* Thesis, Harvard Univ. [Not seen; reported by Stevens and Davis.]

RANKE, OTTO F. (1) *Die Gleichrichter-Resonanztheorie,* München: Lehmann, 1931. (2) Das Massenverhältnis zwischen Membran und Flüssigkeit im Innenohr, *Akust. Zeits.*, 1942, 7, 1–11.

RAWDON-SMITH, A. F. Experimental deafness; further data upon the phenomenon of so-called *auditory fatigue, Brit. J. Psychol.*, 1936, 26, 233–244.

RAWDON-SMITH, A. F., and HAWKINS, J. E., JR. The electrical activity of a denervated ear, *Proc. Roy. Soc. Med.*, 1939, 32, 496–507.

RAYLEIGH, LORD (JOHN WILLIAM STRUTT). On our perception of sound direction, *Phil. Mag.*, 1907, 13, 214–232.

REBOUL, J. A. (1) *Le phénomène de Wever et Bray,* Montpellier, 1937. (2) Théorie des phénomènes mécaniques se passant dans l'oreille interne, *J. physique et de radium,* 1938, 9, 185–194. (3) Remarques sur les théories de l'audition, *Rev. de laryngol.,* 1939, 60, 144–158.

REISSNER, ERNEST. (1) *De auris internae formatione,* Dorpat (Livonia), 1851. (2) Zur Kenntniss der Schnecke im Gehörorgan der Säugethiere und des Menschen, *Arch. f. Anat. Physiol. wiss. Med.,* 1854, 420–427.

RETZIUS, GUSTAV. (1) *Das Gehörorgan der Wirbelthiere,* 1884, II. (2) Die Endigungsweise des Gehörnerven, *Biol. Unters.,* 1892, 3, 29–36. (3) Weiteres über die Endigungsweise des Gehörnerven, *Biol. Unters.,* 1893, 5, 35–38.

RIESZ, R. R. Differential intensity sensitivity of the ear for pure tones, *Phys. Rev.,* 1928, 31, 867–875.

RINNE, H. A. Beitrag zur Physiologie des menschlichen Ohres, *Zeits. f. rat. Med.,* 1865, 24, 12–64.

ROAF, H. E. The analysis of sound waves by the cochlea, *Phil. Mag.,* 1922, 43, 349–354.

ROBERTS, W. H. A two-dimensional analysis of the discrimination of differences in the frequency of vibrations by means of the sense of touch, *J. Franklin Inst.*, 1932, 213, 283–311.

ROEHR, H. Versuche an Meerschweinchen ueber experimentelle Schädigungen in der Schnecke durch reine Pfeifentöne, *Passow-Schaefers Beitr. z. Anat. d. Ohres*, 1912, 5, 390–437.

ROSENZWEIG, M. Discrimination of auditory intensities in the cat, *Amer. J. Psychol.*, 1946, 59, 127–136.

ROSTOSKY, P. Ueber binaurale Schwebungen, *Philos. Stud.*, 1902, 19, 557–598.

RÜEDI, L., and FURRER, W. (1) Acoustic trauma, *Schweiz. Med. Wochenschr.*, 1946, 76, 843–866. (2) Das akustische Trauma, *Pract. otorhino-laryngol.*, 1946, 8.

RUTHERFORD, WILLIAM (1839–1899). (1) *The sense of hearing.* [A lecture at Birmingham, England, Sept. 6, 1886, privately printed.] (2) A new theory of hearing, *J. of Anat. Physiol.*, 1886, 21, 166–168. (3) Tone sensation with reference to the function of the cochlea, *Lancet*, 1898, ii, 389–394, and *Brit. Med. J.*, 1898, ii, 353–358.

SAUL, L. J., and DAVIS, H. Electrical phenomena of the auditory mechanism, *Trans. Amer. Otol. Soc.*, 1932, 22, 137–145.

SCARPA, ANTON. *Anatomische Untersuchungen des Gehörs und Geruchs*, Nürnberg, 1800. [Original Latin edition, 1789.]

SCHAEFER, H., and GÖPFERT, H. Nervenaktionsströme bei Wechselstromreizung, *Pflüg. Arch. ges. Physiol.*, 1936, 238, 404–428.

SCHAEFER, K. L., and ABRAHAM, O. Studien über Unterbrechungstöne, *Pflüg. Arch. ges. Physiol.*, 1901, 83, 207–211; 1901, 85, 536–542; 1902, 88, 475–491.

SCHELHAMMER, GUNTHER C. *De auditu*, liber unus, 1684.

SCHOUTEN, J. F. Synthetic sound, *Philips Tech. Rev.*, 1939, 4, 167–173.

SCHULTZE, MAX. Ueber die Endigungsweise des Hörnerven im Labyrinth, *Arch. f. Anat. Physiol. wiss. Med.*, 1858, 343–381.

SCHULZE, F. A. Die Uebereinstimmung der als Phasenwechseltöne bezeichneten Klangerscheinungen mit der Helmholtzschen Resonanztheorie, *Ann. d. Phys.*, 1914, 45, 283–320.

SCRIPTURE, E. W. The Helmholtz theory of hearing, *Nature*, London, 1922, 109, 518.

SEASHORE, CARL E., ed. The vibrato, *Univ. Iowa Stud. Psychol. Music*, 1932, 1.

SETZEPFAND, W. Zur Frequenzabhängigkeit der Vibrationsempfindung des Menschen, *Zeits. f. Biol.*, 1935, 96, 236–240.

SHAMBAUGH, G. E. (1869–1947). A restudy of the minute anatomy of the structures in the cochlea, *Amer. J. Anat.*, 1907, 7, 245–257.

SHOWER, E. G., and BIDDULPH, R. Differential pitch sensitivity of the ear, *J. Acoust. Soc. Amer.*, 1931, 3, 275–287.

SIEBENMANN, F. Mittelohr und Labyrinth, in Karl von Bardeleben's *Handbuch der Anatomie des Menschen*, 1898, V, part 2, 195–324.

SIVIAN, L. J., and WHITE, S. D. On minimum audible sound fields, *J. Acoust. Soc. Amer.*, 1933, 4, 288–321.

SKOLNICK, A. The upper limit of cutaneous sensitivity to frequency of vibration in the white rat, *J. Exper. Psychol.*, 1938, 22, 273–276.

SMITH, KENDON R. (1) Bone conduction during experimental fixation of the stapes, *J. Exper. Psychol.*, 1943, 33, 96–107. (2) The problem of stimulation deafness; II, Histological changes in the cochlea as a function of tonal frequency, *J. Exper. Psychol.*, 1947, 37, 304–317.

SMITH, KENDON R., and WEVER, E. G. The problem of stimulation deafness; III, The functional and histological effects of a high-frequency stimulus, *J. Exper. Psychol.*, 1949, 39, 238–241.

SMITH, ROBERT. *Harmonics*, 2nd ed., 1759, 56–122. [First ed. 1749, not seen.]

SNOW, W. B. Change of pitch with loudness at low frequencies, *J. Acoust. Soc. Amer.*, 1936, 8, 14–19.

SOLOVCOV, N. O ukoncení sluchového nervu v orgánu Cortiho, *Časopis Lékařů Českých*, 1925, 64, 241–244.

STEIN, STANISLAUS VON. *Die Lehren von den Funktionen der einzelnen Theile des Ohrlabyrinths*, trans. by C. v. Krzywicki, 1894.

STEINBERG, J. C. Positions of stimulation in the cochlea by pure tones, *J. Acoust. Soc. Amer.*, 1937, 8, 176–180.

STEINBERG, J. C., and GARDNER, M. B. The dependence of hearing impairment on sound intensity, *J. Acoust. Soc. Amer.*, 1937, 9, 11–23.

STEPANOW, E. M. (1) Zur Frage über die Function der Cochlea, *Monatsschr. f. Ohrenheilk.*, 1886, 20, 116–124. (2) Experimenteller Beitrag zur Frage ueber die Function der Schnecke, *Monatsschr. f. Ohrenheilk.*, 1888, 22, 85–92.

STEUDEL, U. Über Empfindung und Messung der Lautstärke, *Zeits. Hochfreq. Elektr.*, 1933, 41, 116–128.

STEVENS, S. S. The relation of pitch to intensity, *J. Acoust. Soc. Amer.*, 1935, 6, 150–154.

STEVENS, S. S., and DAVIS, H. *Hearing, its psychology and physiology*, 1938.

STEVENS, S. S., DAVIS, H., and LURIE, M. The localization of pitch perception on the basilar membrane, *J. General Psychol.*, 1935, 13, 297–315.

STEVENS, S. S., and JONES, R. C. The mechanism of hearing by electrical stimulation, *J. Acoust. Soc. Amer.*, 1939, 10, 261–269.

STEVENS, S. S., MORGAN, C. T., and VOLKMANN, J. Theory of the neural quantum in the discrimination of loudness and pitch, *Amer. J. Psychol.*, 1941, 54, 315–335.

STEVENS, S. S., and VOLKMANN, J. The relation of pitch to frequency: a revised scale, *Amer. J. Psychol.*, 1940, 53, 329–353.

STEVENS, S. S., VOLKMANN, J., and NEWMAN, E. B. A scale for the measurement of the psychological magnitude pitch, *J. Acoust. Soc. Amer.*, 1937, 8, 185–190.

STEWART, G. W. (1) Binaural beats, *Psychol. Monog.*, No. 108, 1918, 25, 31–46. (2) The function of intensity and phase in the binaural location of pure tones, II, *Phys. Rev.*, 1920, 15, 432–445.

STOWELL, E. Z., and DEMING, A. F. Aural rectification, *J. Acoust. Soc. Amer.*, 1934, 6, 70–79.

THOMPSON, S. P. (1) On binaural audition, *Phil. Mag.*, 1877, 4, 274–276. (2) Phenomena of binaural audition, Part II, *Phil. Mag.*, 1878, 6, 383–391.

THURAS, A. L. [Unpub., *see* Wegel (2), and Sivian and White.]

THURLOW, W. R. (1) Studies in auditory theory, I, Binaural interaction and the perception of pitch, *J. Exper. Psychol.*, 1943, 32, 17–36. (2) Studies in auditory theory, II, The distribution of distortion in the inner ear, *J. Exper. Psychol.*, 1943, 32, 344–350.

TODD, ROBERT B., and BOWMAN, WILLIAM. *The physiological anatomy and physiology of man*, 1859, II, 63–100.

TOMINAGA, K. Eine neue Theorie des Hörens, *Zentralbl. f. Physiol.*, 1904, 18, 461–466.

TRIMBLE, O. C. Intensity-difference and phase-difference as conditions of stimulation in binaural sound-localization, *Amer. J. Psychol.*, 1935, 47, 264–274.

TRIMMER, J. D., and FIRESTONE, F. A. An investigation of subjective tone by means of the steady tone phase effect, *J. Acoust. Soc. Amer.*, 1937, 9, 24–29.

TROEGER, J. Die Schallaufnahme durch das äussere Ohr, *Phys. Zeits.*, 1930, 31, 26–47.

TROLAND, L. T. Psychophysiological considerations relating to the theory of hearing, *J. Acoust. Soc. Amer.*, 1930, 1, 301–310.

TUNTURI, A. R. (1) Audiofrequency localization in the acoustic cortex of the dog, *Amer. J. Physiol.*, 1944, 141, 397–403. (2) Further afferent connections to the acoustic cortex of the dog, *Amer. J. Physiol.*, 1945, 144, 389–394. (3) A study on the pathway from the medial geniculate body to the acoustic cortex in the dog, *Amer. J. Physiol.*, 1946, 147, 311–319.

TURNBULL, W. W. Pitch discrimination as a function of tonal duration, *J. Exper. Psychol.*, 1944, 34, 302–316.

UPTON, M. Functional disturbances of hearing in guinea pigs after long exposure to an intense tone, *J. General Psychol.*, 1929, 2, 397–412.

VALSALVA, ANTONIO MARIA. *De aure humana tractatus*, Rhenum, 1707.

VANCE, T. F. The lower limit of tonality, *Psychol. Monog.*, 1914, 16, No. 69, 104–114.

VAN DER POL, B. Frequency modulation, *Proc. Inst. Radio Eng.*, 1930, 18, 1194–1205.

VAROLIUS, CONSTANTIUS. *Anatomiae sive de resolutione corporis humani, libri IIII*, Francofurti, 1591.

VESALIUS, ANDREAS. *De humani corporis fabrica, libri septem*, Basileae, 1543.

VOLKMANN, A. W. Nervenphysiologie, in Rudolph Wagner's *Handwörter-buch der Physiologie*, 1844, II, 521–526.

VOLTOLINI, R. Einiges Anatomische aus der Gehörschnecke und über die Function derselben resp. des Gehörorganes, *Virchows Arch. path. Anat. Physiol.*, 1885, 100, 27–41.

WADA, T. Anatomical and physiological studies on the growth of the inner ear of the albino rat, *Amer. Anat. Memoirs* (Wistar Inst. Anat.), No. 10, 1923.

WAETZMANN, ERICH. (1) *Die Resonanztheorie des Hörens*, Braunschweig, 1912. (2) Absorptionsmessungen am Trommelfell mit der Schusterschen Brücke, *Akust. Zeits.*, 1938, 3, 1–6.

WALLER, AUGUSTUS D. (1) A possible part played by the membrana basilaris in auditory excitation, *J. Physiol.*, 1891, 12, xlix-l. (2) *An introduction to human physiology*, 1891, 458–462.

WALZL, E. M., and BORDLEY, J. E. The effect of small lesions of the organ of Corti on cochlear potentials, *Amer. J. Physiol.*, 1942, 135, 351–360.

WATT, HENRY J. (1879–1925). (1) Psychological analysis and theory of hearing, *Brit. J. Psychol.*, 1914, 7, 1–43. (2) *The psychology of sound*, 1917.

WEDELL, C. H., and CUMMINGS, S. B., JR. Fatigue of the vibratory sense, *J. Exper. Psychol.*, 1938, 22, 429–438.

WEGEL, R. L. (1) A study of tinnitus, *Arch. of Otolaryngol.*, 1931, 14, 158–165. (2) Physical data and physiology of excitation of the auditory nerve, *Ann. of Otol., Rhinol. and Laryngol.*, 1932, 41, 740–779.

WEGEL, R. L., and LANE, C. E. The auditory masking of one pure tone by another and its possible relation to the dynamics of the inner ear, *Phys. Rev.*, 1924, 23, 266–285.

WEINBERG, M., and ALLEN, F. On the critical frequency of pulsation of tones, *Phil. Mag.*, 1924, 47, 50–62.

WEVER, E. G. (1) Beats and related phenomena resulting from the simultaneous sounding of two tones, *Psychol. Rev.*, 1929, 36, 402–418, 512–523. (2) Auditory nerve experiments in animals and their relation to hearing, *Laryngoscope*, 1931, 41, 387–391. (3) The physiology of hearing, *Physiol. Revs.*, 1933, 13, 400–425. (4) The width of the basilar membrane in man, *Ann. of Otol., Rhinol. and Laryngol.*, 1938, 47, 37–47. (5) The electrical responses of the ear, *Psychol. Bull.*, 1939, 36, 143–187. (6) The designation of combination tones, *Psychol. Rev.*, 1941, 48, 93–104. (7) The problem of the tonal dip, *Laryngoscope*, 1942, 52, 169–187.

WEVER, E. G., and BRAY, C. W. (1) Auditory nerve impulses, *Science*, 1930, 71, 215. (2) Action currents in the auditory nerve in response to acoustical stimulation, *Proc. Nat. Acad. Sci.*, Washington, 1930, 16, 344–350. (3) Present possibilities for auditory theory, *Psychol. Rev.*, 1930, 37, 365–380. (4) The nature of acoustic response: the relation between sound frequency and frequency of impulses in the auditory nerve, *J. Exper. Psychol.*, 1930, 13, 373–387. (5) The perception of low tones and the resonance-volley theory, *J. of Psychol.*, 1937, 3, 101–114. (6) Distortion in the ear as shown by the electrical responses of the cochlea, *J. Acoust. Soc. Amer.*, 1938, 9, 227–233. (7) The stapedius muscle in relation to sound conduction, *J. Exper. Psychol.*, 1942, 31, 35–43.

WEVER, E. G., BRAY, C. W., and HORTON, G. P. Symposium: Is there localization in the cochlea for low tones? *Ann. of Otol., Rhinol. and Laryngol.*, 1935, 44, 772–776.

WEVER, E. G., BRAY, C. W., and LAWRENCE, M. (1) The locus of distortion in the ear, *J. Acoust. Soc. Amer.*, 1940, 11, 427–433. (2) The origin of combination tones, *J. Exper. Psychol.*, 1940, 27, 217–226. (3) A quantitative study of combination tones, *J. Exper. Psychol.*, 1940, 27, 469–496. (4) The interference of tones in the cochlea, *J. Acoust. Soc. Amer.*, 1940, 12, 268–280. (5) The effect of middle ear pressure upon distortion, *J. Acoust. Soc. Amer.*, 1941, 13, 182–187. (6) The nature of cochlear activity after death, *Ann. of Otol., Rhinol., and Laryngol.*, 1941, 50, 317–329.

WEVER, E. G., BRAY, C. W., and WILLEY, C. F. The response of the cochlea to tones of low frequency, *J. Exper. Psychol.*, 1937, 20, 336–349.

WEVER, E. G., and LAWRENCE, M. (1) Tonal interference in relation to cochlear injury, *J. Exper. Psychol.*, 1941, 29, 283–295. (2) The patterns of response in the cochlea, *J. Acoust. Soc. Amer.*, 1949, 21, 127–134. (3) Unpublished observations.

WEVER, E. G., LAWRENCE, M., and SMITH, K. R. The middle ear in sound conduction, *Arch. of Otolaryngol.*, 1948, 48, 19–35.

WEVER, E. G., and NEFF, W. D. A further study of the effects of partial section of the auditory nerve, *J. Comp. Physiol. Psychol.*, 1947, 40, 217–226.

WEVER, E. G., and SMITH, K. R. The problem of stimulation deafness: I, Cochlear impairment as a function of tonal frequency, *J. Exper. Psychol.*, 1944, 34, 239–245.

WEVER, E. G., and WEDELL, C. H. Pitch discrimination at high frequencies, *Psychol. Bull.*, 1941, 38, 727.

WIEN, M. Ein Bedenken gegen die Helmholtzsche Resonanztheorie des Hörens, *Festschrift Adolph Wüllner*, Leipzig, 1905, 28–35.

WILEY, L. E. A further investigation of auditory cerebral mechanisms, *J. Comp. Neurol.*, 1937, 66, 327–331.

WILKINSON, GEORGE, and GRAY, A. A. *The mechanism of the cochlea*, 1924.

WILLIS, THOMAE. *De anima brutorum*, Londini, 1672, 189–202.

WILSON, H. A., and MYERS, C. S. The influence of binaural phase differences on the localisation of sounds, *Brit. J. Psychol.*, 1906, 2, 363–385.

WINGFIELD, R. C. An experimental study of the apparent persistence of auditory sensations, *J. General Psychol.*, 1936, 14, 136–157.

WITTMAACK, K. (1) Ueber Schädigungen des Gehörs durch Schalleinwirkungen, *Deutsche Otol. Gesellsch., Verh.*, 1907, 16, 239–242; and in more detail in *Zeits. f. Ohrenheilk.*, 1907, 54, 37–80. (2) Eine neue

Stütze der Helmholtz'sche Resonanztheorie, *Pflüg. Arch. ges. Physiol.*, 1907, 120, 249–252. (3) Ueber sekundäre Degenerationen im inneren Ohre nach Akustikusstammverletzungen, *Deutsche Otol. Gesellsch., Verh.*, 1911, 20, 289–296. (4) Demonstration zur Resonanz Theorie, *Acta otolaryngol.*, 1928, 12, 32–40.

WOOLSEY, C. N., and WALZL, E. M. Topical projection of nerve fibers from local regions of the cochlea to the cerebral cortex of the cat, *Bull. Johns Hopkins Hosp.*, 1942, 71, 315–344.

WORONZOW, D. S. Der Einfluss der Ermüdung auf die absolute Refraktärphase des Nerven, *Pflüg. Arch. ges. Physiol.*, 1934, 235, 96–102.

WRIGHTSON, THOMAS (1839–1921), and KEITH, ARTHUR. *An enquiry into the analytical mechanism of the internal ear*, 1918.

YOSHII, U. Experimentelle Untersuchungen ueber die Schädigung des Gehörorgans durch Schalleinwirkung, *Zeits. f. Ohrenheilk.*, 1909, 58, 201–251.

YOUNG, THOMAS. *A course of lectures on natural philosophy*, 1807, I, 301–303, 387 ff.

ZOTH, O. Über eine Modifikation der Ewaldschen Hörhypothese, *Zeits. f. Sinnesphysiol.*, 1923, 55, 179–184.

ZURMUEHL, G. Abhängigkeit der Tonhöhenempfindung von der Lautstärke und ihre Beziehung zur Helmholtzschen Resonanztheorie des Hörens, *Zeits. f. Sinnesphysiol.*, 1930, 61, 40–86.

ZWAARDEMAKER, H. Der Verlust an hohen Tönen mit zunehmendem Alter, *Arch. f. Ohrenheilk.*, 1891, 32, 53–56.

ZWISLOCKI, J. Über die mechanische Klanganalyse des Ohrs, *Experientia*, 1946, 2, 415–417.

INDEX

Abnormalities of hearing, 68, 111, 135, 141, 199, 239, 354
Abraham, 411, 413, 464
Absolute difference limen, 444
  for loudness, 313
  for pitch, 331, 339
Absolute refractory phase, 118, 123, 158
Acoustic tracts, 154, 227
Acoustic trauma, *see* Stimulation deafness
Action currents of nerves, 121, 284
  auditory, 128, 154, 157, 183, 249, 259, 303
  recording of, 125
Adaptation of nerve fibers, 159, 164, 303
Additive character of potentials, 196
Ades, 237, 239, 447, 459, 463
Adrian, 115, 140, 161, 162, 163, 177, 356, 447
Agnew, 421, 460
Albino cat, 136, 141
Alexander, 136, 447
All-or-nothing principle, 115, 127
Allen, 409 467
Alternating currents in nerve excitation, 282, 373
Amplitude modulation, 408
Ampullary organs, 33
Analysis, 10, 14, 26, 51, 76, 83, 92, 117
Anesthesia, 132
  effect on electrical potentials, 141, 156
Antidromic nerve fiber, 162
Apparatus for auditory nerve experiments, 131
Arapova, 372, 447
Arches of Corti, 20, 21, 142
  absence in birds, 32

Arches of Corti, specificity of, 36
Artifacts in auditory nerve experiments, 133
Artificial vowels, 28, 418
Ashcroft, 135, 448
Atrophy of organ of Corti, in albinotic animals, 136
  in cat, 247
  in man, 199
Audioelectric responses, forms of, 134
Auditory area, 192 (*cf.* Cortical areas)
Auditory cortex, 233
Auditory flicker, 408
Auditory nerve, anatomy of, 15, 17, 221
  for the cat, 133
  frequency representation in, 118, 157, 166
  lesions of, 239
  sectioning of, 135, 241
Auditory nerve fibers, courses of, 21, 23, 32, 222, 227
  excitation of, 154, 168
  by electric currents, 373
Auditory nerve impulses, 121 (*see also* Auditory nerve potentials)
  rate of, 77, 157, 163, 165, 288, 303
Auditory nerve potentials, 121, 157, 183, 255, 259, 303
  characteristics of, 137
  discovery of, 128
  distinguished from cochlear potentials, 137
  frequency of, 77, 157, 163, 288, 303
  in higher tracts, 128, 154, 249
  procedures for study of, 131

Auditory nerve potentials, recording of, 125
  synchronization of, 130, 138, 157, 185, 288, 436
Auditory pathways in the brain, 154, 227
Auditory quanta, 35, 51, 351
Auditory radiations, 230, 233
Auditory scale, 190
'Auditory teeth,' 19
Availability of nerve fibers, 293
Ayers, 41, 79, 448
  theory of, 79

Baginsky, 78, 206, 448
Banister, 105, 428, 448, 456
Bard, 237, 448
Barrera, 135, 455
Basilar membrane, 13, 18, 32
  damping of, 37, 50, 105, 110
  mass of, 35, 105, 272
  patterns of response on, 215, 264, 278, 334, 350, 436
  scaling of, 335
  stiffness of, 66, 104, 270
  tension in, 34, 66, 102, 264
  width of, 32, 34, 98
Basilar membrane fibers, interconnection of, 34, 44, 78, 105
  length of, 32, 34, 98
  number of, 36
Bast, 448
Bauhin, 10, 448
Beasley, 421, 448
Beats, uniaural, 375
  binaural, 427, 429, 432
Beat-tone theory, 412
Beauregard, 128, 448
Beck, 128, 448
Békésy, 41, 63, 104, 112, 277, 305, 317, 318, 320, 322, 328, 347, 352, 401, 402, 405, 448
  theory of, 63
Belikoff, 409, 449
Bell, 9, 29, 449
Berendes, 103, 449

Berengario da Carpi, 7, 449
Bezold, 79
Biddulph, 331, 464
Binaural beats, 427, 429, 432
Binaural phenomena, 424
Binaural shift phenomenon, 427, 429
Bird, cochlea of, 32
Bishop, 409, 449
Black, 383, 451
Blair, 449
Blood supply, relation to electrical potentials, 139
Boettcher, 216, 222, 449
Boettcher cells, 20
Bonnier, 40, 41, 80, 449
  theory of, 80
Bordley, 208, 467
Boring, 93, 118, 351, 449
Bowman, 34, 466
Brain stem, auditory connections in, 229
  impulses from, 129
  localization in, 254
Bramwell, 236, 449
Bray, 139, 140, 151, 153, 156, 157, 158, 165, 217, 243, 269, 325, 328, 330, 381, 383, 461, 467
Brecher, 328, 449
Bremer, 450
Breschet, 19, 450
Broca, 81
Bronk, 140, 162, 163, 447
Brown, 163, 177, 450
Brücke, 159, 453
Bryant, 80, 450
Buck, 40, 450
Budde, 358, 450
Bürck, 346, 401, 450
Bunch, 290, 364, 450, 455
Buytendijk, 129, 318, 450

Cairns, 240, 455
Cathodic summation, in nerve excitation, 284
Caton, 128, 450
Cattell, 162, 163, 177, 447, 450

Caussé, 320, 322, 450
Cavity-resonance theories, 10, 11, 12
Central nervous system, anatomy of, 154, 221
    potentials from, 155, 249
    frequency limits of, 155, 436
Cercal organs of insects, 180
Cerebral cortex, 156, 233, 235, 249
Cerebral hemisphere, effect of loss of, 235
Cerebral lesions, 235
Chapin, 421, 450
Chavasse, 320, 322, 450
Chladni, 46, 450
Churcher, 300, 450
Ciocco, 202, 222, 450
Claudius, 21, 31, 450
Claudius cells, 20, 23
Coakley, 451
Cochlea, anatomy of, 7, 17
    anomalies of, 204, 247
    innervation of, 222, 290, 292, 309
    local injury of, 78, 199, 206, 247, 366
    neural projections of, 222, 235
    observations of motion in, 64
Cochlear aqueduct, 275
Cochlear duct, 17, 18, 19
    cross-sectional area of, 275
Cochlear fluid, 8, 275
Cochlear nerve, see Auditory nerve
Cochlear nerve fibers, see Auditory nerve fibers
Cochlear nucleus, 227
    impulses from, 164, 183, 255
Cochlear potentials, 135, 244, 325
    distortion in, 146
    effects of overstimulation on, 210
    in man, 138
    intensity function of, 145, 261
    localization in the cochlea, 219, 349
    source of, 141
Cochlear resonators, identity of, 10, 13, 15, 19, 20, 31, 32, 40

Cochlear resonators, independence of, 34, 44, 78, 105, 108
    specificity of, 36, 67, 108, 194, 197, 350, 394, 412, 438
Cochlear response, see Cochlear potentials
Coiter, 7, 451
Combination tones, 380, 386
    Meyer's theory of, 87
    orders of, 381
    Wrightson's theory of, 92
Conductive deafness, 361
Conductive mechanism, discovery of, 7
Coppée, 155, 254, 284, 304, 451, 458
Corradi, 79
Corti, 19, 30, 451
Corti's membrane, see Tectorial membrane
Cortical areas for hearing, 235, 249
Cortical deafness, 235
Cortical localization of tones, 238, 249
Cortical projections, 233
Cortical radiations, 156
Cotugno, 8, 16, 451
Covell, 383, 451
Cowan, 343, 460
Craik, 447
Cramer, 16, 451
Critical points in excitation, 90, 144, 170
Crowe, 201, 207, 240, 290, 365, 451, 455, 457
Culler, 219, 239, 447, 451
Cummings, 176, 467
Cutaneous nerve fibers, maximum frequency in, 177
Cycle, 443
Cycles, number required for pitch, 346

Dalmatian dogs, 136
Damping, in the cochlea, 37, 50, 105, 110, 402

Damping, principles of, 37, 106, 110, 193, 443
Dandy, 240, 451
Danilewsky, 128, 451
Davis, 136, 156, 157, 163, 183, 208, 255, 259, 303, 304, 322, 323, 335, 342, 357, 391, 451, 452, 454, 461, 464, 465
Deafness, forms of, 361
  from defects of organ of Corti, 136, 141
  from nerve lesions, 135, 239, 361
  from otosclerosis, 68, 362
  in Ménière's disease, 240, 355
  in relation to age, 364
  sensory-neural, 363
Death, effect of on electrical potentials, 139
Decay of response, in a resonator, 37, 194
  in the ear, 402
Decibel, 443
Decorticate animals, hearing in, 236
Decorticate cat, sound localization by, 237, 431
Deiters, 31, 452
Deiters cells, 20, 22, 142
Deming, 412, 466
Dennert, 411, 452
Dentate band, 20
Derbyshire, 157, 304, 391, 452
Difference limen, 444
  absolute, for loudness, 313
    for pitch, 331, 339
  relative, for loudness, 312
    for pitch, 333, 339
  variations of, on quantum theory, 351
Difference tones, 380
Differentiation in the cochlea, 34, 97, 108, 197 (see also Resonance)
Diplacusis, 112, 356
Disharmonic paracusis, 111
Distortion, 310, 329, 381
  in cochlear potentials, 146

Distortion, in hair cells, 151
  locus of, 382
  relation to phase, 421
Distribution of tones over the basilar membrane, 215, 249, 264, 278, 334, 350, 436
Dix, 368, 452
Dorsal acoustic tract, 232
Doupe, 462
Dow, 450
Du Bois Reymond, 282
Dunlap, 94
Dupuy, 128, 448
Duration, effect on loudness, 317
  effect on quality, 346
DuVerney, 12, 452
Dyne, 444

Ebner, 40, 44, 452
Echlin, 163, 178, 452
Ectosylvian gyri, 252
Eddies in the cochlear fluid, 64, 66, 72, 112
Eighth nerve, see Auditory nerve
  sectioning of, 135, 241
Electrical potentials, forms of, 134
Electrical stimulation of the ear, 370, 406
Electrodynamic action of hair cells, 147
Embryological development of the ear, 216
Empedocles, 5
Endolymph, 23
Energy density on basilar membrane, 280
Equal-loudness contours, 306
Erlanger, 123, 449, 452
Esteve, 16, 452
Eustachian tube, 7
Eustachius, 7, 452
Ewald, 40, 41, 45, 341, 432, 452
  theory of, 45
Excitability of nerve fibers, 159, 169
Excitation, phasic character of, 90, 144, 170

Excitatory density of stimulation, 192
Exner, 33, 405, 452, 453
External spiral fibers, 224
External sulcus, 20
External sulcus cells, 20
Eyster, 448

Facial nerve, 226
Fallopius, 7, 453
Fatigue, absence in cochlear response, 140
  auditory, 319
  specificity of, 322
Fechner, 315
Fechner's law, 300
Fessard, 163, 178, 452
Field, 159, 453
Firestone, 421, 450, 466
Fischer, 112, 453
Flanders, 453
Fletcher, 107, 165, 300, 306, 341, 343, 392, 429, 453
Flicker, auditory, 408
Fluid columns, 107, 272
Foà, 130, 453
Focusing principle, in pitch perception, 109, 112 (see also Specificity)
Forbes, 116, 129, 453
Fourier, 26, 453
Fourier series, 26
Fourier's theorem, 26
Fowler, 367, 369, 453
Frank, 69, 453
French, 237, 453
Frequency, 444
  transients of, 404
Frequency-analytic theories, 41, 83
Frequency discrimination, auditory, see Pitch discrimination
  cutaneous, 176
Frequency limits, for the ear, 328
  for single auditory elements, 184
  for the skin, 175
  in higher acoustic tracts, 155, 436
Frequency modulation, 416

Frequency principle, 40, 76, 117
  first established, 130
  limits of operation of, 157
  theoretical basis of, 166, 435
Frequency representation in the auditory nerve, 118, 157, 166
Frequency theories, 40
  frequency-analytic types, 83
  modern developments, 117, 166, 189
  outline, 41
  simple types, 76
Friction, see Damping
Furrer, 357, 464

Galambos, 163, 183, 255, 259, 303, 391, 452, 454, 461
Galen, 6, 454
Galileo, 10, 16, 454
Ganglion cells, 222, 290
  number of, 290, 309, 336
Gardner, 369, 465
Garner, 318, 454
Gasser, 123, 159, 452, 454
Gault, 175
Geffcken, 454
Geldard, 175, 454
Gerard, 156, 454
Gersuni, 372, 447, 454
Gildemeister, 50, 454
Gilmer, 175, 454
Girden, 238, 454
Goebel, 94, 454
Goodfellow, 175, 454
Gotch, 115, 454
Graham, 163, 456
Graphic reconstruction method, 99, 201
Gray, A. A., 102, 105, 110, 348, 359, 439, 455, 468
Gray, C., 458
Gregg, 116, 453
Gross, 451
Gruber, 200, 455
Grüneberg, 136, 455
Grundfest, 159, 454

Guild, 99, 136, 148, 201, 204, 290, 365, 451, 455, 457
Guttman, 135, 455

Habenula perforata, 20, 224
Hair cells, 20, 21
  absence in albinotic animals, 136
  as source of cochlear potentials, 142, 196
  electrodynamic action of, 147
  identified as the sensory cells, 24
  injury by overstimulation, 136, 212
  inner vs. outer, 144, 170
  innervation of, 222, 290, 292, 309
  mode of support of, 23, 142
  result of local atrophy of, 201, 247
  stimulation of, 90, 142, 170
    as phasic, 145
    by electric currents, 372
Haller, 15, 455
Hallpike, 135, 136, 219, 240, 368, 405, 406, 448, 452, 455
Hardesty, 41, 81, 456
  theory of, 81
Hardy, 290, 456
Harmonics, 151, 310, 329, 381
Hartley, 426, 456
Hartline, 163, 456
Hartridge, 94, 105, 405, 406, 455, 456
Hartshorn, 405, 456
Hasse, 32, 40, 41, 43, 456
  theory of, 43
Hawkins, 135, 136, 452, 461
Held, 24, 98, 207, 222, 225, 456
  striae of, 232
Helicotrema, 19
Helmholtz, 25, 104, 109, 351, 375, 382, 412, 418, 438, 456
Helmholtz resonance theory, 25
  early criticisms of, 40, 44
  explanation of beats in, 376
  explanation of modulation in, 413
  modern developments of, 97
  revised form of, 32

Henle, 98
Hensen, 32, 98, 144, 457
Hensen cells, 20, 23
Hermann, 421, 457
High-tone deafness, 201, 365
Higher acoustic tracts, anatomy of, 154, 221
  potentials from, 155, 249
  frequency limits of, 155, 436
Hill, A. V., 283, 284, 286, 457
Hill, S. E., 148, 462
Hoagland, 162, 163, 177, 447, 450, 457
Hodgkin, 284, 457
Hoessli, 144, 457
Hood, 368, 452
Hornbostel, 425, 457
Horton, 210, 457, 468
Hostinsky, 109, 457
Howe, 136, 207, 457
Hughes, 428, 457
Hughson, 136, 207, 325, 457
Hurst, 40, 41, 52, 458
  theory of, 52
Huschke, 19, 21, 458

Implanted-air hypothesis, 5, 8, 11
Incus, discovery of, 7
Independence of cochlear resonators, 34, 44, 78, 105, 108
Induction, 133
Inferior colliculus, 155, 233, 254
  lesions of, 239
Inglis, 458
Ingrassia, 7, 458
Inhibition in nerve action, 255, 391
Innervation of the cochlea, 222, 290, 292, 309
Integration of jnd's, for loudness, 315
  for pitch, 337
Intensity, 445
  limits of, 192
  representation of, 115, 172
  transients of, 400
Intensity-frequency principle, 117, 128, 172

Intensity level, 445
Interference, 151, 383
Intermediate pitches, perception of, 35
Intermittence tone, 411
Internal spiral fibers, 224
Internal sulcus, 20
Internal sulcus cells, 20
Interruption tone, 410
Intraganglionic spiral fibers, 23, 222, 291

Jäderholm, 452
Jeffress, 357, 458
Jenkins, 458
Johnson, E. P., Jr., 220, 458
Johnson, H. M., 238, 458
Jones, I. H., 355, 458
Jones, R. C., 370, 372, 458, 465
Just noticeable difference, 445
  for loudness, 312
  for pitch, 331, 339

Kalischer, 237, 458
Kapell, 429, 460
Katz, 283, 284, 286, 457, 458
Keith, 98, 458
Kellaway, 406, 458
Kemp, 155, 210, 254, 304, 452, 458
Kircher, 10, 458
Kishi, 44, 458
Kleinknecht, 207, 456
Knudsen, 175, 176, 312, 335, 355, 458
Kobrak, 227, 460
Koch, 49, 459
Kock, 312, 459
Kölliker, 21, 23, 31, 35, 459
Koenig, 377, 411, 420, 459
Kotowski, 346, 401, 450
Kreidl, 216, 459
Kryter, 239, 253, 459, 460
Kucharski, 317, 346, 409, 459
Kuile, 40, 41, 55, 144, 459
  theory of, 55

Kurtz, 459
Kwiek, 459

Lane, 270, 387, 427, 433, 459, 467
Larionow, 238, 459
Larsell, J. F., 217, 459
Larsell, O., 217, 459
Lateral lemniscus, 232, 233, 304
  nucleus of, 233
Lateral-line organ, 79
'Law of contrast,' 67, 113
Lawrence, 139, 140, 151, 152, 153, 261, 269, 325, 330, 381, 383, 386, 460, 468
Ledoux, 136, 455
Lehmann, 48, 459
  theory of, 49
Leiri, 94, 459
Lempert, 362, 460
Length, in tuning of the basilar membrane, 32, 98
  of vibrating strings, 97
Lesions, cochlear, 78, 199, 206, 247, 366
  nervous, 235
  subcortical, 239
Lewis, 343, 460
Lewy, 227, 460
Lichte, 346, 401, 450
Licklider, 253, 460
Lifshitz, 318, 460
Limbus, 19
Limen, see Difference limen, Threshold
Lindig, 421, 460
Linearity of cochlear responses, 146, 261
Lipman, 460
Lloyd, 421, 460
Loading of basilar membrane, by cellular masses, 105
  by fluid columns, 107
Localization, in neural tracts and nuclei, 155
  of cochlear potentials, 219, 349

Localization, of responses in the cochlea, 14, 16, 31, 65, 199, 257, 397
of sounds in space, 119, 238, 424
Loesch, 429, 460
Lorente de Nó, 222, 224, 227, 229, 369, 460
Loudness, 89, 299, 445
effect of duration on, 317
equal-loudness contours, 306
Loudness discrimination, 311
Loudness level, 445
Loudness recruitment, 324, 366
Loudness scales, 300
Low-tone acuity with apical atrophies, 204
Low tones, localization of, 206
selective loss of, 203
Lowy, 391, 451, 460
Lucae, 12, 94, 460
Lucas, 447
Lurie, 136, 157, 208, 335, 372, 452, 458, 461, 465
Lux, 107, 461

Macular organs, 13, 33, 420
Magendie, 16, 461
Malleus, discovery of, 7
Marshall, 156, 454
Marx, 210, 461
Masking, 387
Mass, of basilar membrane, 104, 272
of vibrating strings, 97
Mathes, 421, 461
Matthews, 162, 163, 461
Maximum stimulation, principle of, 110, 348, 439
Maximum value of cochlear potentials, 261
Mayer, 408, 461
McCrady, 156, 158, 217, 459, 461
Mechanical resonance of the ear, 269
Medial geniculate bodies, 233
lesions of, 239
Meesters, 318, 450

Membrane hypothesis, 123
Membrane of Corti, see Tectorial membrane
Membrane-resonance theories, 43, 44, 45, 48, 49
outline, 41
Membranous spiral lamina (Basilar membrane), anatomy of, 13, 17, 32
Ménière's disease, 240, 355
Mettler, 239, 447
Metz, 270, 277, 461
Meyer, 40, 41, 60, 370, 461
theory of, 83
Microphonics, 133
Microvolts, 445
Middle ear, discovery of, 7
transmission characteristics of, 277, 382
Middle ear muscles, relation to pitch, 342
Miller, G. A., 318, 454
Miller, R. H., 129, 453
Miller, R. L., 421, 461
Milliseconds, 445
Mills, 236, 461
Minton, 358, 461
Models of the cochlea, Békésy's, 63
Ewald's, 48
Modulation, amplitude, 408
frequency, 416
phase, 422
Modulation index, 417
Monakow, striae of, 232
Moos, 79, 200, 461
Morgan, 352, 452, 461, 465
Morton, 94, 461
Müller, 9, 29, 462
Munk, 462
Munson, 277, 300, 306, 318, 392, 453, 462
'Musical quality,' 28, 419
'Musical shakes,' 38
Myers, 432, 468
Mygind, 94, 462

Natanson, 30, 462
Neff, 135, 243, 462, 468
Nerve, action currents of, 121, 284
  auditory, 128, 154, 157, 183, 249,
    259, 303
  methods of recording, 125, 131
Nerve action, hypothesis of, 123
  variables in, 128
Nerve deafness, 135, 239, 361
Nerve excitation, 159
  by electric currents, 281, 373
  phasic character of, 168
Nerve fibers, 121
  accommodation or adaptation in,
    159, 164, 282, 303
  auditory, courses of, 21, 23, 32,
    222, 227
    level of excitation of, 169
    number active, for tones, 289
    phase of excitation of, 170
    variations among, 168
  degeneration of, 215
  effects of prolonged stimulation
    of, 159
  isolation of single, 161
  refractory phase of, absolute, 118,
    123, 158
    relative, 124
  sensory, 127
Nerve potentials, 121, 284
  auditory, 128, 154, 157, 183, 249,
    259, 303
  recording of, 125, 131
Neural cleft, 22
Neuroacoustic mechanism, 15, 17,
  221
Newman, E. B., 339, 465
Newman, H. W., 462
Nitella cell, 148
Noises, representation of, 33, 419
  thresholds for, 328
Non-analytic frequency theories, see
  Telephone theories
  outline, 41
Non-linearity of the ear, in cochlear
  potentials, 146

Non-linearity of the ear, in percep-
  tion of phase differences, 421
  in perception of pitch, 342
Non-resonance place theories, see
  Traveling wave theories
  outline, 41
Nucleus interstitialis, 232
Nuel, 22, 23, 34, 462

'Occlusion,' 255, 391
O'Connor, 129, 453
Oda, 205, 462
Ohm, 26, 462
Ohm's law, 26, 117
Onset, transients of, 194, 401
Opossum, 158, 217
Organ of Corti, anatomy of, 18, 21,
  105, 142
  defects of, 136, 141, 202
  embryological development of, 216
  injury by overstimulation of, 136,
    212
  size of, 105
Osseous spiral lamina, 8, 13, 18
Ossicles, discovery of, 7
  mass of, 276
Osterhout, 148, 462
Otosclerosis, 68, 362
Outer rods of Corti, 20
  variation in length of, 32
Oval window, discovery of, 7
Overloading, 146, 151 (see also Dis-
  tortion)
Overstimulation, and diplacusis, 357
  effects on inner ear, 136, 142, 151,
    209, 258, 259, 263

Paracusis, 111
Particle velocity, 58, 446
Pasternak, 409, 462
Patterns of action on the basilar
  membrane, 215, 249, 264,
    278, 334, 350, 436
Pattie, 324, 462
Pearce, 322, 462

Perception, theories of, 4, 8
Perceptive deafness, 361
Period of a sound, 445
Peroni, 453
Perrault, 8, 12, 462
Persistence, of tonal sensation, 402
    of vibration, 37, 194
Pfaffmann, 163, 180, 462
Phalangeal cells, 20, 22, 142
Phalangeal process, 20, 22, 142
Phase, 27, 445
    direct perception of, 28, 404, 418
    in modulation, 414, 418
    in sound localization, 425, 428
    of cochlear motions, 65
Phase lag in nerve impulses, 179
Phasic character of excitation, 90,
    144, 170
Phillips, 140, 447
Photoelectric siren, 405
Pillars of Corti, 20, 21, 23
    as resonators, 31
    number of, 35
Pinna reflex, 206
Piper, 129, 462
Pitch, 327
    difference limen for, 331, 339
    limits of, 328
    relation to duration, 346
    relation to intensity, 59, 81, 340
Pitch discrimination, 35, 331
    in decorticate dogs, 237
Pitch scales, 339
Place theory, early forms of, 10, 12,
    15
    Helmholtz's, 25
    membrane-resonance types of, 43
    modern forms of, 97, 189
    outline, 41
    tube-resonance types of, 68
Polarization, of hair cells, 148
    of nerve fibers, 121
Poliak, 234, 462
Pollak, 405, 453
Polvogt, 201, 290, 365, 451, 455

Potentials, additive character of, 196
    (see also Cochlear potentials,
    Nerve potentials)
Pratt, 161, 463
Presbyacusia, 364
Pressure, sound, 445
Pressure-pattern theory, 45
Preyer, 35
Principle of maximum stimulation,
    110, 348, 439
Principle of resemblances, 4, 9
Proetz, 357, 463
Propagation velocity, 58, 446
    for cochlear waves, 70, 73
Pumphrey, 163, 181, 463

Quality, 'musical,' 28, 419
Quanta, auditory, 35, 51, 351

Raab, 237, 463
Radial canals of the cochlea (illus-
    trated, 17, 18), 222
Radial fibers, 222
Raiford, 364, 450
Ramon y Cajal, 227, 463
Ramsdell, 463
Range, of audible frequencies, 102
    of cochlear activity, 258
    of resonance, 32, 37, 67, 108, 194,
        197, 350, 394, 412, 438
Ranke, 41, 69, 441, 463
    theory of, 69
Rawdon-Smith, 135, 163, 181, 219,
    322, 323, 405, 406, 448, 455,
    463
Rayleigh, 426, 427, 463
Reboul, 41, 73, 441, 463
    theory of, 73
Recruitment, 358
Reference intensity, 446
Reference tone, 300, 306
Refractory phase, absolute, 118, 123,
    158, 168
    relative, 124
Regulator neurons, 229
Reissner, 19, 463

Reissner's membrane, 18, 19
  as a resonator, 49
Relative difference limen, 444
  for loudness, 312
  for pitch, 333, 339
Resonance, cavity resonance, 10
  mechanical, of the ear, 269
  physical principles of, 10, 33, 37,
    97, 193
Resonance principle, in the volley
  theory, 193
Resonance theory, early development
  of, 9
  Helmholtz's, 25
  membrane-resonance types of, 43
  modern developments of, 97, 189
  outline, 41
  tube-resonance types of, 68
Resonators, effect of phase shift on,
  404
  in the ear, forms of, 341
  number of, 35
Respiration, effect on electrical po-
  tentials, 139
Resultant displacements theory, 412,
  423
Reticular membrane, 20, 21, 23
Retzius, 24, 98, 224, 463
Riesz, 312, 463
Rinne, 40, 76, 463
  theory of, 76
Rinne test, 205
Rioch, 237, 448
Roaf, 463
Roberts, 176, 464
Robinson, 155, 254, 304, 458
Rods of Corti, 20, 21, 23
  as resonators, 31
  number of, 35
Röhr, 210, 464
Root-mean-square, 446
Rosenthal's canal, 222, 291
Rosenzweig, 237, 464
Rostosky, 432, 464
Round window, discovery of, 7
  in sound transmission, 12, 68

Rüedi, 357, 464
Rutherford, 41, 77, 189, 221, 464
  theory of, 77

Saul, 156, 157, 452, 454, 464
Scala communis cochleae, 204
Scala tympani, 17
  cross-sectional area of, 275
Scala vestibuli, 17
  cross-sectional area of, 275
Scarpa, 17, 21, 464
Scarpa's ganglion (vestibular gang-
  lion), 226
Schaefer, H., 282, 464
Schaefer, K. L., 411, 413, 464
Schelhammer, 8, 464
Schouten, 421, 464
Schultze, 20, 23, 32, 464
Schulze, 421, 464
Scripture, 416, 464
Seashore, 464
Seat of hearing, as the cochlea, 8,
  10, 24
  as the labyrinth, 10, 13, 21
  as the tympanic cavity, 5
Secondary cortical area, 252
Selectivity, see Specificity
Sensation, theories of, 4, 8
Sensitivity, 192, 268
  and interference, 385
  theoretical, 294
Sensory cells, identity of, 24 (see
  also Hair cells)
Sensory-neural deafness, 363
Setzepfand, 175, 464
Shambaugh, 41, 44, 464
  theory of, 44
Shower, 331, 464
Siebenmann, 44, 464
Simple frequency theories, see Tele-
  phone theories
Single auditory elements, impulses
  in, 183
Single-fiber hypothesis, 158
Siren, 36, 405, 416, 420
Sivian, 465

Skolnick, 175, 465
Smith, F. W., 452
Smith, K. R., 136, 211, 259, 362, 465, 468
Smith, R., 412, 465
Snow, 341, 465
Solandt, 283, 286, 457
Solovcov, 223, 465
Sound transmission by the ear, 7, 11, 12, 145, 261, 381 (see also Distortion)
Specific energies, doctrine of, 9, 29, 127
Specificity, of neural connections, 32, 221
of neural excitation, 67, 71, 112
of response in the cochlea, 36, 67, 108, 168, 170, 194, 196, 350, 394, 412, 438
Spectrum level of noise, 394, 446
Spiral fibers, 23, 222, 291
Spiral ligament, 18
size of, 102
Spread of response in the cochlea, 196 (see also Specificity)
Standing waves, 46, 72
Stapedius muscle, discovery of, 7
Stapes, discovery of, 7
fixation of, 68, 362
Stein, 209, 465
Steinberg, 335, 369, 465
Steinbrügge, 79, 200, 461
Stepanow, 79, 200, 206, 465
Steudel, 465
Stevens, 208, 335, 339, 341, 342, 352, 370, 372, 458, 465
Stewart, 428, 432, 466
Stiffness, of basilar membrane, 66, 104, 270
Stimulation deafness, 136, 142, 151, 209, 258, 259, 263
and diplacusis, 357
Stowell, 412, 466
Stretch receptors, 178
Stretched strings, properties of, 97 (see also Resonance)

Stria vascularis, 18, 23
Striae of Held, 232
Striae of Monakow, 232
Strutt (Lord Rayleigh), 426, 427, 463
Sturdy, 447
Subcortical lesions, 239
Subjective equality of jnd's, 315
Submultiple discharge rates, 179, 181, 182
Summation tones, 380
Superior olivary nuclei, 232
Superior temporal convolution, 233
Sylvian fissure, 234
Sympathetic vibration, see Resonance
Synapses, delay at, 155
of cochlear nuclei, 229
Synchronism of responses, in auditory nerve, 130, 138, 157, 185, 288, 436
in central tracts, 155, 436
in cochlear nucleus, 184
in various nerves, 177, 178, 180, 181
limits of, 155, 157, 185, 436
Synthesis of complex sounds, 27, 28, 418

Tectorial membrane, 18, 20, 45, 80, 145
as a resonator, 43, 44, 81
Telephone theories, 76, 77, 79, 80, 81
outline, 41
Temperature, effects on cochlear potentials, 140
Temporal phenomena, 399
Tension, of basilar membrane, 34, 66, 102, 264
of vibrating strings, 97
Tensor tympani muscle, 7, 382
Terminal resonators on the basilar membrane, 114
Tertiary cortical area, 254
Tetanization of nerves, 159

Theories of hearing, cavity-resonance theories, Bauhin, 10
  Perrault, 12
  Willis, 11
  frequency-analytic theories,
    Meyer, 83
    Wrightson, 89
  membrane-resonance theories,
    Ewald, 45
    Hasse, 43
    Koch, 49
    Lehmann, 48
    Shambaugh, 44
    Zoth, 49
  telephone theories, Ayers, 79
    Bonnier, 80
    Hardesty, 81
    Rinne, 76
    Rutherford, 77
    Voltolini, 76
  traveling wave theories, Békésy, 63
    Hurst, 52
    Kuile, 55
    Watt, 61
    Zwislocki, 67
  tube-resonance theories, Ranke, 69
    Reboul, 73
  tuned-element theories, DuVerney, 12
    Helmholtz, 25
  volley theory, 189
Thermal noise, masking by, 392
Thompson, E., 136, 457
Thompson, S. P., 432, 466
Threshold, absence for cochlear potentials, 138
  for nerve potentials, 138
Threshold sensitivity of the ear, 192, 268
Thuras, 270, 466
Thurlow, 343, 349, 466
Time of incidence, in sound localization, 425
Tinnitus, 240, 354

Titchener, 93, 449
Todd, 34, 466
Tominaga, 94, 466
Tonal dip, 363
Tonal interaction, 375
Topographical effects, 219
  for overtones, 349
Touch, 110, 174
Transformation, 151, 380
Transformation principle, 381, 386
Transients, 37, 194, 400
Trapezoid body, 155, 229, 232, 254
Trapezoid nucleus, 229
Traveling wave, 52, 55, 61, 63, 69, 73
Traveling wave theories, 50, 52, 55, 61, 63, 67, 68, 69, 73, 79, 80, 81, 441
  outline, 41
Trimble, 428, 466
Trimmer, 421, 466
Tröger, 270, 466
Troland, 165, 466
Tuberculum acusticum, 227
Tube-resonance theories, 68, 73, 441
  outline, 41
Tuned-element theories, 12, 25
  outline, 41
Tuning in the cochlea, 34, 97, 108, 197 (see also Resonance)
Tunnel fibers, 225
Tunturi, 253, 466
Turnbull, 347, 466
Tympanic lamella, 20, 142
  effects of overstimulation on, 213
Tympanic lip, 19
Tympanic muscles, 7, 11, 382

Upper limit of hearing, 330
Upton, 210, 452, 466

Valsalva, 15, 466
Van der Pol, 466
Vance, 328, 466
Variation tone, 410
Varolius, 7, 466

Velocity, particle, 446
  propagation, 58, 446
  for cochlear waves, 70, 73
Ventral acoustic tract, 155, 232, 254
Ventral cochlear nucleus, 227, 232
Vesalius, 7, 466
Vestibular fibers, 241
Vestibular ganglion (Scarpa's), 226
Vestibular lip, 19
Vestibular nerve, 227
Vibrating string hypothesis, 15, 97
  early criticisms of, 16 (see also
    Resonance, physical princi-
    ples of)
Vibrato, 417
Vibratory sensibility, 174
  theory of, 176
Volkmann, 30, 339, 352, 465, 467
Volley principle, 165, 166
Volley theory, 189
Volokhov, 372, 447, 454
Voltolini, 76, 467
Vortices in the cochlear fluid, 64, 66,
    72, 112

Wada, 216, 467
Waetzmann, 467
Waldeyer, 35
Waller, 40, 41, 79, 467
Walzl, 208, 249, 467, 469
Watt, 40, 41, 61, 467
  theory of, 61
Wave theories, 52, 68
  outline, 41
Weber, E. H., 35
Weber, W., 340
Weber's law, 313
Wedell, 176, 331, 467, 468

Wegel, 148, 270, 298, 335, 355, 387,
    433, 467
Weinberg, 409, 467
Weitz, 175, 454
Wertheimer, 425, 457
Wever, 99, 130, 136, 138, 139, 140,
    151, 152, 153, 156, 157, 158,
    217, 244, 261, 291, 328, 330,
    331, 363, 381, 382, 383, 386,
    460, 461, 465, 467
White, 465
Wien, 110, 468
Wiley, 237, 468
Wilkins, 462
Wilkinson, 102, 107, 468
Willis, 11, 468
Wilson, 432, 468
Wingfield, 409, 468
Witting, 136, 325, 457
Wittmaack, 135, 207, 209, 468
Woolsey, 249, 469
Woronzow, 160, 469
Wright, 240, 455
Wrightson, 40, 41, 89, 469
  theory of, 89

Yanase, 216, 459
Yoshii, 144, 210, 469
Young, 16, 412, 469

Zimmermann, 217, 459
'Zona cochleae,' 15
'Zonae sonorae,' 15
Zoth, 49, 469
Zotterman, 161, 163, 447
Zurmühl, 341, 469
Zwaardemaker, 364, 469
Zwislocki, 67, 469

SOME DOVER SCIENCE BOOKS

SOME DOVER SCIENCE BOOKS

WHAT IS SCIENCE?,
Norman Campbell
This excellent introduction explains scientific method, role of mathematics, types of scientific laws. Contents: 2 aspects of science, science & nature, laws of science, discovery of laws, explanation of laws, measurement & numerical laws, applications of science. 192pp. 5⅜ x 8.   60043-2 Paperbound $1.25

FADS AND FALLACIES IN THE NAME OF SCIENCE,
Martin Gardner
Examines various cults, quack systems, frauds, delusions which at various times have masqueraded as science. Accounts of hollow-earth fanatics like Symmes; Velikovsky and. wandering planets; Hoerbiger; Bellamy and the theory of multiple moons; Charles Fort; dowsing, pseudoscientific methods for finding water, ores, oil. Sections on naturopathy, iridiagnosis, zone therapy, food fads, etc. Analytical accounts of Wilhelm Reich and orgone sex energy; L. Ron Hubbard and Dianetics; A. Korzybski and General Semantics; many others. Brought up to date to include Bridey Murphy, others. Not just a collection of anecdotes, but a fair, reasoned appraisal of eccentric theory. Formerly titled *In the Name of Science*. Preface. Index. x + 384pp. 5⅜ x 8.
20394-8 Paperbound $2.00

PHYSICS, THE PIONEER SCIENCE,
L. W. Taylor
First thorough text to place all important physical phenomena in cultural-historical framework; remains best work of its kind. Exposition of physical laws, theories developed chronologically, with great historical, illustrative experiments diagrammed, described, worked out mathematically. Excellent physics text for self-study as well as class work. Vol. 1: Heat, Sound: motion, acceleration, gravitation, conservation of energy, heat engines, rotation, heat, mechanical energy, etc. 211 illus. 407pp. 5⅜ x 8. Vol. 2: Light, Electricity: images, lenses, prisms, magnetism, Ohm's law, dynamos, telegraph, quantum theory, decline of mechanical view of nature, etc. Bibliography. 13 table appendix. Index. 551 illus. 2 color plates. 508pp. 5⅜ x 8.
60565-5, 60566-3 Two volume set, paperbound $5.50

THE EVOLUTION OF SCIENTIFIC THOUGHT FROM NEWTON TO EINSTEIN,
A. d'Abro
Einstein's special and general theories of relativity, with their historical implications, are analyzed in non-technical terms. Excellent accounts of the contributions of Newton, Riemann, Weyl, Planck, Eddington, Maxwell, Lorentz and others are treated in terms of space and time, equations of electromagnetics, finiteness of the universe, methodology of science. 21 diagrams. 482pp. 5⅜ x 8.
20002-7 Paperbound $2.50

FIVE VOLUME "THEORY OF FUNCTIONS" SET BY KONRAD KNOPP

This five-volume set, prepared by Konrad Knopp, provides a complete and readily followed account of theory of functions. Proofs are given concisely, yet without sacrifice of completeness or rigor. These volumes are used as texts by such universities as M.I.T., University of Chicago, N. Y. City College, and many others. "Excellent introduction . . . remarkably readable, concise, clear, rigorous," *Journal of the American Statistical Association.*

ELEMENTS OF THE THEORY OF FUNCTIONS,
Konrad Knopp
This book provides the student with background for further volumes in this set, or texts on a similar level. Partial contents: foundations, system of complex numbers and the Gaussian plane of numbers, Riemann sphere of numbers, mapping by linear functions, normal forms, the logarithm, the cyclometric functions and binomial series. "Not only for the young student, but also for the student who knows all about what is in it," *Mathematical Journal.* Bibliography. Index. 140pp. 5⅜ x 8.   60154-4 Paperbound $1.50

THEORY OF FUNCTIONS, PART I,
Konrad Knopp
With volume II, this book provides coverage of basic concepts and theorems. Partial contents: numbers and points, functions of a complex variable, integral of a continuous function, Cauchy's integral theorem, Cauchy's integral formulae, series with variable terms, expansion of analytic functions in power series, analytic continuation and complete definition of analytic functions, entire transcendental functions, Laurent expansion, types of singularities. Bibliography. Index. vii + 146pp. 5⅜ x 8.   60156-0 Paperbound $1.50

THEORY OF FUNCTIONS, PART II,
Konrad Knopp
Application and further development of general theory, special topics. Single valued functions. Entire, Weierstrass, Meromorphic functions. Riemann surfaces. Algebraic functions. Analytical configuration, Riemann surface. Bibliography. Index. x + 150pp. 5⅜ x 8.   60157-9 Paperbound $1.50

PROBLEM BOOK IN THE THEORY OF FUNCTIONS, VOLUME 1.
Konrad Knopp
Problems in elementary theory, for use with Knopp's *Theory of Functions*, or any other text, arranged according to increasing difficulty. Fundamental concepts, sequences of numbers and infinite series, complex variable, integral theorems, development in series, conformal mapping. 182 problems. Answers. viii + 126pp. 5⅜ x 8.   60158-7 Paperbound $1.50

PROBLEM BOOK IN THE THEORY OF FUNCTIONS, VOLUME 2,
Konrad Knopp
Advanced theory of functions, to be used either with Knopp's *Theory of Functions*, or any other comparable text. Singularities, entire & meromorphic functions, periodic, analytic, continuation, multiple-valued functions, Riemann surfaces, conformal mapping. Includes a section of additional elementary problems. "The difficult task of selecting from the immense material of the modern theory of functions the problems just within the reach of the beginner is here masterfully accomplished," *Am. Math. Soc.* Answers. 138pp. 5⅜ x 8.
60159-5 Paperbound $1.50

THE RISE OF THE NEW PHYSICS (formerly THE DECLINE OF MECHANISM),
A. d'Abro
This authoritative and comprehensive 2-volume exposition is unique in scientific publishing. Written for intelligent readers not familiar with higher mathematics, it is the only thorough explanation in non-technical language of modern mathematical-physical theory. Combining both history and exposition, it ranges from classical Newtonian concepts up through the electronic theories of Dirac and Heisenberg, the statistical mechanics of Fermi, and Einstein's relativity theories. "A must for anyone doing serious study in the physical sciences," *J. of Franklin Inst.* 97 illustrations. 991pp. 2 volumes.
20003-5, 20004-3 Two volume set, paperbound $5.50

THE STRANGE STORY OF THE QUANTUM, AN ACCOUNT FOR THE GENERAL READER OF THE GROWTH OF IDEAS UNDERLYING OUR PRESENT ATOMIC KNOWLEDGE, *B. Hoffmann*
Presents lucidly and expertly, with barest amount of mathematics, the problems and theories which led to modern quantum physics. Dr. Hoffmann begins with the closing years of the 19th century, when certain trifling discrepancies were noticed, and with illuminating analogies and examples takes you through the brilliant concepts of Planck, Einstein, Pauli, de Broglie, Bohr, Schroedinger, Heisenberg, Dirac, Sommerfeld, Feynman, etc. This edition includes a new, long postscript carrying the story through 1958. "Of the books attempting an account of the history and contents of our modern atomic physics which have come to my attention, this is the best," H. Margenau, Yale University, in *American Journal of Physics.* 32 tables and line illustrations. Index. 275pp. 5⅜ x 8.
20518-5 Paperbound $2.00

GREAT IDEAS AND THEORIES OF MODERN COSMOLOGY,
Jagjit Singh
The theories of Jeans, Eddington, Milne, Kant, Bondi, Gold, Newton, Einstein, Gamow, Hoyle, Dirac, Kuiper, Hubble, Weizsäcker and many others on such cosmological questions as the origin of the universe, space and time, planet formation, "continuous creation," the birth, life, and death of the stars, the origin of the galaxies, etc. By the author of the popular *Great Ideas of Modern Mathematics.* A gifted popularizer of science, he makes the most difficult abstractions crystal-clear even to the most non-mathematical reader. Index.
xii + 276pp. 5⅜ x 8½. 20925-3 Paperbound $2.50

GREAT IDEAS OF MODERN MATHEMATICS: THEIR NATURE AND USE,
Jagjit Singh
Reader with only high school math will understand main mathematical ideas of modern physics, astronomy, genetics, psychology, evolution, etc., better than many who use them as tools, but comprehend little of their basic structure. Author uses his wide knowledge of non-mathematical fields in brilliant exposition of differential equations, matrices, group theory, logic, statistics, problems of mathematical foundations, imaginary numbers, vectors, etc. Original publications, appendices. indexes. 65 illustr. 322pp. 5⅜ x 8. 20587-8 Paperbound $2.25

THE MATHEMATICS OF GREAT AMATEURS, *Julian L. Coolidge*
Great discoveries made by poets, theologians, philosophers, artists and other non-mathematicians: Omar Khayyam, Leonardo da Vinci, Albrecht Dürer, John Napier, Pascal, Diderot, Bolzano, etc. Surprising accounts of what can result from a non-professional preoccupation with the oldest of sciences. 56 figures. viii + 211pp. 5⅜ x 8½. 61009-8 Paperbound $2.00

College Algebra, H. B. Fine
Standard college text that gives a systematic and deductive structure to algebra; comprehensive, connected, with emphasis on theory. Discusses the commutative, associative, and distributive laws of number in unusual detail, and goes on with undetermined coefficients, quadratic equations, progressions, logarithms, permutations, probability, power series, and much more. Still most valuable elementary-intermediate text on the science and structure of algebra. Index. 1560 problems, all with answers. x + 631pp. 5⅜ x 8. 60211-7 Paperbound $2.75

Higher Mathematics for Students of Chemistry and Physics, J. W. Mellor
Not abstract, but practical, building its problems out of familiar laboratory material, this covers differential calculus, coordinate, analytical geometry, functions, integral calculus, infinite series, numerical equations, differential equations, Fourier's theorem, probability, theory of errors, calculus of variations, determinants. "If the reader is not familiar with this book, it will repay him to examine it," *Chem. & Engineering News.* 800 problems. 189 figures. Bibliography. xxi + 641pp. 5⅜ x 8.   60193-5 Paperbound $3.50

Trigonometry Refresher for Technical Men, A. A. Klaf
A modern question and answer text on plane and spherical trigonometry. Part I covers plane trigonometry: angles, quadrants, trigonometrical functions, graphical representation, interpolation, equations, logarithms, solution of triangles, slide rules, etc. Part II discusses applications to navigation, surveying, elasticity, architecture, and engineering. Small angles, periodic functions, vectors, polar coordinates, De Moivre's theorem, fully covered. Part III is devoted to spherical trigonometry and the solution of spherical triangles, with applications to terrestrial and astronomical problems. Special time-savers for numerical calculation. 913 questions answered for you! 1738 problems; answers to odd numbers. 494 figures. 14 pages of functions, formulae. Index. x + 629pp. 5⅜ x 8. 20371-9 Paperbound $3.00

Calculus Refresher for Technical Men, A. A. Klaf
Not an ordinary textbook but a unique refresher for engineers, technicians, and students. An examination of the most important aspects of differential and integral calculus by means of 756 key questions. Part I covers simple differential calculus: constants, variables, functions, increments, derivatives, logarithms, curvature, etc. Part II treats fundamental concepts of integration: inspection, substitution, transformation, reduction, areas and volumes, mean value, successive and partial integration, double and triple integration. Stresses practical aspects! A 50 page section gives applications to civil and nautical engineering, electricity, stress and strain, elasticity, industrial engineering, and similar fields. 756 questions answered. 556 problems; solutions to odd numbers. 36 pages of constants, formulae. Index. v + 431pp. 5⅜ x 8.   20370-0 Paperbound $2.25

Introduction to the Theory of Groups of Finite Order, R. Carmichael
Examines fundamental theorems and their application. Beginning with sets, systems, permutations, etc., it progresses in easy stages through important types of groups: Abelian, prime power, permutation, etc. Except 1 chapter where matrices are desirable, no higher math needed. 783 exercises, problems. Index. xvi + 447pp. 5⅜ x 8.   60300-8 Paperbound $3.00

AN INTRODUCTION TO THE GEOMETRY OF N DIMENSIONS,
D. H. Y. Sommerville
An introduction presupposing no prior knowledge of the field, the only book in English devoted exclusively to higher dimensional geometry. Discusses fundamental ideas of incidence, parallelism, perpendicularity, angles between linear space; enumerative geometry; analytical geometry from projective and metric points of view; polytopes; elementary ideas in analysis situs; content of hyper-spacial figures. Bibliography. Index. 60 diagrams. 196pp. 5⅜ x 8.
60494-2 Paperbound $1.50

ELEMENTARY CONCEPTS OF TOPOLOGY, P. Alexandroff
First English translation of the famous brief introduction to topology for the beginner or for the mathematician not undertaking extensive study. This unusually useful intuitive approach deals primarily with the concepts of complex, cycle, and homology, and is wholly consistent with current investigations. Ranges from basic concepts of set-theoretic topology to the concept of Betti groups. "Glowing example of harmony between intuition and thought," David Hilbert. Translated by A. E. Farley. Introduction by D. Hilbert. Index. 25 figures. 73pp. 5⅜ x 8.
60747-X Paperbound $1.25

ELEMENTS OF NON-EUCLIDEAN GEOMETRY,
D. M. Y. Sommerville
Unique in proceeding step-by-step, in the manner of traditional geometry. Enables the student with only a good knowledge of high school algebra and geometry to grasp elementary hyperbolic, elliptic, analytic non-Euclidean geometries; space curvature and its philosophical implications; theory of radical axes; homothetic centres and systems of circles; parataxy and parallelism; absolute measure; Gauss' proof of the defect area theorem; geodesic representation; much more, all with exceptional clarity. 126 problems at chapter endings provide progressive practice and familiarity. 133 figures. Index. xvi + 274pp. 5⅜ x 8.
60460-8 Paperbound $2.00

INTRODUCTION TO THE THEORY OF NUMBERS, L. E. Dickson
Thorough, comprehensive approach with adequate coverage of classical literature, an introductory volume beginners can follow. Chapters on divisibility, congruences, quadratic residues & reciprocity. Diophantine equations, etc. Full treatment of binary quadratic forms without usual restriction to integral coefficients. Covers infinitude of primes, least residues. Fermat's theorem. Euler's phi function, Legendre's symbol, Gauss's lemma, automorphs, reduced forms, recent theorems of Thue & Siegel, many more. Much material not readily available elsewhere. 239 problems. Index. I figure. viii + 183pp. 5⅜ x 8.
60342-3 Paperbound $1.75

MATHEMATICAL TABLES AND FORMULAS,
compiled by Robert D. Carmichael and Edwin R. Smith
Valuable collection for students, etc. Contains all tables necessary in college algebra and trigonometry, such as five-place common logarithms, logarithmic sines and tangents of small angles, logarithmic trigonometric functions, natural trigonometric functions, four-place antilogarithms, tables for changing from sexagesimal to circular and from circular to sexagesimal measure of angles, etc. Also many tables and formulas not ordinarily accessible, including powers, roots, and reciprocals, exponential and hyperbolic functions, ten-place logarithms of prime numbers, and formulas and theorems from analytical and elementary geometry and from calculus. Explanatory introduction. viii + 269pp. 5⅜ x 8½.
60111-0 Paperbound $1.50

NUMERICAL SOLUTIONS OF DIFFERENTIAL EQUATIONS,
H. Levy & E. A. Baggott
Comprehensive collection of methods for solving ordinary differential equations of first and higher order. All must pass 2 requirements: easy to grasp and practical, more rapid than school methods. Partial contents: graphical integration of differential equations, graphical methods for detailed solution. Numerical solution. Simultaneous equations and equations of 2nd and higher orders. "Should be in the hands of all in research in applied mathematics, teaching," *Nature.* 21 figures. viii + 238pp. 5⅜ x 8. 60168-4 Paperbound $1.85

ELEMENTARY STATISTICS, WITH APPLICATIONS IN MEDICINE AND THE BIOLOGICAL SCIENCES, *F. E. Croxton*
A sound introduction to statistics for anyone in the physical sciences, assuming no prior acquaintance and requiring only a modest knowledge of math. All basic formulas carefully explained and illustrated; all necessary reference tables included. From basic terms and concepts, the study proceeds to frequency distribution, linear, non-linear, and multiple correlation, skewness, kurtosis, etc. A large section deals with reliability and significance of statistical methods. Containing concrete examples from medicine and biology, this book will prove unusually helpful to workers in those fields who increasingly must evaluate, check, and interpret statistics. Formerly titled "Elementary Statistics with Applications in Medicine." 101 charts. 57 tables. 14 appendices. Index. vi + 376pp. 5⅜ x 8. 60506-X Paperbound $2.25

INTRODUCTION TO SYMBOLIC LOGIC,
S. Langer
No special knowledge of math required — probably the clearest book ever written on symbolic logic, suitable for the layman, general scientist, and philosopher. You start with simple symbols and advance to a knowledge of the Boole-Schroeder and Russell-Whitehead systems. Forms, logical structure, classes, the calculus of propositions, logic of the syllogism, etc. are all covered. "One of the clearest and simplest introductions," *Mathematics Gazette.* Second enlarged, revised edition. 368pp. 5⅜ x 8. 60164-1 Paperbound $2.25

A SHORT ACCOUNT OF THE HISTORY OF MATHEMATICS,
W. W. R. Ball
Most readable non-technical history of mathematics treats lives, discoveries of every important figure from Egyptian, Phoenician, mathematicians to late 19th century. Discusses schools of Ionia, Pythagoras, Athens, Cyzicus, Alexandria, Byzantium, systems of numeration; primitive arithmetic; Middle Ages, Renaissance, including Arabs, Bacon, Regiomontanus, Tartaglia, Cardan, Stevinus, Galileo, Kepler; modern mathematics of Descartes, Pascal, Wallis, Huygens, Newton, Leibnitz, d'Alembert, Euler, Lambert, Laplace, Legendre, Gauss, Hermite, Weierstrass, scores more. Index. 25 figures. 546pp. 5⅜ x 8. 20630-0 Paperbound $2.75

INTRODUCTION TO NONLINEAR DIFFERENTIAL AND INTEGRAL EQUATIONS,
Harold T. Davis
Aspects of the problem of nonlinear equations, transformations that lead to equations solvable by classical means, results in special cases, and useful generalizations. Thorough, but easily followed by mathematically sophisticated reader who knows little about non-linear equations. 137 problems for student to solve. xv + 566pp. 5⅜ x 8½. 60971-5 Paperbound $2.75

A SOURCE BOOK IN MATHEMATICS,
D. E. Smith
Great discoveries in math, from Renaissance to end of 19th century, in English translation. Read announcements by Dedekind, Gauss, Delamain, Pascal, Fermat, Newton, Abel, Lobachevsky, Bolyai, Riemann, De Moivre, Legendre, Laplace, others of discoveries about imaginary numbers, number congruence, slide rule, equations, symbolism, cubic algebraic equations, non-Euclidean forms of geometry, calculus, function theory, quaternions, etc. Succinct selections from 125 different treatises, articles, most unavailable elsewhere in English. Each article preceded by biographical introduction. Vol. I: Fields of Number, Algebra. Index. 32 illus. 338pp. 5⅜ x 8. Vol. II: Fields of Geometry, Probability, Calculus, Functions, Quaternions. 83 illus. 432pp. 5⅜ x 8.
60552-3, 60553-1 Two volume set, paperbound $5.00

FOUNDATIONS OF PHYSICS,
R. B. Lindsay & H. Margenau
Excellent bridge between semi-popular works & technical treatises. A discussion of methods of physical description, construction of theory; valuable for physicist with elementary calculus who is interested in ideas that give meaning to data, tools of modern physics. Contents include symbolism; mathematical equations; space & time foundations of mechanics; probability; physics & continua; electron theory; special & general relativity; quantum mechanics; causality. "Thorough and yet not overdetailed. Unreservedly recommended," *Nature* (London). Unabridged, corrected edition. List of recommended readings. 35 illustrations. xi + 537pp. 5⅜ x 8. 60377-6 Paperbound $3.50

FUNDAMENTAL FORMULAS OF PHYSICS,
ed. by D. H. Menzel
High useful, full, inexpensive reference and study text, ranging from simple to highly sophisticated operations. Mathematics integrated into text—each chapter stands as short textbook of field represented. Vol. 1: Statistics, Physical Constants, Special Theory of Relativity, Hydrodynamics, Aerodynamics, Boundary Value Problems in Math, Physics, Viscosity, Electromagnetic Theory, etc. Vol. 2: Sound, Acoustics, Geometrical Optics, Electron Optics, High-Energy Phenomena, Magnetism, Biophysics, much more. Index. Total of 800pp. 5⅜ x 8.
60595-7, 60596-5 Two volume set, paperbound $4.75

THEORETICAL PHYSICS,
A. S. Kompaneyets
One of the very few thorough studies of the subject in this price range. Provides advanced students with a comprehensive theoretical background. Especially strong on recent experimentation and developments in quantum theory. Contents: Mechanics (Generalized Coordinates, Lagrange's Equation, Collision of Particles, etc.), Electrodynamics (Vector Analysis, Maxwell's equations, Transmission of Signals, Theory of Relativity, etc.), Quantum Mechanics (the Inadequacy of Classical Mechanics, the Wave Equation, Motion in a Central Field, Quantum Theory of Radiation, Quantum Theories of Dispersion and Scattering, etc.), and Statistical Physics (Equilibrium Distribution of Molecules in an Ideal Gas, Boltzmann Statistics, Bose and Fermi Distribution. Thermodynamic Quantities, etc.). Revised to 1961. Translated by George Yankovsky, authorized by Kompaneyets. 137 exercises. 56 figures. 529pp. 5⅜ x 8½.
60972-3 Paperbound $3.50

CHANCE, LUCK AND STATISTICS: THE SCIENCE OF CHANCE,
Horace C. Levinson
Theory of probability and science of statistics in simple, non-technical language.
Part I deals with theory of probability, covering odd superstitions in regard to
"luck," the meaning of betting odds, the law of mathematical expectation,
gambling, and applications in poker, roulette, lotteries, dice, bridge, and other
games of chance. Part II discusses the misuse of statistics, the concept of statistical probabilities, normal and skew frequency distributions, and statistics applied to various fields—birth rates, stock speculation, insurance rates, advertis-
ing, etc. "Presented in an easy humorous style which I consider the best kind of
expository writing," Prof. A. C. Cohen, Industry Quality Control. Enlarged
revised edition. Formerly titled *The Science of Chance*. Preface and two new
appendices by the author. xiv + 365pp. 5⅜ x 8.   21007-3 Paperbound $2.00

BASIC ELECTRONICS,
prepared by the U.S. Navy Training Publications Center
A thorough and comprehensive manual on the fundamentals of electronics.
Written clearly, it is equally useful for self-study or course work for those with
a knowledge of the principles of basic electricity. Partial contents: Operating
Principles of the Electron Tube; Introduction to Transistors; Power Supplies
for Electronic Equipment; Tuned Circuits; Electron-Tube Amplifiers; Audio
Power Amplifiers; Oscillators; Transmitters; Transmission Lines; Antennas and
Propagation; Introduction to Computers; and related topics. Appendix. Index.
Hundreds of illustrations and diagrams. vi + 471pp. 6½ x 9¼.
61076-4 Paperbound $2.95

BASIC THEORY AND APPLICATION OF TRANSISTORS,
prepared by the U.S. Department of the Army
An introductory manual prepared for an army training program. One of the
finest available surveys of theory and application of transistor design and
operation. Minimal knowledge of physics and theory of electron tubes required.
Suitable for textbook use, course supplement, or home study. Chapters: Introduction; fundamental theory of transistors; transistor amplifier fundamentals;
parameters, equivalent circuits, and characteristic curves; bias stabilization;
transistor analysis and comparison using characteristic curves and charts; audio
amplifiers; tuned amplifiers; wide-band amplifiers; oscillators; pulse and switching circuits; modulation, mixing, and demodulation; and additional semi-
conductor devices. Unabridged, corrected edition. 240 schematic drawings,
photographs, wiring diagrams, etc. 2 Appendices. Glossary. Index. 263pp.
6½ x 9¼.   60380-6 Paperbound $1.75

GUIDE TO THE LITERATURE OF MATHEMATICS AND PHYSICS,
N. G. Parke III
Over 5000 entries included under approximately 120 major subject headings of
selected most important books, monographs, periodicals, articles in English,
plus important works in German, French, Italian, Spanish, Russian (many
recently available works). Covers every branch of physics, math, related engineering. Includes author, title, edition, publisher, place, date, number of
volumes, number of pages. A 40-page introduction on the basic problems of
research and study provides useful information on the organization and use of
libraries, the psychology of learning, etc. This reference work will save you
hours of time. 2nd revised edition. Indices of authors, subjects, 464pp. 5⅜ x 8.
60447-0 Paperbound $2.75

MATHEMATICAL PHYSICS, *D. H. Menzel*
Thorough one-volume treatment of the mathematical techniques vital for classical mechanics, electromagnetic theory, quantum theory, and relativity. Written by the Harvard Professor of Astrophysics for junior, senior, and graduate courses, it gives clear explanations of all those aspects of function theory, vectors, matrices, dyadics, tensors, partial differential equations, etc., necessary for the understanding of the various physical theories. Electron theory, relativity, and other topics seldom presented appear here in considerable detail. Scores of definition, conversion factors, dimensional constants, etc. "More detailed than normal for an advanced text . . . excellent set of sections on Dyadics, Matrices, and Tensors," *Journal of the Franklin Institute.* Index. 193 problems, with answers. x + 412pp. 5⅜ x 8.   60056-4 Paperbound $2.50

THE THEORY OF SOUND, *Lord Rayleigh*
Most vibrating systems likely to be encountered in practice can be tackled successfully by the methods set forth by the great Nobel laureate, Lord Rayleigh. Complete coverage of experimental, mathematical aspects of sound theory. Partial contents: Harmonic motions, vibrating systems in general, lateral vibrations of bars, curved plates or shells, applications of Laplace's functions to acoustical problems, fluid friction, plane vortex-sheet, vibrations of solid bodies, etc. This is the first inexpensive edition of this great reference and study work. Bibliography, Historical introduction by R. B. Lindsay. Total of 1040pp. 97 figures. 5⅜ x 8.   60292-3, 60293-1 Two volume set, paperbound $6.00

HYDRODYNAMICS, *Horace Lamb*
Internationally famous complete coverage of standard reference work on dynamics of liquids & gases. Fundamental theorems, equations, methods, solutions, background, for classical hydrodynamics. Chapters include Equations of Motion, Integration of Equations in Special Gases, Irrotational Motion, Motion of Liquid in 2 Dimensions, Motion of Solids through Liquid-Dynamical Theory, Vortex Motion, Tidal Waves, Surface Waves, Waves of Expansion, Viscosity, Rotating Masses of Liquids. Excellently planned, arranged; clear, lucid presentation. 6th enlarged, revised edition. Index. Over 900 footnotes, mostly bibliographical. 119 figures. xv + 738pp. 6⅛ x 9¼.   60256-7 Paperbound $4.00

DYNAMICAL THEORY OF GASES, *James Jeans*
Divided into mathematical and physical chapters for the convenience of those not expert in mathematics, this volume discusses the mathematical theory of gas in a steady state, thermodynamics, Boltzmann and Maxwell, kinetic theory, quantum theory, exponentials, etc. 4th enlarged edition, with new material on quantum theory, quantum dynamics, etc. Indexes. 28 figures. 444pp. 6⅛ x 9¼.
60136-6 Paperbound $2.75

THERMODYNAMICS, *Enrico Fermi*
Unabridged reproduction of 1937 edition. Elementary in treatment; remarkable for clarity, organization. Requires no knowledge of advanced math beyond calculus, only familiarity with fundamentals of thermometry, calorimetry. Partial Contents: Thermodynamic systems; First & Second laws of thermodynamics; Entropy; Thermodynamic potentials: phase rule, reversible electric cell; Gaseous reactions: van't Hoff reaction box, principle of LeChatelier; Thermodynamics of dilute solutions: osmotic & vapor pressures, boiling & freezing points; Entropy constant. Index. 25 problems. 24 illustrations. x + 160pp. 5⅜ x 8.   60361-X Paperbound $2.00

APPLIED OPTICS AND OPTICAL DESIGN,
A. E. Conrady
With publication of vol. 2, standard work for designers in optics is now complete for first time. Only work of its kind in English; only detailed work for practical designer and self-taught. Requires, for bulk of work, no math above trig. Step-by-step exposition, from fundamental concepts of geometrical, physical optics, to systematic study, design, of almost all types of optical systems. Vol. 1: all ordinary ray-tracing methods; primary aberrations; necessary higher aberration for design of telescopes, low-power microscopes, photographic equipment. Vol. 2: (Completed from author's notes by R. Kingslake, Dir. Optical Design, Eastman Kodak.) Special attention to high-power microscope, anastigmatic photographic objectives. "An indispensable work," *J., Optical Soc. of Amer.* Index. Bibliography. 193 diagrams. 852pp. 6⅛ x 9¼.
60611-2, 60612-0 Two volume set, paperbound $8.00

MECHANICS OF THE GYROSCOPE, THE DYNAMICS OF ROTATION,
R. F. Deimel, Professor of Mechanical Engineering at Stevens Institute of Technology
Elementary general treatment of dynamics of rotation, with special application of gyroscopic phenomena. No knowledge of vectors needed. Velocity of a moving curve, acceleration to a point, general equations of motion, gyroscopic horizon, free gyro, motion of discs, the damped gyro, 103 similar topics. Exercises. 75 figures. 208pp. 5⅜ x 8.
60066-1 Paperbound $1.75

STRENGTH OF MATERIALS,
J. P. Den Hartog
Full, clear treatment of elementary material (tension, torsion, bending, compound stresses, deflection of beams, etc.), plus much advanced material on engineering methods of great practical value: full treatment of the Mohr circle, lucid elementary discussions of the theory of the center of shear and the "Myosotis" method of calculating beam deflections, reinforced concrete, plastic deformations, photoelasticity, etc. In all sections, both general principles and concrete applications are given. Index. 186 figures (160 others in problem section). 350 problems, all with answers. List of formulas. viii + 323pp. 5⅜ x 8.
60755-0 Paperbound $2.50

HYDRAULIC TRANSIENTS,
G. R. Rich
The best text in hydraulics ever printed in English . . . by former Chief Design Engineer for T.V.A. Provides a transition from the basic differential equations of hydraulic transient theory to the arithmetic integration computation required by practicing engineers. Sections cover Water Hammer, Turbine Speed Regulation, Stability of Governing, Water-Hammer Pressures in Pump Discharge Lines, The Differential and Restricted Orifice Surge Tanks, The Normalized Surge Tank Charts of Calame and Gaden, Navigation Locks, Surges in Power Canals—Tidal Harmonics, etc. Revised and enlarged. Author's prefaces. Index. xiv + 409pp. 5⅜ x 8½.
60116-1 Paperbound $2.50

Prices subject to change without notice.

Available at your book dealer or write for free catalogue to Dept. Adsci, Dover Publications, Inc., 180 Varick St., N.Y., N.Y. 10014. Dover publishes more than 150 books each year on science, elementary and advanced mathematics, biology, music, art, literary history, social sciences and other areas.